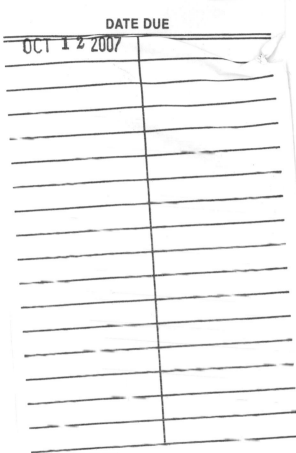

Exploring the Biological Contributions to Human Health

Does Sex Matter?

Committee on Understanding the Biology of
Sex and Gender Differences

Theresa M. Wizemann and Mary-Lou Pardue, *Editors*

Board on Health Sciences Policy

INSTITUTE OF MEDICINE

NATIONAL ACADEMY PRESS
Washington, D.C.

NATIONAL ACADEMY PRESS • 2101 Constitution Avenue, N.W. • Washington, DC 20418

NOTICE: The project that is the subject of this report was approved by the Governing Board of the National Research Council, whose members are drawn from the councils of the National Academy of Sciences, the National Academy of Engineering, and the Institute of Medicine. The members of the committee responsible for the report were chosen for their special competences and with regard for appropriate balance.

Support for this project was provided by the U.S. Department of Health and Human Services (Office on Women's Health, National Institutes of Health Office of Research on Women's Health, National Institute of Environmental Health Sciences, National Institute on Drug Abuse, National Institute of Mental Health, U.S. Food and Drug Administration, Centers for Disease Control and Prevention), the National Science Foundation, the Environmental Protection Agency, the National Aeronautics and Space Administration, the Society for Women's Health Research, the Research Foundation for Health and Environmental Effects, Ortho-McNeil/Johnson & Johnson, and the Unilever United States Foundation. The views presented in this report are those of the Committee on Understanding the Biology of Sex and Gender Differences and are not necessarily those of the funding organizations.

Library of Congress Cataloging-in-Publication Data

Institute of Medicine (U.S.). Committee on Understanding the Biology of Sex and Gender Differences.
  Exploring the biological contributions to human health : does sex matter? / Committee on Understanding the Biology of Sex and Gender Differences ; Theresa M. Wizemann and Mary-Lou Pardue, editors.
      p. ; cm.
Includes bibliographical references and index.
  ISBN 0-309-07281-6 (hardcover)
  1. Sex differences. 2. Sex factors in disease.
  [DNLM: 1. Sex Factors. 2. Genetics, Biochemical. 3. Health. 4.
Research Design—standards. 5. Sex Characteristics. QZ 53 I59e 2001]
  I. Wizemann, Theresa M. II. Pardue, Mary Lou. III. Title.
  QP81.5 .I56 2001
  616'.001'57846—dc21
                        2001002537

Additional copies of this report are available for sale from the National Academy Press, 2101 Constitution Avenue, N.W., Box 285, Washington, DC 20055. Call (800) 624-6242 or (202) 334-3313 (in the Washington metropolitan area), or visit the NAP's home page at **www.nap.edu.** The full text of this report is available at **www.nap.edu.**

For more information about the Institute of Medicine, visit the IOM home page at **www.iom.edu.**

Cover photograph: Human X and Y Chromosomes (magnified 35,000 times). Source: Biophoto Associates, Photo Researchers, Inc.

*"Knowing is not enough; we must apply.
Willing is not enough; we must do."*
—Goethe

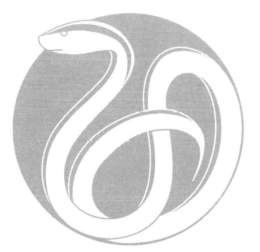

INSTITUTE OF MEDICINE

Shaping the Future for Health

THE NATIONAL ACADEMIES

National Academy of Sciences
National Academy of Engineering
Institute of Medicine
National Research Council

The **National Academy of Sciences** is a private, nonprofit, self-perpetuating society of distinguished scholars engaged in scientific and engineering research, dedicated to the furtherance of science and technology and to their use for the general welfare. Upon the authority of the charter granted to it by the Congress in 1863, the Academy has a mandate that requires it to advise the federal government on scientific and technical matters. Dr. Bruce M. Alberts is president of the National Academy of Sciences.

The **National Academy of Engineering** was established in 1964, under the charter of the National Academy of Sciences, as a parallel organization of outstanding engineers. It is autonomous in its administration and in the selection of its members, sharing with the National Academy of Sciences the responsibility for advising the federal government. The National Academy of Engineering also sponsors engineering programs aimed at meeting national needs, encourages education and research, and recognizes the superior achievements of engineers. Dr. William A. Wulf is president of the National Academy of Engineering.

The **Institute of Medicine** was established in 1970 by the National Academy of Sciences to secure the services of eminent members of appropriate professions in the examination of policy matters pertaining to the health of the public. The Institute acts under the responsibility given to the National Academy of Sciences by its congressional charter to be an adviser to the federal government and, upon its own initiative, to identify issues of medical care, research, and education. Dr. Kenneth I. Shine is president of the Institute of Medicine.

The **National Research Council** was organized by the National Academy of Sciences in 1916 to associate the broad community of science and technology with the Academy's purposes of furthering knowledge and advising the federal government. Functioning in accordance with general policies determined by the Academy, the Council has become the principal operating agency of both the National Academy of Sciences and the National Academy of Engineering in providing services to the government, the public, and the scientific and engineering communities. The Council is administered jointly by both Academies and the Institute of Medicine. Dr. Bruce M. Alberts and Dr. William A. Wulf are chairman and vice chairman, respectively, of the National Research Council.

COMMITTEE ON UNDERSTANDING THE BIOLOGY OF SEX AND GENDER DIFFERENCES

MARY-LOU PARDUE (*Chair*), Boris Magasanik Professor, Department of Biology, Massachusetts Institute of Technology, Cambridge

DANIEL L. AZARNOFF, President, D. L. Azarnoff Associates, and Senior Vice President, Clinical/Regulatory Affairs, Cellegy Pharmaceuticals, South San Francisco

SHERI BERENBAUM, Professor, Department of Physiology, Southern Illinois University School of Medicine, Carbondale

KAREN J. BERKLEY, McKenzie Professor, Program in Neuroscience, Florida State University, Tallahassee

ANNE FAUSTO-STERLING, Professor of Biology and Women's Studies, Senior Fellow, Francis Wayland Collegium, Brown University, Providence

DANIEL D. FEDERMAN, Senior Dean for Alumni Relations and Clinical Teaching, Carl W. Walter Professor of Medicine and Medical Education, Harvard Medical School, Boston

BARBARA ANN GILCHREST, Professor and Chairman, Department of Dermatology, Boston University, Boston

MELVIN M. GRUMBACH, Edward B. Shaw Professor of Pediatrics, University of California San Francisco School of Medicine, San Francisco

SHIRIKI KUMANYIKA, Associate Dean, Health Promotion and Disease Prevention, Center for Clinical Epidemiology and Biostatistics, University of Pennsylvania School of Medicine, Philadelphia

JUDITH H. LaROSA, Professor, Department of Preventive Medicine and Community Health, State University of New York Downstate Medical Center at Brooklyn, Brooklyn

MICHAEL D. LOCKSHIN, Director, Barbara Volcker Center for Women and Rheumatic Disease, Hospital for Special Surgery, and Professor of Medicine, Weill College of Medicine of Cornell University, New York

JILL PANETTA, Senior Research Scientist, Research Manager, Lilly Center for Women's Health, Eli Lilly & Company, Indianapolis

CARMEN SAPIENZA, Professor of Pathology, Temple University School of Medicine, Philadelphia

SALLY E. SHAYWITZ, Professor of Pediatrics, Yale University School of Medicine, New Haven

JOHN G. VANDENBERGH, Professor, Department of Zoology, North Carolina State University, Raleigh

Reviewers

This report has been reviewed in draft form by individuals chosen for their diverse perspectives and technical expertise, in accordance with procedures approved by the National Research Council's (NRC's) Report Review Committee. The purpose of this independent review is to provide candid and critical comments that will assist the institution in making its published report as sound as possible and to ensure that the report meets institutional standards for objectivity, evidence, and responsiveness to the study charge. The review comments and draft manuscript remain confidential to protect the integrity of the deliberative process. We wish to thank the following individuals for their review of this report:

LESLIE Z. BENET, Professor, Department of Biopharmaceutical Sciences, University of California, San Francisco

DAVID P. CREWS, Ashbel Smith Professor of Zoology and Psychology, University of Texas at Austin

ALICE EAGLY, Professor, Department of Psychology, Northwestern University, Evanston, IL

SHERINE E. GABRIEL, Director, Center for Patient Oriented Research, Mayo Clinic, Rochester, MN

JANET S. HYDE, Chair, Department of Psychology, University of Wisconsin at Madison

ELEANOR E. MACCOBY, Professor Emeritus, Department of Psychology, Stanford University, Stanford

Although the reviewers listed above have provided many constructive comments and suggestions, they were not asked to endorse the conclusions or recommendations, nor did they see the final draft of the report before its release. The review of this report was overseen by **ELIZABETH BARRETT-CONNOR**, Professor and Chief, Division of Epidemiology, University of California, San Diego, appointed by the Institute of Medicine, and **BARBARA CALEEN HANSEN**, Professor of Physiology and Director, Obesity and Diabetes Research Center, University of Maryland School of Medicine at Baltimore, appointed by the NRC's Report Review Committee, who were responsible for making certain that an independent examination of this report was carried out in accordance with institutional procedures and that all review comments were carefully considered. Responsibility for the final content of this report rests entirely with the authoring committee and the institution.

Preface

Does sex matter? Almost anyone would answer "yes" to this simple question. However, subsumed within this question are two much more difficult questions: When does sex matter? and How does sex matter? These two questions define the task undertaken by the Committee on Understanding the Biology of Sex and Gender Differences. This committee was charged with evaluating the current scientific understanding of the answers to these questions with respect to their influence on human health.

Specifically, the committee was charged with considering biology at the cellular, developmental, organ, organismal, and behavioral levels. The goal, as in all studies of biology, is to understand the organism in terms of all of the interactions that occur between levels within the organism as well as the mutual interactions between the organism and its environment. This was a broad charge, which required a committee made up of individuals drawn from a wide range of subfields of biology and medicine. We have learned much from each other and from a number of invited speakers specializing in fields in which the committee did not have expertise. We also made an extensive survey of the relevant literature.

The most obvious and best-studied differences between the sexes are in the reproductive systems. Much less work has been done on sex differences in nonreproductive areas of biology, and this is where the committee has focused its efforts. Differences are much less expected in nonreproductive areas of biology, but differences do occur, and some of these differences have important consequences. Understanding these differences makes it possible to design health care more effectively for individuals, both males and females.

An additional and more general reason for studying differences between the sexes is that these differences, like other forms of biological variation, can offer important insights into underlying biological mechanisms. An often-quoted piece of advice to those studying biology is to "cherish your exceptions." These exceptions traditionally include organisms with mutations and organisms from different species that accomplish the same goal in slightly modified ways. Only relatively recently has it been recognized that sexual variations are as important as these exceptions in providing similarities and contrasts that can reveal important details about the processes involved.

This is an especially opportune time to take stock of what is known about differences and similarities in the basic biology of the sexes, because in the last few years biological research has acquired an arsenal of powerful tools that can be used to answer new questions. Reviews like the one presented in this report juxtapose knowledge from different subfields, create new connections between subfields, and inevitably, raise new questions. The arsenal of new tools enables us to answer questions that only a short time ago seemed impossible to answer.

The picture that emerges from the study described in this report shows that there are numerous sex differences in nonreproductive tissues. Some of these differences can be explained by what we now know. Some are unexplained and point to important questions for future study. Some are large and have known effects on the health of individuals; these differences have immediate consequences in terms of health care. Some of the differences are small, with no known effects on health, but they may provide clues that can be used to solve new biological questions. This report provides a broad view of the research and issues that the committee considered. It is, of necessity, a summary with a small number of examples chosen to illustrate the points that we make and to convey the interesting science that is being done in these areas.

Sex does matter. It matters in ways that we did not expect. Undoubtedly, it also matters in ways that we have not begun to imagine.

Mary-Lou Pardue, Ph.D.
Chair

Acknowledgments

The committee is indebted to the experts in many scientific disciplines who presented informative talks to the committee and participated in lively discussions (see Appendix A). In addition, the committee is grateful to the members of the scientific community who made themselves available by phone and e-mail for consultation and technical advice.

The committee also wishes to thank the Institute of Medicine staff who contributed to the report. Theresa Wizemann has done a superb job as study director. Thelma Cox has taken very good care of the committee, in spite of severe weather conditions at two of the meetings that presented challenges to her management skills. Sarah Pitluck provided able assistance in the early part of the study and Dalia Gilbert assisted in the later stages. Kathi Hanna, Michael Hayes, and Michael Edington provided helpful style guidance and technical editing. Valerie Setlow helped guide the early development stages of the project. The committee thanks Andrew Pope, Director of the Board on Health Sciences Policy for his continuing interest in this work and guidance throughout the process.

Many thanks go to Bruce Alberts, President of the National Academy of Sciences and Chair of the National Research Council, and Ken Shine, President of the Institute of Medicine, for advice and guidance in focusing the task. Thanks also go to the staff of the National Research Council Board on Biology for helpful suggestions and nominations of committee members and reviewers.

This report was made possible by the generous support of 14 sponsors: U.S. Department of Health and Human Services (Office on Women's Health, National Institutes of Health Office of Research on Women's

Health, National Institute of Environmental Health Sciences, National Institute on Drug Abuse, National Institute of Mental Health, U.S. Food and Drug Administration, Centers for Disease Control and Prevention), the National Science Foundation, the Environmental Protection Agency, the National Aeronautics and Space Administration, the Society for Women's Health Research, the Research Foundation for Health and Environmental Effects, Ortho-McNeil/Johnson & Johnson, and the Unilever United States Foundation. Special thanks go to Phyllis Greenberger of the Society for Women's Health Research, Vivian Pinn of the National Institutes of Health Office of Research on Women's Health, and Susan Wood, formerly of the Office on Women's Health of the U.S. Department of Health and Human Services for their persistence and vision in developing the proposal for this study.

Contents

TABLES, FIGURES, AND BOXES

Tables

Figures

Boxes

Abstract

One of the most compelling reasons for looking at what is known about the biology of sex differences is that there are striking differences in human disease that are not explained at this time.

Being male or female is an important basic human variable that affects health and illness throughout the life span. Differences in health and illness are influenced by individual genetic and physiological constitutions, as well as by an individual's interaction with environmental and experiential factors. The incidence and severity of diseases vary between the sexes and may be related to differences in exposures, routes of entry and the processing of a foreign agent, and cellular responses. Although in many cases these sex differences can be traced to the direct or indirect effects of hormones associated with reproduction, differences cannot be solely attributed to hormones. Therefore, sex should be considered when designing and analyzing studies in all areas and at all levels of biomedical and health-related research.

The study of sex differences is evolving into a mature science. There is now sufficient knowledge of the biological basis of sex differences to validate the scientific study of sex differences and to allow the generation of hypotheses with regard to health. The next step is to move from the descriptive to the experimental phase and establish the conditions that must be in place to facilitate and encourage the scientific study of the mechanisms and origins of sex differences. Naturally occurring variations in sex differentiation can provide unique opportunities to obtain a better understanding of basic differences and similarities between and within the sexes.

Barriers to the advancement of knowledge about sex differences in health and illness exist and must be eliminated. Scientists conducting research on sex differences are confronted with an array of barriers to progress, including ethical, financial, sociological, and scientific factors.

The committee provides scientific evidence in support of the conclusions presented above and makes recommendations to advance the understanding of sex differences and their effects on health and illness.

Executive Summary

The explosion in the growth of new biological information over the past decade has made it increasingly apparent that many normal physiological functions—and, in many cases, pathological functions—are influenced either directly or indirectly by sex-based differences in biology (also referred to throughout this report as *sex differences*).

In recent years, considerable attention has been given to the differences and similarities between females and males (1) at the *societal* level by researchers evaluating how individual behaviors, lifestyles, and surroundings affect one's biological development and health and (2) at the level of the *whole organism* by clinicians and applied researchers investigating the component organs and systems of humans. However, scientists have paid much less attention to the direct and intentional study of these differences at the basic *cellular* and *molecular* levels. Where data are available, they have often been a by-product of other areas of research. Historically, the research community assumed that beyond the reproductive system such differences do not exist or are not relevant.

Scientific evidence of the importance of sex[1] differences throughout the life span abounds. Investigators are now positioned to take this work

---

[1]The committee defines *sex* as the classification of living things, generally as male or female according to their reproductive organs and functions assigned by the chromosomal complement, and *gender* as a person's self-representation as male or female, or how that person is responded to by social institutions on the basis of the individual's gender presentation. Gender is shaped by environment and experience.

1

to the next level, at which the mechanisms and origins of such differences can be explored. This will allow scientists and clinicians to understand the implications of these differences for human health. The critical questions to be answered are

- How can information on sex differences be translated into preventive, diagnostic, and therapeutic practice?
- How can the new knowledge about and understanding of biological sex differences and similarities most effectively be used to positively affect patient outcomes and improve health and health care?

SCOPE OF THE REPORT

In November 1999, the Institute of Medicine (IOM) formed the Committee on Understanding the Biology of Sex and Gender Differences in response to combined requests from a consortium of public and private sponsors. The committee members brought expertise from a broad array of disciplines in basic and applied biomedical research. In general, the sponsors asked the committee to evaluate and consider the current understanding of sex differences and determinants at the biological level. Specifically, they asked that the following issues be addressed:

- the knowledge base on and research priorities for animal and cellular models that could be used to determine when sex and gender differences exist and when they are relevant to biological functioning at the cellular, developmental, organ, organismal, and behavioral levels;
- current and potential barriers to the conduct of valid and productive research on sex and gender differences and their determinants, including ethical, financial, sociological, and scientific factors; and
- strategies that can be used to overcome such barriers and promote the acceptance of this research by the scientific community and the general public.

The committee was not charged with the task of preparing a definitive text on all known differences and similarities between the sexes but, rather, was charged with considering factors and traits that characterize and differentiate males and females across the life span and that underlie sex differences in health (including genetic, biochemical, physiological, physical, and behavioral elements). Thus, the focus of this report is on sex-based differences, versus similarities, as they are more likely to successfully demonstrate the need for further research and lead to greater understanding of the significance of sex in human biology and health. Moreover, despite the influence of pregnancy, parity, and parenthood on the manifestation of some diseases and health outcomes, this report does not directly address these issues, as they are deserving of separate and more in-depth attention.

On the basis of its review, the committee arrived at a series of findings and conclusions and developed recommendations that are designed to facilitate scientific endeavors in this area, take advantage of new opportunities in basic and applied research, and fill identified research gaps.

OVERARCHING CONCLUSIONS

Three common, recurring messages emerged as the committee addressed its primary task (reviewing and evaluating the current state of knowledge about sex differences in health and illness and scientific evidence related to sex differences in health and illness) and as it met with scientific experts across diverse disciplines.

- **Sex matters.** Sex, that is, being male or female, is an important basic human variable that should be considered when designing and analyzing studies in all areas and at all levels of biomedical and health-related research. Differences in health and illness are influenced by individual genetic and physiological constitutions, as well as by an individual's interaction with environmental and experiential factors. The incidence and severity of diseases vary between the sexes and may be related to differences in exposures, the routes of entry and the processing of a foreign agent, and cellular responses. Although in many cases these sex differences can be traced to the direct or indirect effects of hormones associated with reproduction, differences cannot be solely attributed to hormones.
- **The study of sex differences is evolving into a mature science.** There is now sufficient knowledge of the biological basis of sex differences to validate the scientific study of sex differences and to allow the generation of hypotheses. The next step is to move from the descriptive to the experimental and to establish the conditions that must be in place to facilitate and encourage the scientific study of the mechanisms and origins of sex differences. Naturally occurring variations in sexual differentiation and development can provide unique opportunities to obtain a better understanding of basic differences and similarities between and within the sexes.
- **Barriers to the advancement of knowledge about sex differences in health and illness exist and must be eliminated.** Scientists conducting research on sex differences are confronted with an array of barriers to progress, including ethical, financial, sociological, and scientific factors.

After considering the data and examples presented throughout this report, the committee expects that the public, scientific, and policy communities alike will agree that the understanding of sex differences in health and illness merits serious scientific inquiry in all aspects of biomedical and health-related research. Some of the answers have been stumbled upon fortuitously. Until the question of sex, however, is routinely asked and the results—positive or negative—are routinely reported, many opportunities to obtain a better understanding of the pathogenesis of disease and to advance human health will surely be missed.

FINDINGS AND RECOMMENDATIONS

Every Cell Has a Sex

The biological differences between the sexes have long been recognized at the biochemical and cellular levels. Rapid advances in molecular biology have revealed the genetic and molecular bases of a number of sex-based differences in health and human disease, some of which are attributed to sexual genotype—XX in the female and XY in the male. Genes on the sex chromosomes can be expressed differently between males and females because of the presence of either single or double copies of the gene and because of several other phenomena: of different meiotic effects, X-chromosome inactivation, and genetic imprinting. The inheritance of either a male or a female genotype is further influenced by the source (maternal or paternal) of the X chromosome. The relative roles of the sex chromosome genes and their expressions explain X-chromosome-linked diseases and are likely to illuminate the reasons for the heterogeneous expression of some diseases within and between the sexes.

These findings argue that there are multiple, ubiquitous differences in the basic cellular biochemistries of males and females that can affect an individual's health. Many of these differences do not necessarily arise as a result of differences in the hormonal regime to which males and females are exposed but are a direct result of the genetic differences between the two sexes. Thus, the committee makes the following recommendation:

RECOMMENDATION 1: Promote research on sex at the cellular level.

The committee recommends that research be conducted to

   • **determine the functions and effects of X-chromosome- and Y-chromosome-linked genes in somatic cells as well as germ-line cells;**
   • **determine how genetic sex differences influence other levels of biological organization (cell, organ, organ system, organism), including susceptibility to disease; and**
   • **develop systems that can identify and distinguish between the effects of genes and the effects of hormones.**

Sex Begins in the Womb

Sex differences of importance to health and human disease occur throughout the life span, although their specific expression varies at different stages of life. Some differences originate in events occurring in the intrauterine environment, where developmental processes differentially organize tissues for later activation in the male or female. In the prenatal period, sex determination and differentiation occur in a series of sequential processes governed by genetic and environmental factors. During the prepubertal period, behavioral and hormonal changes manifest the secondary sexual characteristics that reinforce the sexual identity of the individual through adolescence and into adulthood. Hormonal events occurring in puberty lay a framework for biological differences that persist through life and contribute to the variable onset and progression of disease in males and females. It is important to study sex differences at all stages of the life cycle, relying on animal models of disease and including sex as a variable in basic and clinical research designs.

RECOMMENDATION 2: Study sex differences from womb to tomb.

The committee recommends that researchers and those who fund research focus on the following areas:

- **inclusion of sex as a variable in basic research designs,**
- **expansion of studies to reveal the mechanisms of intrauterine effects, and**
- **encouragement of studies at different stages of the life span to determine how sex differences influence health, illness, and longevity.**

Sex is an important marker of individual variability. Some of this sex-related variability results from events that occur in the intrauterine environment but that do not materialize until later in life. Current research varies in its level of attention to these matters.

The committee acknowledges that inclusion of people, animals, or cells and tissues of both sexes in all studies is not always feasible or appropriate. Rather, the committee is urging researchers to regard sex, that is, being male or female, as an important basic human variable that should be considered when designing, analyzing, and reporting findings from studies in all areas and at all levels of biomedical research. Statistical methods can be used to evaluate the effect of sex without necessarily doubling the sample size of every study. In addition, it is particularly important that researchers revisit and revise approaches to studying whole-animal physiology in light of what has been learned in the past decade about major sex differences.

RECOMMENDATION 3: Mine cross-species information.

• **Researchers should choose models that mirror human sex differences and that are appropriate for the human conditions being addressed.** Given the interspecies variation, the mechanisms of sex differences in nonhuman primates may be the best mimics for some mechanisms of sex differences in humans. Continued development of appropriate animal models, including those involving nonhuman primates, should be encouraged and supported under existing regulations and guidelines (see the Guide for the Care and Use of Laboratory Animals [National Research Council, 1996]).

• **Researchers should be alert to unexpected phenotypic sex differences resulting from the production of genetically modified animals.**

Sex Affects Behavior and Perception

Basic genetic and physiological differences, in combination with environmental factors, result in behavioral and cognitive differences between males and females. Sex differences in the brain, sex-typed behavior and gender identity, and sex differences in cognitive ability should be studied at all points in the life span. Hormones play a role in behavioral and cognitive sexual dimorphism but are not solely responsible. In addition, sex differences in the perception of pain have important clinical implications. Research is needed on the natural variations between and within the sexes in behavior, cognition, and perception, with expanded investigation of sex differences in brain organization and function. To better understand the influences and roles of factors that may lead to sex differences, the committee makes the following recommendations:

RECOMMENDATION 4: Investigate natural variations.

• **Examine genetic variability, disorders of sex differentiation, reproductive status, and environmental influences to better understand human health.**

Naturally occurring variations provide useful models that can be used to study the influences and origins of a range of factors that influence sex differences.

RECOMMENDATION 5: Expand research on sex differences in brain organization and function.

New technologies make it possible to study sex-differential environmental and behavioral influences on brain organization and function and to recognize modulators of brain organization and function. Innovative ways to expand the availability of and reduce the cost of new technologies need to be explored.

Sex Affects Health

Males and females have different patterns of illness and different life spans, raising questions about the relative roles of biology and environment in these disparities. Dissimilar exposures, susceptibilities, and responses to initiating agents and differences in energy storage and metabolism result in variable responses to pharmacological agents and the initiation and manifestation of diseases such as obesity, autoimmune disorders, and coronary heart disease, to name a few. Understanding the bases of these sex-based differences is important to developing new approaches to prevention, diagnosis, and treatment.

RECOMMENDATION 6: Monitor sex differences and similarities for all human diseases that affect both sexes.

Investigators should

- consider sex as a biological variable in all biomedical and health-related research; and
- design studies that will
  - control for exposure, susceptibility, metabolism, physiology (cycles), and immune response variables;
  - consider how ethical concerns (e.g., risk of fetal injury) constrain study designs and affect outcomes; and
  - detect sex differences across the life span.

The Future of Research on Biological Sex Differences: Challenges and Opportunities

Being male or female is an important fundamental variable that should be considered when designing and analyzing basic and clinical research. Historically, the terms *sex* and *gender* have been loosely, and sometimes inappropriately, used in the reporting of research results, a situation that should be remedied through further clarification. Conducting studies that account for sex differences might require innovative designs, methods, and model systems, all of which might require additional resources. Studies relying on biological materials would benefit from a determination and disclosure of the sex of origin of the material, and clinical researchers should attempt to identify the endocrine status of research subjects. Longitudinal studies should be designed to allow analysis of data by sex. Once studies are conducted, data regarding sex differences, or the lack thereof, should be readily available in the scientific literature. Interdisciplinary efforts are needed to conduct research on sex differences.

RECOMMENDATION 7: Clarify use of the terms *sex* and *gender*.

Researchers should specify in publications their use of the terms *sex* and *gender*. To clarify usage and bring some consistency to the literature, the committee recommends the following:

- **In the study of human subjects, the term *sex* should be used as a classification, generally as male or female, according to the reproductive organs and functions that derive from the chromosomal complement.**
- **In the study of human subjects, the term *gender* should be used to refer to a person's self-representation as male or female, or how that person is responded to by social institutions on the basis of the individual's gender presentation.**
- **In most studies of nonhuman animals the term *sex* should be used.**

RECOMMENDATION 8: Support and conduct additional research on sex differences.

Because differences between the sexes are pervasive across all subdisciplines of biology, all research sponsors should encourage research initiatives on sex differences. Research sponsors and peer-review committees should recognize that research on sex differences may require additional resources.

RECOMMENDATION 9: Make sex-specific data more readily available.

Journal editors should encourage researchers to include in their reports descriptions of the sex ratios of the research population and to specify the extent to which analyses of the data by sex were included in the study. If there is no effect (absence of a sex difference), that should be stated in the results. When designing or updating databases of scientific journal articles and other information, informatics developers should devise ways of reliably accessing sex-specific data.

RECOMMENDATION 10: Determine and disclose the sex of origin of biological research materials.

The origin and sex chromosome constitutions of cells or tissue cultures used for cell biological, molecular biological, or biochemical experiments should be stated when they are known. Attempts should be made to discern the sex of origin when it is unknown. Journal editors should encourage inclusion of such information in Materials and Methods sections as standard practice.

RECOMMENDATION 11: Longitudinal studies should be conducted and should be constructed so that their results can be analyzed by sex.

The health status of males and females can vary considerably, both within and between the sexes, across the life span—from intrauterine development to old age. Most longitudinal studies have been designed with specific disease end points, thereby precluding consideration of many other relevant developmental issues and other diseases, disorders, and conditions.

RECOMMENDATION 12: Identify the endocrine status of research subjects (an important variable that should be considered, when possible, in analyses).

Data on cycles (menstrual, circadian, etc.) are often lacking. Most studies do not define which part of the cycle participants were in at the time of study, note participants only by age and not whether they are pre- or postmenopausal, or are based on only one cycle.

RECOMMENDATION 13: Encourage and support interdisciplinary research on sex differences.

Interdisciplinary research is generally accepted as valuable and important. Opportunities for interdisciplinary collaboration to enhance the understanding of sex differences, however, have not been fully realized. The committee recommends the continued development of interdisciplinary research programs and strategies for more effective communication and cooperation to achieve the following goals:

- synergy between and among basic scientists, epidemiologists, social scientists, and clinical researchers;
- enhanced collaboration across medical specialties; and
- better translational—or bench-to-bedside—research and interlevel integration of data (cellular, to animal, to human).

RECOMMENDATION 14: Reduce the potential for discrimination based on identified sex differences.

The committee noted that, historically, studies on race, ethnicity, age, nationality, religion, and sex have sometimes led to discriminatory practices. The committee believes, therefore, that these historical practices should be taken into consideration so that they will not be repeated. The past should not limit the future of research but should serve as a guide to its use. Ethical research on the biology of sex differences is essential to the advancement of human health and should not be constrained.

SUMMARY

Despite the progress made in focusing on women's health research and including women in clinical trials, such research will have limited value unless the underlying implications—that is, the actual differences between males and females that make such research so critical—are systematically studied and elucidated. Such research can enhance the basis for interpreting the results of separate studies with males and females, helping to clarify findings of no essential sex differences and suggesting mechanisms to be pursued when sex differences are found.

BOX 1
Summary of Barriers to Progress in Research on Sex Differences

Terminology

• There is inconsistent and often confusing use of the terms *sex* and *gender* in the scientific literature and popular press.

Research Tools and Resources

• The conduct of research on sex differences and longitudinal research may require more complex studies and additional resources.
• Information on sex differences can be difficult to glean from the published literature.
• Useful information on the sex of origin of cell and tissue culture material is often lacking in the literature.
• There is a lack of data from longitudinal studies encompassing different diseases, disorders, and conditions across the life span.
• There is a lack of consideration of hormonal variability.

Interdisciplinary and Collaborative Research

• The application of federal regulations is not uniform.
• Opportunities for interdisciplinary collaboration have been underused.

Non-Health-Related Implications of Research on Sex Differences in Health

• There is a lack of awareness that the consequences of genetics and physiology may be amenable to change.
• The finding of sex differences can lead to discriminatory practices.

BOX 2
Summary of Recommendations

Recommendations for Research

- Promote research on sex at the cellular level.
- Study sex differences from womb to tomb.
- Mine cross-species information.
- Investigate natural variations.
- Expand research on sex differences in brain organization and function.
- Monitor sex differences and similarities for all human diseases that affect both sexes.

Recommendations for Addressing Barriers to Progress

- Clarify use of the terms *sex* and *gender*.
- Support and conduct additional research on sex differences.
- Make sex-specific data more readily available.
- Determine and disclose the sex of origin of biological research materials.
- Conduct and construct longitudinal studies so that the results can be analyzed by sex.
- Identify the endocrine status of research subjects.
- Encourage and support interdisciplinary research on sex differences.
- Reduce the potential for discrimination based on identified sex differences.

1
Introduction

There has been an explosion in the growth of new biological information over the past decade, in large part because of the development of
highly advanced techniques that can be used to study the cellular and
molecular mechanisms of normal and abnormal human biology.[1] As a
result, it has become increasingly apparent that many normal physiological functions—and, in many cases, pathological functions—are influenced
either directly or indirectly by sex-based differences in biology (also referred to throughout this report as *sex differences*).

Scientific evidence of the importance of sex[2] differences throughout
the life span abounds. Investigators are now positioned to take this work
to the next level, at which the mechanisms and origins of such differences

---

[1]*Biology* is defined as the study of life and living organisms (*Dorland's Illustrated Medical Dictionary*, 1994; *Stedman's Medical Dictionary*, 1995). Given that no living organism carries out its life alone and that there is no such thing as a null environment (void of any influ-ence), the committee defines *biology*, for the purposes of this report, to include the genetic, molecular, biochemical, hormonal, cellular, physiological, behavioral, and psychosocial as-pects of life.

[2]The committee defines *sex* as the classification of living things, generally as male or female according to their reproductive organs and functions assigned by the chromosomal complement, and *gender* as a person's self-representation as male or female, or how that person is responded to by social institutions on the basis of the individual's gender presen-tation. Gender is shaped by environment and experience. See additional discussion later in this chapter.

can be explored. This will allow scientists and clinicians to understand the implications of these differences for human health.

Although many specific questions beg to be asked, the critical underlying question to be answered is this:

How and when do the basic biological differences between males and females matter to the overall health of boys and girls or men and women?

This is a complex question, the answer to which is not easily derived. There is no such thing as a pure biological effect, just as there is no such thing as a null environment (one void of any influence). The "biology" of a given individual therefore includes genetic, physiological, and hormonal effects as well as the environmental, behavioral, and societal influences that shape that individual.

The question presented above might therefore be better phrased as follows:

How can information on sex differences be translated into preventative, diagnostic, and therapeutic practice? How can the new knowledge about and understanding of biological sex differences and similarities most effectively be used to positively affect patient outcomes and improve health and health care?

Answers to these questions will help reshape the biomedical and health-related research conducted in the future.

SCOPE OF THE REPORT

In November 1999, the Institute of Medicine (IOM) formed the Committee on Understanding the Biology of Sex and Gender Differences in response to combined requests from a consortium of public and private sponsors.[3] In general, the sponsors asked that the IOM committee evaluate and consider the current understanding of sex differences and determinants at the biological level.

Specifically, the sponsors asked the committee to address the following issues:

- the knowledge base on and research priorities for animal and cel-

---

[3]U.S. Department of Health and Human Services (Office on Women's Health, National Institutes of Health Office of Research on Women's Health, National Institute of Environmental Health Sciences, National Institute on Drug Abuse, National Institute of Mental Health, U.S. Food and Drug Administration, Centers for Disease Control and Prevention); National Science Foundation, Environmental Protection Agency, National Aeronautics and Space Administration, Society for Women's Health Research, Research Foundation for Health and Environmental Effects, Ortho-McNeil/Johnson & Johnson; Unilever United States Foundation.

lular models that could be used to determine when sex and gender differences exist and when they are relevant to biological functioning at the cellular, developmental, organ, organismal, and behavioral levels;

• current and potential barriers to the conduct of valid and productive research on sex and gender differences and their determinants, including ethical, financial, sociological, and scientific factors; and

• strategies that can be used to overcome such barriers and promote the acceptance of this research by the scientific community and the general public.

The committee's charge was not to prepare a definitive text on all known differences between the sexes but, rather, to consider factors and traits that characterize and differentiate males and females across the life span and that underlie sex differences in health (including behavioral, biochemical, genetic, physical, and physiological elements).

The committee members brought expertise from a broad array of disciplines in basic and applied biomedical research, including behavioral science, cellular biology, clinical research, developmental psychology, developmental and reproductive biology, epidemiology, genetics, health sciences policy, immunology, molecular biology, neuroscience, pathology, pharmacology, physiology, women's health, and zoology.

Focusing the Analysis on Biology Across the Life Span

After critical review of the task and a discussion with the study sponsors at the first meeting, the committee acknowledged the potentially broad scope that a comprehensive analysis of sex and gender differences in health would have. This is evidenced by the expansive National Institutes of Health (NIH) report *Agenda for Research on Women's Health for the 21st Century* (National Institutes of Health, Office of Research on Women's Health, 1999a–f), a six-volume report that synthesizes the proceedings of four scientific workshops that were held in 1996 and 1997 and that included presentations and testimony from more than 1,500 scientific experts, policy makers, and public participants. The resulting document is a survey of ongoing research on women's health, and five overarching themes recur throughout: (1) "Women's health is expanding into the larger concept of gender-specific medicine," (2) "Research on women's health must include the full biological life cycle of the woman," (3) "Multidisciplinary research is essential," (4) "The importance of social and behavioral science to research on women's health is unquestionable," and (5) "The collection of first-hand information from women [is needed] to correct male models of normal function and of pathophysiology of disease" (National Institutes of Health, Office of Research on Women's Health, 1999a, p. 13–14).

With its inventory of current research, the NIH report served as a resource for the IOM committee, whose charge extended beyond assessment of women's health to assessment of basic biological differences between males and females that affect human health. It was agreed that another inventory of current research was not needed and was not part of the committee's task.

Thus, in addressing its charge, the committee identified and assessed examples of basic biological differences between males and females. It evaluated these differences as they vary over the continuum of the life span of the individual, in addition to how they relate to the understanding of human disease and health in both males and females. The committee considered how biological function is shaped by experiential influences and identified areas in which additional research would be important to improve the overall understanding of the relationship between sex and human health.

The committee also discusses animal (including human) and cellular models in the context of the different examples of sex differences. In light of the evolving understanding of the important role of sex in biological development and the onset of disease, it is particularly important that researchers revisit and revise approaches to studying whole-animal physiology.

The focus of this report is on sex-based differences, versus sex-based similarities, as they are more likely to successfully demonstrate the need for further research and lead to greater understanding of the significance of sex in human biology and health.

Moreover, despite the influence of pregnancy, parity, and parenthood on the manifestation of some diseases and health outcomes, this report does not directly address these issues, as they are deserving of separate and more in-depth attention.

Social status, and the value (or lack thereof) of males or females in certain families or populations, can have a profound effect on health. Low social status, absence of freedoms, limited or no access to health care including family planning and hormone treatments, and poor quality of care are particularly important issues for the health of women in certain cultures and may have a greater impact on their overall health than biology. As the focus of this report is the health consequences of biologically-based differences between the sexes, these issues are not addressed here. Discussion of some of these issues can be found in *In Her Own Right: The Institute of Medicine's Guide to Women's Health Issues* (Benderly, 1997) and *In Her Lifetime: Female Morbidity and Mortality in Sub-Saharan Africa* (Institute of Medicine, 1996).

BOX 1-1
Definitions

Sex: The classification of living things, generally as male or female according to their reproductive organs and functions assigned by chromosomal complement.

Gender: A person's self-representation as male or female, or how that person is responded to by social institutions based on the individual's gender presentation. Gender is rooted in biology and shaped by environment and experience.

Biology: The study of life and living organisms (*Dorland's Illustrated Medical Dictionary*, 1994; *Stedman's Medical Dictionary*, 1995), including the genetic, molecular, biochemical, hormonal, cellular, physiological, behavioral, and psychosocial aspects of life.

Defining the Terms *Sex* and *Gender*

The committee clarified, for its own purposes, how the terms *sex* and *gender* would be used throughout the course of the study and the report (see Box 1-1). Therefore, using these definitions to discuss differences between males and females, the committee refers to *sex differences* when the differences appear to have primarily biological origins and to *gender differences* when they appear to be expressed in response to social influences. The committee acknowledges, however, that it is impossible to know a priori the causes for a particular difference between males and females. Nevertheless, this distinction does have value by signifying that society responds to individuals on the basis of their sex and gender. Males and females differ not only in their basic biology but also in the ways that they interact with and are treated in society.

With respect to sex, humans are generally dimorphic. With some exceptions, individuals are either chromosomally XX and developmentally female or chromosomally XY and developmentally male. In defining sex, it is important to distinguish between "genetic sex" and "phenotypic sex," since disorders such as the adrenogenital syndrome and the androgen-insensitivity mutation (*Tfm*) give rise to phenotypes that seem to contradict an individual's genetic sex.

In contrast, gender is a continuum. An individual may display characteristics considered more typical of the opposite sex, and a person's sense of gender may change over the course of a lifetime. Gender identity and gender role affect individual activities, exposures, and access to care, all of which can affect health and all of which vary widely across cultures.

The *American Medical Association Manual of Style* (Iverson, 1998) defines sex as the biological characteristics of males and females. The American Medical Association (AMA) acknowledges that gender includes more than sex and is a cultural indicator of an individual's personal and social status. The World Health Organization (WHO) (1998b) defines *sex* as "genetic/physiological or biological characteristics of a person which indicates whether one is female or male" and defines *gender* as referring to "women's and men's roles and responsibilities that are socially determined" (p. 10). WHO notes that "gender is related to how we are perceived and expected to think and act as women and men because of the ways society is organized" (p. 10). The committee's chosen definitions are in line with those of AMA and WHO.

Although such definitions are helpful, two committee members argued that they imply that the idea of biological difference suggests a predominance of physiology, with a subsequent fine-tuning by environment.[4] Moreover, the two committee members were concerned that dividing biological and environmental events into separate spheres could make researchers less likely to ask solid mechanistic questions about, for example, how diet and mechanical stress affect bone development.

To illustrate, a variety of factors, including behavioral habits, hormones, genetics, and environmental influences, affect the development of bone mass. Some of these are generally understood to be internal to the organism (genes and hormones), and some are generally understood to be external. In one sense, some might be called "sex related" and others might be called "gender related." Closer examination, however, shows that this distinction is less clear-cut. Exercise and body weight, for example, both contribute to bone formation. In the United States, current conventions promote extreme thinness as an appropriate body image for young girls, whereas vigorous weight-bearing exercises are still less commonly performed by girls and young women than by boys. Both of these factors result in difference in weight-bearing impacts on bones and thus contribute to differences in the development of bone mass. In other words, culture and behavior (gender) become contributing causes to differences in bone mass between males and females (sex).

Some questions that might be addressed at the developmental and molecular levels include the following: Does mechanical stress activate particular genes in osteoclasts or osteoblasts? How is physical stress translated into cellular, bone-shaping activity (via hormones? via other types of receptors?). (For examples of model systems that study mechanical stress and bone development, see Cullen et al. [2000], Marie and Zerath

---

[4]Two committee members raised concerns that the definitions adopted by the full committee were appropriate but that the subsequent analysis did not fully put the definition into action.

[2000], Mosley [2000], Pedersen et al. [1999].) Does diet affect circulating hormone levels, the synthesis or turnover of hormone receptors on critical cell types in the bone, or other aspects of bone metabolism? More theoretically, these questions ask how social gender intersects with bone development at the molecular and cellular levels.

The ability to look at sex and gender as part of a single system in which social elements act with biological elements to produce the body has important consequences for medical treatment. In this example, when more is understood about the mechanism of bone formation—including how the many factors interact to either promote or impede bone development—researchers and clinicians can begin to formulate an arsenal of new approaches to increase bone mass well before menopause.

This example illustrates how biological questions that are posed as a result of an approach that examines how factors outside the body are translated into differences between male and female bodies will break new scientific ground.

Throughout the report, the committee presents data—where available—that genes, physiology, and the physical and social environments operate in concert to produce a phenotype. Researchers are just beginning to unravel these complex interactions, revealing how these factors work together to produce differences between males and females that provide many new opportunities for investigation.

SEX DIFFERENCES BEYOND THE REPRODUCTIVE SYSTEM

Although an individual can be characterized initially by the presence of particular reproductive organs, sex differences encompass much more than that. Evidence suggests that the distinct anatomy and physiology that develop as a result of having been dealt two X chromosomes (XX) or an X chromosome and a Y chromosome (XY) at fertilization can have a much broader influence on an individual's health than was previously thought. Although it is anatomically obvious why only males develop prostate cancer and only females get ovarian cancer, it is not at all obvious why, for example, females are more likely than males to recover language ability after suffering a left-hemisphere stroke (Shaywitz et al., 1995) or why females have a far greater risk than males of developing life-threatening ventricular arrhythmias in response to a variety of potassium channel-blocking drugs (Ebert et al., 1998).

Recent research has shed some light on these puzzles. In the case of stroke, for example, functional magnetic resonance imaging has shown that females rely on both sides of the brain for certain aspects of language, whereas males predominantly rely on the left hemisphere (Shaywitz et al., 1995). In the case of drug-induced arrhythmias, data suggest that sex steroid hormones influence the activities of specific cardiac ion channels (Ebert et al., 1998).

Differences in the prevalence and severity of a broad range of diseases, disorders, and conditions exist between the sexes (for additional examples, see Box 1-2). Some of the variations appear to be influenced by physiological differences, such as the role of sex hormones in cardiovascular disease and osteoporosis, or by experiential and environmental differences, such as smoking habits or exposure to the sun's ultraviolet rays as a result of one's occupation, recreational activities, or clothing styles. Observations such as these are important to the development of an understanding of the etiology of and optimal approaches to the diagnosis and treatment of specific diseases, with the ultimate goal being improvement of the health of both sexes. It is important to remember, however, that physiological factors and experiential factors do not act independently and cannot be neatly compartmentalized. Moreover, the distinction between the origins of these differences—biological environment versus social environment—can be valuable as well as a hindrance.

For some disparities in incidence and manifestation, such as for some of the autoimmune diseases, there are far fewer clues, experiential or biological, to explain the observed differences. The relapsing intermittent form of multiple sclerosis, for example, occurs predominantly in females but has a more severe effect on males (Noseworthy et al., 2000).

Differences between the sexes may be modest, yet they may still result in important outcomes. Small absolute differences between the sexes may result in large differences in health and illness among members of the general population. In addition, small differences between the sexes may be informative in providing an understanding of the underlying mechanisms of normal and pathological functions.

Sex Variability

Biologists study variability as part of life, and many biological variables, for example, age and family history, affect health. The committee considered such variables for which data were available and relevant to the discussion. Ultimately, however, this report is about the influence of sex—one of the most basic human variables—on health.

In addition to variability between the sexes, there is also considerable variability within each sex. Factors such as race and ethnicity may affect health as well. A striking aspect of some sex differences is the consistency with which they appear across populations with vastly different health status profiles and environmental circumstances.

A simple example of variability within populations is height. On average, males are taller than females. This is apparent across all cultures and has been for thousands of years. Although it is partially dictated by parentage, height is also influenced by environmental factors, such as nutrition (Valian, 1998).

In other cases, sex differences vary among populations, giving clues to their dependence on the interplay of sex and other variables. Obesity is a condition for which the differences between sexes varies by ethnicity. Females are generally more likely than males to be obese, but the sex difference is much more striking in some ethnic groups and even varies among subgroups within ethnic groups (see Chapter 5). Recent studies with animals indicate that alterations in hormonal and nutritional exposures during fetal development can result in variability in health and illness among males and among females (Barker, 2000; Nathanielsz, 1999; vom Saal et al., 1999). Age and reproductive status add to variability in health and illness within the sexes as well.

Most of the discussion so far has been of "typical" males and females, that is, those with the expected XY or XX sex chromosome constitution and the corresponding expected developmental characteristics. Although sexual dimorphism (two, and only two, distinct forms of sex, male or female) at all levels is the "rule," exceptions are more common than most people realize, resulting in chromosomal, gonadal, hormonal, or genital deviations from the chromosomal, gonadal, hormonal, or genital constitution of a "typical" male or female (Blackless et al., 2000). Study of these exceptions can shed light not only on the clinical implications for individuals with a mixed sex genotype (genetic makeup) or phenotype (visible properties of a person) but also on the role of sex in normal development.

EVOLVING RESEARCH POLICY

In recent years, considerable attention has been given to the differences and similarities between females and males (1) at the *societal* level by researchers evaluating how individual behaviors, lifestyles, and surroundings affect one's biological development and health and (2) at the level of the *whole organism* by clinicians and applied researchers investigating the component organs and systems of humans. However, scientists have paid much less attention to the direct and intentional study of these differences at the basic *cellular* and *molecular* levels. Where data are available, they have often been a by-product of other research. Historically, the research community assumed that beyond the reproductive system such differences do not exist or are not relevant. (One example is the lack of consideration of the sex of origin of cells and tissues used in research [see Chapter 6].)

The conjoint study of males and females to explore sex differences is not a well-established convention in scientific practice. Since World War II and until relatively recently, clinical research was conducted primarily

BOX 1-2
Examples of Sex Differences Beyond the Reproductive System

Differences Associated with the Sex Chromosomes

Males have only one X chromosome, and thus, their cells have only one copy of each X-chromosome-specific gene. Females have two X chromosomes, but their cells approach the same status of male cells by a special mechanism called X-chromosome inactivation. Early in the development of female cells, most cells inactivate one of their two X chromosomes, leaving only one set of X-chromosome genes able to function in that cell and its progeny. (Some genes, however, escape inactivation [see Chapter 2].) The initial decision of which X chromosome to inactivate appears to be random. As a result, each female is made up of mixed populations of cells, some containing X-chromosome genes inherited from her mother and some containing genes from her father.

These mixed populations provide a safety net for females who get a deleterious X-chromosome gene from one parent. A striking example of this safety net is seen with incontinentia pigmenti (IP), a skin disorder seen in females, but not males, as affected males die in utero or shortly after birth. In this case, the mutated gene causes cell death. Male embryos and male infants carrying the gene undergo extensive cell death and do not survive. In female embryos with one copy of the gene, cells in which the gene for the disease is on the active X chromosome die, but the dead cells are replaced by cells expressing the functional gene from the other X chromosome. As a result, females survive and most of their cells express the functional gene. Some of the other cells remain, and it is this minority population that causes the blisters and warty lesions characteristic of IP (Francis and Sybert, 1997; Goldsmith and Epstein, 1999).

Differences in Immune Function

Females have a more aggressive immune response to infectious challenge but are also more likely than males to develop autoimmune diseases, such as thyroiditis or lupus.

Hashimoto thyroiditis is an overwhelmingly female disease (10:1) in humans, but experimental models of thyroiditis in mice and rats are not sex discrepant.

Systemic lupus erythematosus is a predominantly female disease (6-9:1) in humans; its severity is similar in females and males. In experimental mice, it is female predominant in some strains, sex neutral in others, and male predominant in still others; and its severity is greater in the affected sex.

Fetal cells circulate in the bloodstreams of women who have been pregnant. In women with scleroderma, they circulate in much greater quantities and for far longer periods of time (decades) than they do in healthy women.

with men. As described below, there have been both conceptual and practical deterrents to the inclusion of women and a tendency to underreport rather than highlight sex differences that might bring about possible scientific insights. As a result, the medical community lacks useful, comparable data on conditions that occur disproportionately, that manifest dif-

Gonadal hormones markedly affect immune and inflammatory cell responses, but men and women respond similarly to infection.

Vaccinations induce higher antibody levels in females than males; arthritis as a complication of vaccination is more common in females (see Chapter 5).

Differences in Symptoms, Type, and Onset of Cardiovascular Disease

Men begin to experience heart attacks, on average, 10 years earlier than women and have a better 1-year postattack survival rate than women. Symptoms of heart attack show distinct sex differences: most men experience acute, crushing chest pain, whereas most women experience shortness of breath and fatigue as well as chest pain (see Chapter 5).

Differences in Response to Toxins

Although it is likely that the rate of lung cancer among females is on the rise largely because younger women are smoking more, it may also be the case that females are predisposed biologically to the adverse effects of the toxins in cigarettes. Women are at a 1.2- to 1.7-fold higher risk than men for all major types of lung cancer at every level of exposure to cigarette smoke. Variations in factors such as smoking history and body size do not account for the increased risk. Recent data suggest that sex differences in metabolism or gene expression may underlie these differences in cancer risk (Guinee et al., 1995; Manton, 2000; Shriver et al., 2000; Tseng et al., 1999).

Differences in Brain Organization

Men and women differ in brain organization for language. Men rely on the left inferior frontal gyrus to carry out language tasks, such as determining if two nonsense words rhyme. Women use both the left and the right inferior gyri to carry out the same task. Interestingly, men and women perform the task equally accurately and equally rapidly. This may protect women who suffer a left-sided stroke from experiencing decrements in their language performance.

Differences in Pain

Females are more sensitive than males to nociceptive (potentially or frankly damaging) stimuli, including those that occur in internal organs. Added to this greater sensitivity of females is a higher prevalence of many painful disorders in females. Recent studies with humans show that kappa-opioid drugs are more effective analgesics in young adult women than in young adult men (see Chapter 4) (Berkley and Holdcroft, 1999; Gear et al.,1999).

ferently, or that require different approaches to diagnosis and treatment in males and females. For many years it was assumed that males, particularly Caucasian males, provided the "norm" or "standard," and there was a tendency to view females as being "deviant or problematic, even in studying diseases that affect both sexes" (Institute of Medicine, 1994, p.

8). Unfortunately, although some reports now treat males and females as being different, but equally "normal," the habit of viewing the male as the norm or baseline can still be found in the current medical literature (Nicolette, 2000).

Over the past several decades, the women's health movement has successfully worked toward achieving a significant increase in the amount of research conducted on women's health issues. Critics argue that the majority of such research has focused on reproductive health. Still others suggest that the pendulum has swung too far in the direction of studies focusing on women, with researchers now collecting data exclusively on females without including the corresponding data on males. Nevertheless, the study of sex-based differences in biology has yielded information beneficial to the health of both males and females.

The justification for excluding females from clinical studies arose partially from efforts to protect them. Protection of human research subjects emerged as a policy issue after World War II with the issuance of the Nuremberg Code of Ethics in 1949, which outlined the basic moral, ethical, and legal requirements of conducting research with human subjects (McCarthy, 1994; U.S. Government Printing Office, 1949). This landmark document led the way for a series of protectionist policies, including human subject protections issued by the U.S. Public Health Service in 1966 that were revised repeatedly and that were ultimately rewritten and published as the policy guidelines for the entire U.S. Department of Health, Education, and Welfare in 1971 and again, with more stringent federal regulations, in 1974 (45 CFR 46, May 30, 1974).

These efforts were spurred by a series of alarming adverse events, including those caused by thalidomide and diethylstilbestrol (DES), and the exposure of abusive and unethical research practices, such as the Tuskegee syphilis study and the use of U.S. servicemen during World War II as research subjects in studies of the effects of mustard agents and lewisite (a poison gas) (Institute of Medicine, 1993, 1994).

Although none of these provisions excluded specific subpopulations from clinical research, the policies stated that subjects who were vulnerable because of physical, mental, or social circumstances must not be exploited. Hence, few women were included, as pregnant women and their fetuses were grouped into the category of "vulnerable populations" (45 CFR 46, subpart B; Institute of Medicine, 1994). Thus, although the thalidomide and DES incidents were not related to the participation of women in clinical trials, they fostered an aversion to involving women who were or who could become pregnant in any drug-related research (Institute of Medicine, 1994). (Although both thalidomide and DES were successfully tested in clinical trials, the side effects were not apparent until the approved drugs were used widely by pregnant women, who were not part of the clinical trial population.)

In 1977 the U.S. Food and Drug Administration (FDA) issued guidelines recommending that pharmaceutical companies exclude women in their childbearing years from phase I clinical studies (studies with healthy subjects to evaluate the safety of a new drug) (U.S. Food and Drug Administration, 1977). In addition, the U.S. Department of Health and Human Services established in 1991 that "no pregnant woman may be involved as a subject in an activity . . . unless the purpose of the activity is to meet the health need of the mother and the fetus will be placed at risk only to the minimum extent necessary to reach such needs" (45 CFR 46.207).

Scientifically, women were excluded as clinical research participants because (1) there was a general belief among clinical researchers that men and women will not differ significantly in response to treatment in most situations, and (2) the inclusion of women introduces additional variables (in the form of hormonal cycles) and decreases the homogeneity of the study population (Institute of Medicine, 1994). Ironically, even as it was acknowledged that the female hormonal cycle is a significant confounding variable and test substances might respond unpredictably to hormonal fluctuations, it was nonetheless widely believed that men and women were similar enough that it was acceptable to then treat women with therapies developed solely on the basis of the results of studies performed with men as research subjects (Haseltine and Jacobson, 1997).

The policy of exclusion continued into the mid-1980s, when, in 1985, the U.S. Public Health Service Task Force on Women's Health Issues concluded that health care for women and the quality of health information available to women had been compromised by the historical lack of research on women's health issues (U.S. Public Health Service, 1985). In response, NIH issued a new policy in 1986 that encouraged the inclusion of women in clinical research, requested justification for the exclusion of women, and suggested evaluation of the data for differences by sex. A 1990 investigation by the U.S. General Accounting Office (GAO), however, found that the guidelines were not being implemented with any regularity (U.S. General Accounting Office, 1990).

With government and public interest in the composition of study populations escalating, NIH created a new office, the Office of Research on Women's Health (ORWH), and issued a stronger policy statement on the inclusion of women and minorities in clinical studies. In 1993, with the passage of the National Institutes of Health Revitalization Act (P.L. 103-43), ORWH was authorized statutorily and the guidelines for inclusion of women and minorities became law. That same year, FDA lifted the 1977 restrictions on the inclusion of women in their childbearing years in phase I clinical trials and encouraged analysis of clinical data by sex but did not require inclusion of both sexes in clinical trials (Merkatz et al., 1993). In 1998, FDA published the final rule, Investigational New Drug

Applications and New Drug Applications (U.S. Department of Health and Human Services, 1998). This rule allows the agency to refuse to file any new drug application that does not appropriately analyze safety and efficacy data by sex.

In 2000, GAO reassessed NIH's progress in conducting research on women's health in the decade since publication of the 1990 GAO report. GAO reported that NIH has made "significant progress in implementing a strengthened policy in including women in clinical research," treating the inclusion of women and minorities as a matter of scientific merit in the review process for extramural research (U.S. General Accounting Office, 2000, p. 2). However, the GAO report noted that less progress has been made in encouraging analysis of the data by sex.

NIH agreed with GAO's overall conclusion. With regard to the criticism that NIH has not ensured the analysis of the data by sex, NIH raised concerns that GAO had included in its review unpublished reports based on research that had occurred before the new requirements were enacted (Kirschstein, 2000). The reports referred to in the GAO audit (which were subsequently published [Montgomery and Sherif, 2000; Vidaver et al., 2000]) looked at articles published between 1993 and 1998 in select journals and found that few, if any, data from research funded under the 1993 mandate for the inclusion of women in clinical trials would have been available or published within that period (Pinn, 2000).

Despite the progress made in focusing on women's health research and including women in clinical trials, such research will have limited value unless the underlying implications—that is, the actual differences between males and females that make such research so critical—are systematically studied and elucidated. Such research can enhance the basis for interpreting the results of separate studies with males and females, helping to clarify findings of no essential sex differences, and suggesting mechanisms to be pursued when sex differences are found. The availability of mechanistic explanations is also critical for the effective use of current knowledge, that is, indicating where existing research done only with a male population or only with a female population is most or least likely to be directly applicable to both sexes.

ORGANIZATION OF REPORT

Chapters 2 to 5 give specific, in-depth examples of sex differences and discuss how those differences influence the health of both individual males and individual females. The information is presented at increasing levels of organizational complexity, from the cellular level, to the whole-organism level, to the response of the organism to its environment. Specifically, Chapter 2 describes the basic genetic, cellular, and molecular differences between the sexes. Chapter 3 provides background information on the development and changes of the whole human across the life span. Chapter 4 presents examples of how basic genetic and physiological differences between males and females might produce phenotypic differences. Chapter 5 looks into the response of the individual to external agents encountered purposefully (e.g., food or medications) or coincidentally (e.g., infectious agents or ultraviolet radiation). Discussions of animal (including human) and cellular research models of human conditions appear throughout the report, generally in conjunction with a particular example. Finally, Chapter 6 addresses overarching barriers to valid and productive research on sex and gender differences as they relate to health and discusses the challenges and opportunities that lie ahead in this emerging field of research. The report includes four appendixes to provide the reader with additional information: Appendix A discusses data sources and committee methods, Appendix B describes physiological and pharmacological differences between the sexes, Appendix C includes a glossary, and Appendix D includes IOM committee and staff biographies.

The examples used throughout the report were chosen to demonstrate that sex differences occur across a wide variety of interrelated disciplines. The use of a particular example is not meant to imply that research in that area is more important or should have priority over research in other areas.

In each chapter, on the basis of its review, the committee arrived at a series of findings and conclusions and developed recommendations that are designed to facilitate scientific endeavors in this area, take advantage of new opportunities in basic and applied research, and fill identified research gaps.

2

Every Cell Has a Sex

ABSTRACT

The biological differences between the sexes have long been recognized at the biochemical and cellular levels. Rapid advances in molecular biology have revealed the genetic and molecular bases of a number of sex-based differences in health and human disease, some of which are attributed to sexual genotype—XX in the female and XY in the male. Genes on the sex chromosomes can be expressed differently between males and females because of the presence of either single or double copies of the gene and because of the phenomena of different meiotic effects, X inactivation, and genetic imprinting. The inheritance of either a male or a female genotype is further influenced by the source (maternal or paternal) of the X chromosome. The relative roles of the sex chromosome genes and their expression explains X-chromosome-linked disease and is likely to illuminate the reasons for heterogeneous expression of some diseases within and between the sexes.

The notion that there are biological differences between the sexes is most evident and comfortable when it is applied to the reproductive system. However, sex differences have been identified or suggested at many levels of biological organization, from biochemical to behavioral. For the majority of the population, as well as a substantial fraction of scientists, not all known differences are obvious, and not all of those that have been suggested or suspected are easily explainable in biological terms.

In terms of genetic mechanisms, two general models attempt to explain how an individual's genes give rise to sex differences (Figure 2-1). In the first model, a series of critical hormone-responsive genes, shared by both males and females, are influenced differently in the alternative hormonal milieus of the male or female throughout their life spans, thus leading to or contributing to the many differences observed between the sexes. In the second model (which is not necessarily exclusive of the first one), one or more genes, located on the sex chromosomes and thus expressed differently in the two sexes, encode proteins involved in rate-limiting or rate-influencing steps in biochemical or physiological pathways that are critical to establishing differences between the sexes.

The purpose of this chapter is twofold: (1) to describe those differences that exist between males and females at the biochemical and cellular levels and that result directly from the defining genotypic difference between male and female mammals, namely, an XY (male) sex chromosome constitution versus an XX (female) sex chromosome constitution, and (2) to describe how males and females may transmit to their offspring genetic information that is the same but that is transmitted at different observed phenotypic or genotypic ratios. This information will then serve as a foundation for consideration of the onset of sex differences during development and throughout life in response to both intrinsic and extrinsic exposures.

SEX AND THE HUMAN GENOME

Males and females have partially different genomes. Viewed from a purely reductionist standpoint, many differences between the male and female sexes are predicted to be rooted in differences between the genetic contents of male and female cells and differences in the expression of those genetic contents. As the complete DNA sequence of the human genome has now been determined, it is important to place the discussions of this chapter into the context of the human genome.

The human genome contains, by current measurements, a little more than 3 billion base pairs of DNA (Lander, 1996; National Human Genome Research Institute, 2000). Earlier estimates predicted an estimated 50,000 to 100,000 different genes (National Human Genome Research Institute, 2000). The most recent estimates, based on the current drafts of the human genome sequence, suggest that there are approximately 30,000 human genes (International Human Genome Sequencing Consortium, 2001; Venter et al., 2001). However, this lower figure may be a minimum estimate because it is derived using an algorithm that identifies genes on the basis of their similarity to a modest sized panel of already characterized human genes.

The hallmark of human biology is variation, and much of the observed variation both within and between the sexes is encoded within the

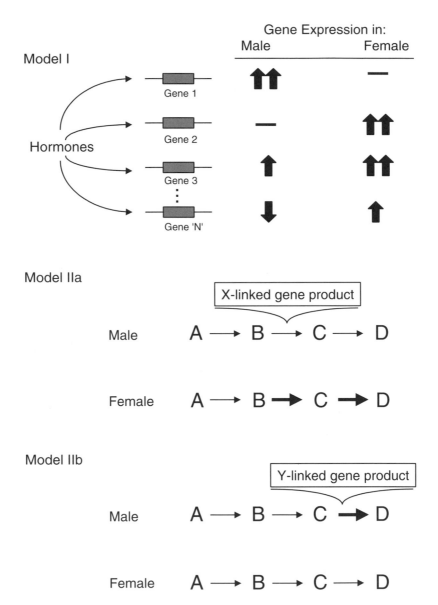

FIGURE 2-1 Schematic representation of two general models used to explain sex differences in gene expression. In Model I, hormones in males and females differentially influence the level of expression of different genes (Gene 1 to Gene N) in the genome. Arrows indicate the direction and the magnitude of the effect. In Model II, a rate-limiting step in various pathways (e.g., metabolic or signal transduction pathways) is encoded by or influenced by an X- or Y-chromosome-linked gene that shows dosage differences between males and females. Thus, the net amounts of Products C and D differ between the sexes.

human genome. At the DNA level, an estimated 1 of every 1,300 bases on the autosomes (non-sex-determining chromosomes) differs between any two individuals (International SNP Map Working Group, 2001; Nickerson et al., 1998; Venter et al., 2001). In other words, the genomes of individuals may differ at some 4 to 6 million base positions. Some of these differences will lead to gene products that are functionally distinct, for example, receptors that differ in their affinity or rate of turnover, enzymes that differ in their steady-state levels, and genes that differ in their degree of hormone responsiveness. Although ongoing studies of human DNA variation will soon provide a more robust estimate, one can calculate from previous studies of enzyme variation and more recent investigations of gene variation (Zwick et al., 2000) that the precise composition and functioning of thousands of proteins will differ between any two individuals.

Notwithstanding this degree of population-level variation in the DNA sequence, most of the genes in the genome are thought to not differ in either sequence or level of expression as a simple consequence of the sex of the individual. However, as will be illustrated more fully in the following sections, there are three types of genes (see also Box 2-1) in which an individual's sex per se is likely to play a role.

First, genes on the Y chromosome are expressed only in males, and many of these have no counterpart on the X chromosome or autosomes; thus, expression of these genes will be limited to males.

Second, some genes on the X chromosome are expressed at higher levels in females than in males. Although the process of X-chromosome inactivation equalizes the effective dosage of most X-chromosome genes between male and female cells by inactivating one of the two X chromosomes in female cells, not all genes on the inactivated X chromosome

---

BOX 2-1
Genetic Factors That May Differentially Affect the
Basic Biochemistry of Male and Female Cells

Female specific:
- expression of some genes from both X chromosomes,
- defect in initiation or maintenance of X-chromosome inactivation, and
- changes in estrogen-responsive genes (e.g., the HER2 gene in breast cancer) in germ-line or somatic cells.

Male specific:
- X-chromosome-linked recessive mutations,
- expression of Y-chromosome-specific genes, and
- changes in androgen-responsive genes in germ-line or somatic cells.

respond to this mechanism. The relatively few genes that are not equalized can have significant effects on the phenotypes of cells.

Third, the expression of many genes is likely to be influenced by hormonal differences between the two sexes. For example, some of these may be genes whose expression is limited to sexually dimorphic tissues or cell types (e.g., the ovary, testis, prostate, and breast), whereas others may be globally expressed but subject to hormonal regulation in different tissues or at different times during development (see Chapter 3).

Although only a limited number of genes have been examined to date, from the standpoint of sexual dimorphism, new approaches to quantification of the expression of genes in different samples on a genome-wide basis promise to change this. DNA arrays, or "gene chips," containing tens of thousands of human genes can be queried to compare their levels of expression between different tissues or different sexes under a variety of physiological or hormonal conditions (Lander, 1996; Lockhart and Winzeler, 2000). Such studies will yield a large database of gene expression data. More difficult will be determination of the relative effects of differences in gene expression on the characteristic phenotypic differences seen between males and females. Nonetheless, this new technology with DNA arrays promises to provide a comprehensive functional view of the genome in different cellular states, and studies that address differences in expression throughout the male and female genomes should reap a rich harvest.

BASIC MOLECULAR GENETICS:
WHAT IS THE POTENTIAL FOR DIFFERENCES
BETWEEN THE SEXES?

The issue of whether there should be genetic differences in basic cellular biochemistry between female and male cells (as a direct result of sex chromosome constitution rather than hormonal influences) (see Figure 2-1 and Box 2-1) is often approached from two opposing perspectives. Geneticist Jacques Monod's famous adage that "What's true of *Escherichia coli* is true of an elephant" represents the point of view that genes have been conserved over time and among species. This view has had extraordinary staying power in molecular biology and genetics, and if "yeast" was substituted for "*E. coli,*" the statement would have even greater vitality. If the basic biochemistries of organisms separated by a billion years of evolution are so similar, then (so goes the logic) why should one expect that males and females within the *same* species should exhibit important differences in their basic biochemistries? An opposing perspective acknowledges that the majority of human disease-causing mutations exhibit dominant or semidominant effects (McKusick, 2000). Thus, a change in the activity of a single gene can have a large effect on the organism that

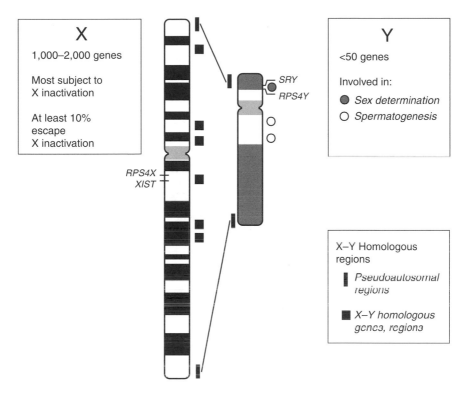

FIGURE 2-2 Comparison of gene contents and gene organizations on the X and Y chromosomes (see text for details).

carries that gene. Because the sex chromosomes comprise approximately 5 percent of the total human genome (Figure 2-2), there is the potential for 1 in 20 biochemical reactions to be differentially affected in male versus female cells. From this standpoint, it is difficult to imagine that male and female cells will not differ in at least some aspects of basic biochemistry, given the complexity of most biological pathways.

Males Have a Y Chromosome, Females Do Not

The male genome differs from the female genome in the number of X chromosomes that it contains, as well as by the presence of a Y chromosome. It is the overriding presence of a gene on the Y chromosome (*SRY*) that results in development of the male gonadal phenotype. However, apart from causing the dramatic divergence from the female developmental pathway (which the indeterminate gonad would otherwise follow and which has been discussed in a number of reviews [Hiort and

Holterhus, 2000, Sinclair, 1998; Vilain and McCabe, 1998]), it was long considered a valid biological question to ask whether the Y chromosome carried any genes of "importance." The paucity and nature of traits that were thought, by genetic criteria, to segregate with the Y chromosome ("hairy ears," for example [Dronamraju, 1964]) tended to reinforce the notion that the Y chromosome encoded the male gonadal phenotype (Koopman et al., 1991), one or more genes involved in male fertility (Lahn and Page, 1997), the HY male transplantation antigen (Wachtel et al., 1974), and not much else. Surprisingly, recent studies show that the Y chromosome carries some genes that are involved in basic cellular functions and that are expressed in many tissues (Lahn and Page, 1997).

Cytologically, the Y chromosome consists of two genetically distinct parts (Figure 2-2). The most distal portion of the Y-chromosome short arm (Yp) is shared with the most distal portion of the X-chromosome short arm (Xp) and normally recombines with its X-chromosome counterpart during meiosis in males. This region is called the "pseudoautosomal region" because loci in this region undergo pairing and exchange between the two sex chromosomes during spermatogenesis, just as genes on autosomes exchange between homologues. There is also a second pseudoautosomal region involving sequences on the distal long arms of the sex chromosomes (Watson et al., 1992) (Figure 2-2). The remainder of the Y chromosome (the Y-chromosome-specific portion) does not recombine with the X chromosome and strictly comprises "Y-chromosome-linked DNA" (although some of the nonrecombining part of the Y chromosome retains residual homology to X-chromosome-linked genes, reflecting the shared evolutionary history of the two sex chromosomes [see below]). The pseudoautosomal region(s) reflects the role of the Y chromosome as an essential pairing homologue of the X chromosome during meiosis in males (Rappold, 1993), whereas the Y-chromosome-specific region, including the testis-determining factor gene, *SRY*, provides the chromosomal basis of sex determination.

The Y chromosome is one of the smallest human chromosomes, with an estimated average size of 60 million base pairs, which is less than half the size of the X chromosome. Cytologically, much of the long arm (Yq) is heterochromatic and variable in size within populations, consisting largely of several families of repetitive DNA sequences that have no obvious function. A significant proportion of the Y-chromosome-specific sequences on both Yp and Yq are, in fact, homologous (but not identical) to sequences on the X chromosome. These sequences, although homologous, should not be confused with the pseudoautosomal regions. Pseudoautosomal sequences may be identical on the X and Y chromosomes, reflecting their frequent meiotic exchange, whereas the sequences on Yp and Yq homologous with the Y and X chromosomes are more distantly related to each other, reflecting their divergence from a common ancestral chromosome (Lahn and Page, 1999).

Only about two dozen different genes are encoded on the Y chromosome (although some are present in multiple copies). Unlike collections of genes that are located on the autosomes and the X chromosome and that reflect a broad sampling of different functions without any obvious chromosomal coherence, Y-chromosome-linked genes demonstrate functional clustering and can be categorized into only two distinct classes (Lahn and Page, 1997). One class consists of genes that are homologous to X-chromosome-linked genes and that are, for the most part, expressed ubiquitously in different tissues. Some of these genes are involved in basic cellular functions, thus providing a basis for functional differences between male and female cells. For example, the ribosomal protein S4 genes on the X and Y chromosomes encode slightly different protein isoforms (Watanabe et al., 1993); thus, ribosomes in male cells will differ characteristically from ribosomes in female cells, setting up the potential for widespread biochemical differences between the sexes. The second class of Y-chromosome-linked genes consists of Y-chromosome-specific genes that are expressed specifically in the testis and that may be involved in spermatogenesis (Figure 2-2). Deletion or mutation of some of these genes has been implicated in cases of male infertility, but otherwise, these genes have no obvious phenotypic effects (Kent-First et al., 1999; McDonough, 1998).

Females Have Two X Chromosomes, Males Have One

Male and female genomes also differ in the other sex chromosome, the X chromosome, in that females have twice the dose of X-chromosome-linked genes that males have. The X chromosome consists of approximately 160 million base pairs of DNA (about 5 percent of the total haploid genome) and encodes an estimated 1,000 to 2,000 genes (Figure 2-2). By the nature of X-chromosome-linked patterns of inheritance, females can be either homozygous or heterozygous for X-chromosome-linked traits, whereas males, because they have only a single X chromosome, are hemizygous. Of those X-chromosome-linked genes known to date, most are X chromosome specific; only pseudoautosomal genes and a few genes that map outside of the pseudoautosomal region have been demonstrated to have functionally equivalent Y-chromosome homologues (Willard, 2000).

Products of X-chromosome-linked genes, like those on the autosomes, are involved in virtually all aspects of cellular function, intermediary metabolism, development, and growth control. Although many are responsible for general cellular functions and are expressed widely in different tissues, others are specific to particular tissues or particular time points during development, and several are known to be responsible for steps in gonadal differentiation (Pinsky et al., 1999).

X-Chromosome Inactivation Compensates for Differences in Gene Dosage

The twofold difference between males and females in the dosage of genes on the X chromosome is negated at many loci by the process of X-chromosome inactivation (Figure 2-3). X-chromosome inactivation is, on

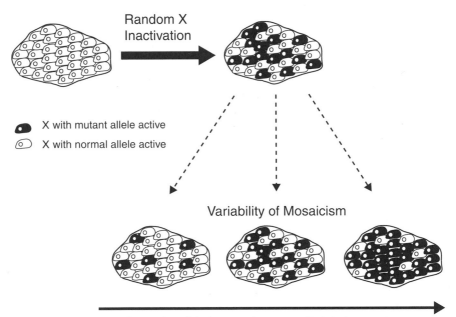

FIGURE 2-3 Schematic representation of X-chromosome inactivation in female somatic cells. Inactivation early in development is believed to be random, with an equal probability a priori that the maternal or paternal X chromosome will be active or inactive. Females are therefore epigenetic mosaics. However, the distribution of cells that express alleles from one or the other X chromosome can vary widely in different tissues or individuals. Inter- or intraindividual variation in the expression of one allele at X-chromosome-linked loci may result from selection against cells that express a particular allele (such as a mutant *G6PD* [glucose-6-phosphate dehydrogenase] allele) or stochastic variation in the proliferation of cells, in which one or the other X chromosome has been inactivated. The phenotype observed in females heterozygous for X-chromosome-linked traits can also vary widely, with an increasing level of clinical expression or increasing severity correlating with the proportion of cells expressing a mutant allele from the active X chromosome. Variations between females may also occur as the result of differences in the levels at which particular X-chromosome-linked genes may escape inactivation or become reactivated as cells age (Wareham et al., 1987).

a cytological level, a large-scale process in which one of the two X chromosomes becomes heterochromatic. The end result of this process can be seen under the microscope as the Barr chromatin body in the nucleus of the female cells. X-chromosome inactivation is associated with extensive silencing of genes on the affected X chromosome and occurs in almost every cell of XX females but does not occur in XY males. The one documented exception to this rule occurs, reciprocally, in reproductive cells; the single X chromosome of males becomes heterochromatic in spermatocytes, whereas both X chromosomes are thought to be active in primary oocytes. This unusual characteristic in which both X chromosomes are active in a single cell also occurs very early in the development of female embryos. Because the process of X-chromosome inactivation is not completed until near the time of implantation (reviewed by Willard [2000]), there is a preimplantation developmental window during which there may be basic differences in cellular chemistry between female and male embryos. It is unknown whether the differences in gene expression that have been shown to occur (Gutierrez-Adan et al., 2000; Latham et al., 2000) or that may occur during this period influence the establishment of additional differences between the sexes during the postimplantation or postnatal periods.

In any case, the simple fact of X-chromosome inactivation leads to two levels of difference between males and females. The first is that XX cells must operate whatever cellular machinery is required to initiate and establish the inactivation of an X chromosome in all mitotically active cells and also (perhaps) to actively maintain the inactive state of one X chromosome in terminally differentiated cells first. The second level of difference is superimposed on the first and is a property of populations of XX cells: females, by virtue of not inactivating the same X chromosome in every cell, are "epigenetic mosaics."

X-Chromosome-Based Differences Between Cells

There has been substantial recent progress in understanding the biochemistry and molecular biology of the X-chromosome inactivation process. These advances have been described in detail in several recent reviews (Heard et al., 1997; Willard, 2000), but the overall conclusion relevant to this report is that genes involved in the initiation, establishment, or maintenance of the X-chromosome inactivation process are or have been expressed in every somatic cell of females. Although some of the genes in the X-chromosome inactivation pathway may be expressed at some level or at some time in males (Daniels et al., 1997; Ray et al., 1997), the overall process that results in the cytologically visible heterochromatization of an entire chromosome is a fundamentally "female" characteristic, whether considered in vivo or in vitro. Here, then, is a basic biochemical process that is a fundamental consequence of having two X chromosomes. The biochemical results of the process can be measured and quantified in the tissues of individual females or in cells in culture dishes. The process affects genes that are involved in many important metabolic processes as well as genes that are known to be important in the regulation of expression of other genes (Amir et al., 1999; Melcher et al., 2000).

Because there is a stochastic or random component in the choice of which of the two X chromosomes is inactivated (Puck and Willard, 1998), individual females have two epigenetically distinct populations of cells: those in which the maternally derived X chromosome remains active and those in which the paternally derived X chromosome remains active (Figure 2-3). By contrast, males have only an active maternally derived X chromosome in all of their cells.

This X-chromosome-based, female-specific mosaicism is often invoked as the reason for much of the dramatic sex differences observed in the severities of recessive X-chromosome-linked disease phenotypes (McKusick, 2000). All cells of XY males must suffer the consequences of a mutation in an X-chromosome-linked gene, but only that fraction of a female's cells that carry the mutation on the active X chromosome will be affected. Such situations have resulted, in some cases, in strong somatic selection against cells that bear the mutation on the active X chromosome and thus avoidance (or minimization) of the disease phenotype (Belmont, 1996; Willard, 2000).

It should be noted that the stochastic nature of the initial choice of which X chromosome to inactivate can be influenced by many factors. Environmental, epigenetic, and genetic factors have all been demonstrated to influence the X-chromosome inactivation pattern (the proportion of a female's cells with a designated active X chromosome) of individual females (Puck and Willard, 1998). The relative importance of each may be different in different individuals, to the extent that all sisters within an individual family may show nearly identical patterns of X-chromosome inactivation, whereas identical twins in other families may exhibit wide variations in the proportions of their cells that have one or the other active X chromosome.

Not all of the genes on the X chromosome respond to the inactivation process by transcriptional silencing (Willard, 2000). This fact may lead secondarily to biochemical differences between XX cells and XY cells. As many as 10 to 15 percent of X-chromosome-linked genes have been identified as being expressed from the inactive X chromosome, at least in cells in culture, and are therefore said to "escape" X-chromosome inactivation (Carrel et al., 1999). Some of these are transcribed from both the active and the inactive X chromosome at similar levels, whereas others appear to be transcribed from the inactive X chromosome at reduced, but still significant, levels (Carrel and Willard, 1999; Fisher et al., 1990). Regardless of the level at which such genes escape X-chromosome inactivation, it is likely that XX cells will produce higher levels of gene product from some of these loci than XY cells will. It has been suggested that some of these differences may lead to sex-specific levels of risk for certain diseases, such as the suspected relationship between gastrin-releasing peptide receptor and smoking-related lung cancer (Shriver et al., 2000). Gastrin-releasing peptide is expressed by both the active and the inactive X chromosomes, and elevated levels of gastrin-releasing peptide are hypothesized to be associated with an elevated risk of lung cancer in women who smoke.

An interesting genomic consideration resulting from the study of genes that escape X-chromosome inactivation is that their distribution along the X chromosome is not random. A higher proportion of the genes on the short arm of the X chromosome than on the long arm of the X chromosome escape X-chromosome inactivation (Carrel et al., 1999). This issue may reflect the different evolutionary histories of the X-chromosome arms (Lahn and Page, 1999) but may also be related to whether particular X-chromosome-linked genes have homologues on the Y chromosome (Jegalian and Page, 1998). It is of some interest that the particular genes that escape inactivation appear to differ among different females (Carrel and Willard, 1999), thus providing additional avenues for differences between and within the sexes. It is unknown whether there are significant population variations in patterns of inactivation and thus X-chromosome-linked gene expression.

The X-Chromosome Dosage Matters

In general, the possible effect(s) of any variant in an X-chromosome-linked gene may differ between the sexes for a variety of reasons, as outlined below.

• **Gene dosage.** For genes that are specific to the X chromosome and that escape X-chromosome inactivation, female cells (with two X chromosomes) may contain higher levels of the gene product than male cells, which have only a single X chromosome. Depending on the cellular role of the particular gene product, this dosage difference may have more pervasive effects on the expression of other genes in the genome. For example, a twofold change in the level of an X-chromosome-linked transcription factor might lead to dramatic effects on the levels of genes regulated by that transcription factor.

• **Mosaicism.** For genes that are subject to X-chromosome inactivation, most females are mosaics of two cell populations, one expressing alleles on the paternally inherited X chromosome and one expressing alleles on the maternally inherited X chromosome (see below). Thus, expression of an X-chromosome-linked phenotype is often much more variable in females than in males.

• **Hemizygosity.** Because males have only a single X chromosome, functional variants cannot be "masked" by a second X chromosome. Thus, males often demonstrate a clearer, more common, or more extreme version of the variant phenotype than females do.

• **X-chromosome-linked dominant traits.** A dramatic example of the effect of male hemizygosity for X-chromosome-linked traits involves X-chromosome-linked dominant mutations that are lethal in males in utero and that are therefore evident only in females. For example, X-chromosome-linked incontinentia pigmenti is a relatively benign dermatological condition in females, but it is lethal in males who inherit a mutant allele (Smahi et al., 2000).

Differences Between Male and Female Cells That Have Not Been Linked to Sex Chromosomes

The incidence of a number of diseases whose etiologies cannot be traced to the sex chromosomes differ dramatically between males and females (McKusick, 2000). Although the basis for these differences in incidence is most often ascribed to hormonal influences, the possibility that other genetic differences are at fault cannot be discounted.

EFFECTS OF PARENTAL IMPRINTING ON THE EXPRESSION OF GENETIC INFORMATION

The discovery that some genes are expressed only from the maternal allele and that others are expressed only from the paternal allele, a phenomenon called "genomic imprinting" (reviewed by Tilghman [1999]), reinforces the concept that there are multiple biochemical differences between the gametogenic cells of males and females and that these differences may affect the expression of genetic information in the next generation.

Because autosomes are transmitted equally to both sexes, it is not predicted that inheritance of imprinted genetic information on the autosomes should have a differential effect on male versus female offspring. The situation is different for sex chromosomes. Imprinting-related differences between the sexes do exist for the X chromosome. Males have only a maternal X chromosome, but females have both a maternal X chromosome and a paternal X chromosome; therefore, X-chromosome-linked genes that pass through the paternal germ line have the potential to affect the phenotype of female offspring but not that of male offspring. In this regard, there is direct evidence that the imprinting process affects the expression of alleles in females at the *Xist* locus (a gene that is critical to the process of X-chromosome inactivation and that is expressed primarily from the paternal allele in some extraembryonic cells) in females (reviewed by Lyon [1999]).

There is also indirect evidence that imprinting affects the expression of a locus on Xp that has female-specific effects on cognitive and behavioral phenotypes. The latter evidence is derived from studies of patients with Turner syndrome, who have inherited only one X chromosome (XO) from either the mother or the father (Skuse et al., 1997). These findings may have broader implications for cognitive function or behavior in males and females because males inherit only a maternal X chromosome, whereas females inherit both a maternal X chromosome and a paternal X chromosome.

UNEXPECTED OR NONOBVIOUS SEX DIFFERENCES

Sex-Specific Meiotic Effects

Although the basic mechanism of meiosis, the creation of haploid gametes from diploid precursors, is universal, there are both quantitative and qualitative differences between males and females in the production of gametes. These differences have characteristic effects on the ways that males and females drive the evolutionary process, as well as the mechanisms by which diseases that result from genetic defects are manifest.

The three most important differences between males and females in the gametogenic process are as follows: (1) the number of stem cell divisions that occur to give rise to the germ cell population, (2) the timing of the first and second meiotic divisions, and (3) the number of gametes produced from each primary germ cell.

The male produces billions of sperm from a population of stem cells that continue to divide throughout the entire adult life. In contrast, the female produces a relatively small number of ova (~500) from a limited population of oocytes that arise early in embryogenesis. These oocytes are arrested at the meiotic prophase from fetal life until ovulation, which may occur as many as 50 years after the initiation of meiosis. This simple numerical difference in the number of stem cell divisions between the two sexes dictates that most mutations resulting from errors in DNA replication take place in the male germ line (Haldane, 1935), although the magnitude of this difference and whether additional factors may contribute are subjects of debate (Hurst and Ellegren, 1998). On the other hand, the protracted length of time that an individual ovum may be arrested at the meiotic prophase is correlated with the fact that aneuploidy (gain or loss of one or more chromosomes) resulting from nondisjunction (improper separation of chromosomes at nuclear division) occurs much more frequently through the female germ line than through the male germ line (Hassold et al., 2000).

Although all four products of meiosis in the male have the potential to become functional sperm, each primary oocyte gives rise to only a single ovum. Additional differences in the meiotic process are found in the observed rate of recombination and the consequent length of the human genetic map obtained by measurement with chromosomes from females compared with those obtained by measurement with chromosomes from males. In general, there is more recombination over the autosomes during female meiosis than during male meiosis (Broman et al., 1998). Only the comparatively small, "pseudoautosomal" portion of the X and Y chromosomes recombine during male meiosis, but the rate of recombination in this region is approximately 10 times greater than the rate of recombination in this region during female meiosis (Hunt and LeMaire, 1992; Rappold, 1993).

Sex-of-Offspring-Specific Transmission Ratio Distortion

In a number of instances the inheritance of alleles from heterozygous parents does not appear to be equal between male and female offspring (Naumova et al., 1998; Pardo-Manuel de Villena et al., 2000; Siracusa et al., 1991; see also Sapienza [1994] for a review). Such sex-specific biases in the inheritance of genetic information are not expected per se (especially in the case of autosomal loci) but may be due to a number of causes, including meiotic drive, preferential cosegregation of sex chromosomes with one of a pair of homologous chromosomes, preferential fertilization, and preferential death of the embryo of one sex. These biases that are specific to the sex of the offspring have been observed as a result of transmission through both male and female parents (reviewed by Sapienza [1994]). As a practical matter, it is important to consider the source and magnitude of any observed inheritance biases because they may affect the mapping and identification of genetic traits that are more prevalent in one sex than the other. An interesting side effect of sex-of-offspring-specific transmission ratio distortion is that the observed frequencies of alleles at some loci may differ between the sexes.

GENETICS AS A TOOL

Genetics has long been an important tool for the dissection of biological mechanisms. Its use, however, has been limited by the investigator's ability to find appropriate mutant phenotypes and then to identify the gene and gene product responsible for producing the phenotype. Recently, an array of genetic techniques has greatly expanded the power of genetics. These techniques exploit the ability to clone specific genes and modify their sequences to destroy or modify the gene product. This modified sequence is then inserted into the genome of an intact animal or cultured cell to determine the effect on the phenotype. The details of introducing transgenes vary with species, but in the most successful cases, the transgene can exactly replace the resident gene. In other cases, transgenes cannot be specifically targeted and the resident gene may still be present; thus, the types of questions that can be asked are more limited.

Transgenic techniques have overcome several problems of conventional genetics. They greatly speed study because there is a direct link between the gene used in the experiment and the phenotype. The investigator can precisely specify the gene modification rather than depend on random mutagenesis, making it possible to focus not only on a specific gene but also on a particular feature of that gene. For example, by removing the domain responsible for phosphorylation, one can study its role in the parent protein.

Two classes of important genes are difficult to study by conventional genetics. The first class is redundant genes, such as families of genes that all fulfill the same function. It is unlikely that random mutagenesis will knock out all members of even a very small family of genes, but targeted transgenes can easily achieve this to allow study of the action of this gene family. A second class of important genes includes those that produce lethal phenotypes or that have effects in one developmental stage that preclude study of their activity in a later stage. Techniques that allow the transgene to be specifically inactivated in a tissue of choice offer ways to bypass these problems because the gene can be expressed normally except in the tissue where it is being studied. Similar techniques can be used to drive inappropriate expression of a gene in specific tissues where the inappropriate expression can be informative.

Transgenic techniques can also be used to construct model systems to meet specific requirements. For example, mouse transgenic systems are being used in many laboratories as models for human genetic diseases and for cancer studies. The models need not be restricted to mouse genes but can also contain transgenes of human origin to study specific interactions. The increasing number of mice being bred to carry transgenes of interest makes it possible to rapidly test gene interactions by breeding different transgenic animals. Despite the power of these new techniques, however, interpretation of experimental results is not always straightforward. For example, the manipulations involved with introducing the new DNA sequence can sometimes introduce unexpected genetic changes, either at the locus under study or at unrelated loci. In addition, identical transgene or knockout models may have variable phenotypes, depending on the strain's background (just as for "normal" mutant alleles).

FINDINGS AND RECOMMENDATIONS

Findings

Males and females have partially different genomes:

- The Y chromosome carries genes that are involved in basic cellular functions and that are expressed in many different tissues.
- In females, the majority of genes on one of the two X chromosomes are silenced in every cell. This inactivation makes each female a functional mosaic because some cells express one X chromosome and others cells express the other one. The advantages of heterozygosity can be amplified by selection against cells in which the active X chromosome carries a detrimental allele.
- Some genes on the inactive X chromosome are not silenced, leading to higher levels of their products in female cells.
- Female cells must have cellular machinery to establish and maintain the inactivation of the X chromosome.
- Male and female germ cells differentially imprint the genetic information to be transmitted to their progeny.

These findings argue that there are multiple, ubiquitous differences in the basic cellular biochemistry of males and females that can affect an individual's health. Many of these differences do not necessarily arise as a result of differences in the hormonal environment of the male and female but are a direct result of the genetic differences between the two sexes.

Recommendation

RECOMMENDATION 1: Promote research on sex at the cellular level.

The committee recommends that research be conducted to

- **determine the functions and effects of X-chromosome- and Y-chromosome-linked genes in somatic cells as well as germ-line cells,**
- **determine how genetic sex differences influence other levels of biological organization (cell, organ, organ system, organism), including susceptibility to disease, and**
- **develop systems that can identify and distinguish between the effects of genes and the effects of hormones.**

The phenotypic differences between males and females are determined, initially, by genes on the sex chromosomes. Sex chromosome-linked genes can be expressed in both germ-line and somatic cells and could influence an individual's phenotype, including disease susceptibility, at many levels.

3

Sex Begins in the Womb

ABSTRACT

*Sex differences of importance to health and human disease occur through-
out the life span, although the specific expression of these differences varies
at different stages of life. Some differences originate in events occurring in
the intrauterine environment, where developmental processes differentially
organize tissues for later activation in the male or female. In the prenatal
period, sex determination and differentiation occur in a series of sequential
processes governed by genetic and environmental factors. During the pubertal period, behavioral and hormonal changes manifest the secondary
sexual characteristics that reinforce the sexual identity of the individual
through adolescence and into adulthood. Hormonal events occurring in
puberty lay a framework for biological differences that persist through life
and that contribute to variable onset and progression of disease in males
and females. It is important to study sex differences at all stages of the life
cycle, relying on animal models of disease and including sex as a variable in
basic and clinical research designs.*

All human individuals—whether they have an XX, an XY, or an atypi-
cal sex chromosome combination—begin development from the same
starting point. During early development the gonads of the fetus remain
undifferentiated; that is, all fetal genitalia are the same and are phenotypi-
cally female. After approximately 6 to 7 weeks of gestation, however, the
expression of a gene on the Y chromosome induces changes that result in
the development of the testes. Thus, this gene is singularly important in

inducing testis development. The production of testosterone at about 9 weeks of gestation results in the development of the reproductive tract and the masculinization (the normal development of male sex characteristics) of the brain and genitalia. In contrast to the role of the fetal testis in differentiation of a male genital tract and external genitalia in utero, fetal ovarian secretions are not required for female sex differentiation. As these details point out, the basic differences between the sexes begin in the womb, and this chapter examines how sex differences develop and change across the lifetime. The committee examined both normal and abnormal routes of development that lead individuals to become males and females and the changes during childhood, reproductive adulthood, and the later stages of life.

BIOLOGY OF SEX

One of the basic goals of biologists is to explain observed variability among and within species. Why does one individual become infected when exposed to a microbiological agent when another individual does not? Why does one individual experience pain more acutely than another? Sex is a prime variable to which such differences can be ascribed. No one factor is responsible for variability, but rather, a blend of genetic, hormonal, and experiential factors operating at different times during development result in the phenotype called a human being.

As suggested by the reproductive processes of some species and punctuated by recent successful efforts at cloning of some species, sexual reproduction is not necessary for species perpetuation. Debate exists on why sexual reproduction has evolved. Most biologists agree that it increases the variability upon which evolutionary selection can operate; for example, variability would allow some offspring to escape pathogens and survive to reproduce. This theory is not without its critics (Barton and Charlesworth, 1998). The contribution of genetics to sex differences has been described in Chapter 2. Here the focus is more on the endocrine and experiential bases for the development and expression of sex as a phenotype.

Different species of vertebrate animals have evolved different pathways to determine sex, but it is interesting that in all cases two sexes emerge with distinctly different roles in the social and reproductive lives of the animals (Crews, 1993; Francis, 1992). In all vertebrates the genetic basis of sex is determined by meiosis, a process by which paired chromosomes are separated, resulting in the formation of an egg or sperm, which are then joined at fertilization. Variations in the phenotypic characteristics of the different sexes are determined during development by internal chemical signals. The process can be influenced by external factors such as maternal endocrine dysfunction or endocrine disrupters, as well as fetal endocrine disorders and exogenous medications (Grumbach and Conte, 1998).

Nongenomic Sexual Differentiation and Sexual Flexibility

Nongenomic sexual differentiation has evolved in several species of fishes and reptiles. In these species, sex results from external signals. For example, temperature during embryogenesis is the cue acting on autosomal genes to result in adult males and females in several species. In many species of flounder, for instance, elevated temperatures of the water in which the larval fish develop results in a higher proportion of males (Yamamoto, 1999). Similarly, in several turtle species the incubation temperature of the eggs influences the sex ratio of the animals (Crews et al., 1989).

In some species, sex determination can be delayed until well after birth or the sex can even change after the birth of an organism. One fascinating study found that several species of fish develop sexual phenotypes as a result of the fish's social rank in a group (Baroiller et al., 1999; Warner, 1984). The blue-headed wrasse is a polygynous coral reef fish with three phenotypes that vary in size, coloration, reproductive organs, physiology, and behavior (Godwin et al., 1996; Warner and Swearer, 1991). These phenotypes are females, initial-phase males, and terminal-phase males. As a result of changes in the social role, a fish can progress rapidly through these phenotypes. Upon the disappearance of a terminal-phase male, the behavior of the largest female in the group converts to male-like behavior in minutes and the fish shows full gonadal changes in days.

The belted sandfish (*Serranus subligarius*) stands out as one of the most remarkable demonstrations of vertebrate sexual flexibility. This coastal marine fish is a simultaneous hermaphrodite (Cheek et al., 2000). Its gonads produce both sperm and eggs, and each fish has the reproductive tract anatomies of both sexes simultaneously. Within minutes each individual can show three alternative mating behaviors—that is, female, courting male, or streaker male—along with the appropriate external color changes (Cheek et al., 2000). A streaker male awaits the peak moment during the courtship of male and female morphs and then streaks in to release sperm at the moment of spawning. The sperm compete with the courting male's sperm. Partners can switch between male and female roles within seconds and may take turns fertilizing each other's eggs. The frequency with which an individual plays the female or male role is, in part, a function of size. Larger fish are more likely to play the male role more often.

In contrast, mammalian sex determination is more directly under the control of a single internal event: fertilization. Under normal conditions, the direction of sexual development is initiated and determined by the presence or absence of a Y chromosome.

Intrauterine Environment

In mammals, once genetic sex has been determined and the fetus begins its development, the fetal environment, especially hormones, can result in significant modifications of the genetically based sex. The effect of prenatal hormones on later anatomy, physiology, and behavior are most clearly demonstrated in several animals showing the "intrauterine position effect" (vom Saal et al., 1999). In litter-bearing mammals such as mice, rats, gerbils, and pigs, each pup shares the uterus with several others, some of which are of a different sex. Significant differences among females occur if the fetus is located between two males or with a male on one side or with no male on either side. Testosterone is produced by fetal males and can masculinize adjacent females to various degrees. Thus, not only do individuals vary as a result of genetic variability, but they can also vary as a result of prenatal hormonal organizational effects (see additional discussion in Chapter 4). Extensive studies with the female mouse have revealed that adult anatomical structures, such as the genitalia and sexually dimorphic parts of the brain, and the rate of reproductive development vary as a result of proximity to males in the womb (Vandenbergh and Huggett, 1995).

Studies with animals suggest that hormonal transfer between fetuses can influence later anatomical, physiological, and behavioral characteristics. Some data from studies with humans, recently summarized by Miller (1998), suggest that a similar phenomenon occurs in mixed-sex twins. His review of the literature reveals a number of characteristics apparently influenced by transmission of testosterone from the male twin to the female twin. For example, (1) dental asymmetry is also a characteristic of females with male co-twins (the right jaw of the male has larger teeth) (Boklage, 1985), (2) spontaneous otoacoustic emissions are at an intermediate level in females with male co-twins (the rates of clicking sounds produced in the cochlea usually differ between males and females) (McFadden, 1993), and (3) the level of sensation seeking appears to be higher in females with male co-twins than in those without male co-twins (Resnick et al., 1993). These studies suggest that, as in rodent models, testosterone transferred to human female fetuses can have masculinizing effects on anatomical, physiological, and behavioral traits.

In humans, the metabolic stress of pregnancy increases the incidence of gestational diabetes in susceptible women. Transgenerational passage of diabetes may contribute to the higher incidence of impaired glucose tolerance, obesity, and hypertension in the offspring of diabetic mothers and to the prevalence of diabetes in such human communities as the Pima Indians (Cho et al., 2000; Silverman et al., 1995). This passage of a disease condition across generations by non-genome-dependent mechanisms emphasizes the importance of good maternal care and health during pregnancy. Although males will also be affected by a hyperglycemic environment during fetal life and will themselves have an increased risk of diabetes in adulthood, they do not provide the womb environment during the critical phases of fetal development of the next generation. Thus, males do not pass the tendency across generations (Cho et al., 2000; Nathanielsz, 1999; Silverman et al., 1995).

Low birth weight or small body size at birth as a result of reduced intrauterine growth are associated with increased rates of coronary heart disease and non-insulin-dependent diabetes in adult life (reviewed by Barker [2000]). The "fetal origins hypothesis" proposes that undernutrition during critical periods of fetal growth can force the fetus to adapt by altering cardiovascular, metabolic, or endocrine functions to survive. (Note that debate continues as to whether the association is truly causal [Kramer, 2000; The Lancet, 2001; Lumey, 2001].) These changes, such as redistribution of blood flow, changes in the production of fetal and placental hormones involved in growth, and metabolic changes, can permanently change the function and structure of the body. For example, offspring who were exposed in utero to maternal famine during the first trimester of development had higher total cholesterol and low-density lipid cholesterol levels and a higher ratio of low-density lipid to high-density lipid cholesterol levels, all of which are risk factors for heart disease (Roseboom et al., 2000). This altered lipid profile persisted even after adjustments for adult lifestyle factors such as smoking, socioeconomic status, or use of lipid-lowering drugs. Male offspring had higher rates of obesity at age 19 years, but maternal malnutrition during early gestation was associated with a higher prevalence of obesity in 50-year-old women (Ravelli et al., 1999).

Such permanent alterations in body structure or functions may have effects on future generations as well. Studies show that when a female fetus is undernourished and subsequently of low birth weight, the permanent physiological and metabolic changes in her body can lead to reduced fetal growth and raised blood pressure in her offspring (Barker at al., 2000; Stein and Lumey, 2000). Furthermore, in birth cohorts of males with spina bifida who had been exposed to prenatal famine, the relative risk of death was 2.5-fold greater than that in similarly affected female offspring (Brown and Susser, 1997). These traits in the offspring were not affected by the father's size at birth.

EARLY DEVELOPMENT

The remarkable accumulation of knowledge over the past five decades and new and continuing insights in the field of sex determination and sex differentiation represent major landmarks in biomedical science. No aspect of prenatal development is better understood. Advances in embryology, steroid biochemistry, molecular and cell biology, cytogenetics, genetics, endocrinology, immunology, transplantation biology, and the behavioral sciences have contributed to the understanding of sexual anomalies in humans and to the improved clinical management of individuals with these disorders. Major contributions to this understanding have stemmed from studies of patients with abnormalities of sex determination and differentiation and the recent advances emanating from molecular genetics. These advances, considered together, illustrate that a failure in any of the sequential stages of sexual development, whether the cause is genetic or environmental, can have a profound effect on the sex phenotype of the individual and can lead to complete sex reversal, various degrees of ambisexual development, or less overt abnormalities in sexual function that first become apparent after sexual maturity (Grumbach and Conte, 1998; Wilson, 1999).

Sex Determination

Sex determination and sex differentiation are sequential processes that involve successive establishment of chromosomal sex in the zygote at the moment of conception, determination of gonadal (primary) sex by the genetic sex, and determination of phenotypic sex by the gonads. At puberty the development of secondary sexual characteristics reinforces and provides more visible phenotypic manifestations of the sexual dimorphism. *Sex determination* is concerned with the regulation of the development of the primary or gonadal sex, and *sex differentiation* encompasses the events subsequent to gonadal organogenesis. These processes are regulated by at least 70 different genes that are located on the sex chromosomes and autosomes and that act through a variety of mechanisms including those that involve organizing factors, gonadal steroids and peptide hormones, and tissue receptors. Mammalian embryos remain sexually undifferentiated until the time of sex determination.

An important point is that early embryos of both sexes possess indifferent common primordia that have an inherent tendency to feminize unless there is active interference by masculinizing factors (Grumbach and Conte, 1998).

It has been known for more than four decades that a testis-determining locus, *TDF* (testis-determining factor), resides on the Y chromosome. About 10 years ago, the testis-determining gene was found to be the *SRY* (sex-determining region Y) gene (Ferguson-Smith and Goodfellow, 1995; Koopman, 1999; Koopman et al., 1991; O'Neill and O'Neill, 1999; Sinclair et al., 1990; Swain and Lovell-Badge, 1999), which is the primary sex determinant, as it is the inducer of differentiation of the indifferent gonad into testes and hence is the inducer of male sexual development. SRY is expressed in 46,XY gonads in Sertoli cell progenitors at the stage of sex cord formation, but unlike the mouse, in which SRY expression is brief, SRY mRNA persists in Sertoli cells at 18 weeks of gestation (Hanley et al., 2000). As discussed in Chapter 2, the human SRY gene is located on the short arm of the Y chromosome and comprises a single exon that encodes a protein of 204 amino acids including a 79-residue conserved DNA bending and DNA binding domain: the HMG (high-mobility-group) box.

The mechanisms involved in the translation of genetic sex into the development of a testis or an ovary are now understood in broad terms (Figure 3-1).

It is known that a variety of autosomal and X-chromosome-linked genes, literally a cascade of genes that exert complex gene dosage balancing activities, are involved in testis determination. All major sex-determining genes have been shown to be subject to a dosage effect. In the human, the SRY protein is detected at an early age of gonadal differentiation in XY embryos, where it induces Sertoli cell differentiation. In the human adult, it is present in both Sertoli and germ cells. In embryonic and fetal life, the evidence suggests that the SRY gene product regulates gene expression in a cell-autonomous manner. The precise molecular mechanisms by which SRY triggers testis development are unknown, nor is it yet known how SRY is regulated. The genetic sex of the zygote is established by fertilization of a normal ovum by an X-chromosome- or Y-chromosome-bearing sperm.

Genes Contributing to Sex Determination

Apart from SRY, a number of autosomal and X-chromosome-linked genes have been identified and have a critical role in male or female sex determination, the testis- and ovary-determining cascades (Roberts et al., 1999) (Table 3-1). In the human, heterozygous mutations or deletion of the Wilm's tumor (WT1) gene located on chromosome 11p13 results in urogenital malformations as well as Wilm's tumors. Knockout of the WT1 gene in mice results in apoptosis of the metanephric blastema, with the resultant absence of the kidneys and gonads. Thus, WT1, a transcriptional regulator, appears to act on metanephric blastema early in urogenital development.

SF-1 (steroidogenic factor-1) is an orphan nuclear receptor involved in transcriptional regulation. It is expressed in both the male and the female urogenital ridges as well as steroidogenic tissues, where it is re-

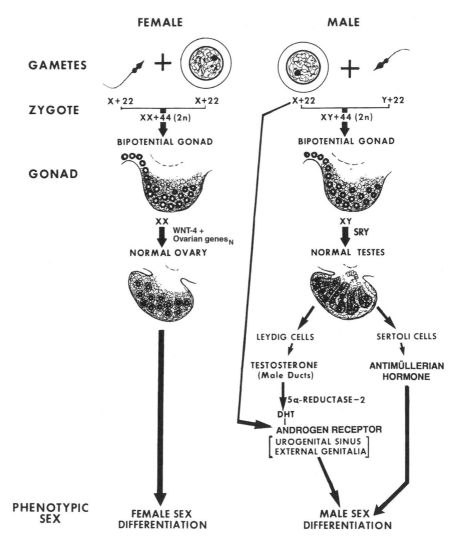

FIGURE 3-1   From genotype to phenotype: a diagrammatic representation of human sex determination and differentiation. Intrinsic or extrinsic factors adversely affecting any stage of these processes can lead to anomalies of sex. Source: Grumbach and Conte (1998, Figure 29-28, p. 1329). Reprinted, with permission, from M. M. Grumbach and F. A. Conte. 1998. *In: Williams Textbook of Endocrinology*, 9th ed. J. D. Wilson, D. W. Foster, H. M. Kronenberg, and P. R. Larsen, eds. Philadelphia: W. B. Saunders Co. Copyright by W. B. Saunders Company, Philadelphia.

TABLE 3-1 Some Genes Involved in Human Sex Determination

Gene	Chromosome Localization	Family	Function	Phenotype of Mutations
SRY	Yp11	HMG protein	Transcription factor	XY gonadal dysgenesis (sex reversal)
WT1	11p13	Zinc finger protein	Transcription factor	Dysgenetic male pseudohermaphrodism and XY gonadal dysgenesis
SF-1	9q33	Orphan nuclear receptor	Transcription factor	Heterozygous mutation: XY gonadal dysgenesis and adrenal failure
DAX-1	Xp21.3	Orphan nuclear receptor	Transcription factor	Duplication: XY gonadal dysgenesis
SOX-9	17q24	HMG protein	Transcription factor	Camptomelic dysplasia with XY gonadal dysgenesis
DMRT-1 (DMRT-2?)	9p24.3	DM domain	Transcription factor	XY gonadal dysgenesis
WNT-4	1p32-36	Secreted glycoprotein	Extracellular signaling	Duplication: XY gonadal dysgenesis

quired for the synthesis of, for example, testosterone and estrogen, and in Sertoli cells, where it regulates the anti-müllerian hormone gene (Parker et al., 1999). SF-1 is encoded by the mammalian homologue of the *Drosophila melanogaster* gene (*FTZ-F1*). Knockout of the *Sf-1* gene in mice results in apoptosis of the genital ridge cells that give rise to the adrenals and gonads and, thus, a lack of gonadal and adrenal morphogenesis in both males and females. A heterozygous mutation in the human gene encoding SF-1 causes XY sex reversal (Achermann et al., 1999), which results in individuals with normal female external genitalia, streak-like gonads containing sparse and poorly differentiated tubules, and the failure of adrenal development. WT1 and SF-1 appear to play important roles in the differentiation of the genital ridge from the intermediate mesoderm. WT1 and SF-1 are expressed when the indifferent gonadal ridge first differentiates at 32 days postovulation in both female and male embryos (Hanley et al., 1999).

XY gonadal dysgenesis with resulting female differentiation has occurred in 46,XY individuals with intact *SRY* function but with duplication of Xp21, leading to a double dose of the *DAX-1* (dosage-sensitive sex reversal congenital adrenal hypoplasia congenital-critical region on the X chromosome, gene 1) gene. On the other hand, a mutation or deletion of *DAX-1* in XY individuals results in X-linked congenital adrenal hypoplasia and hypogonadotropic hypogonadism but not an abnormality in testis differentiation. Similarly, duplication of the *DAX-1* gene on one X chromosome appears not to affect ovarian morphogenesis or function in 46,XX females. Targeted disruption of the *Dax-1* gene in mice does not affect ovarian development. It has been suggested that *Dax-1* is an "anti-testis" factor rather than an ovary-determining gene. *SRY* and *Dax-1* appear to act antagonistically in gonadal dysgenesis (Parker et al., 1999; Roberts et al., 1999). *Dax-1* expression is detected in the primate gonadal ridge days before the peak expression of *SRY* (Hanley et al., 2000).

Camptomelic dysplasia is a skeletal dysplasia associated with sex reversal because of gonadal dysgenesis in about 60 percent of affected 46,XY individuals. A gene for a camptomelic dysplasia, *SOX-9*, has been localized to 17q24.3–25.1. The products of *SOX* genes (for the *SRY*-related HMG-box gene), as a rule, are more than 50 percent identical to those of *SRY* genes at the amino acid level in the HMG-box region (Koopman, 1999). In the human, *SOX-9* transcripts are present in the gonadal ridge of both male and female embryos (Hanley et al., 2000).

XY individuals with 9p– or 10q– deletions as well as patients with 1p32–36 duplications exhibit gonadal dysgenesis and male pseudohermaphrodism, which suggests that autosomal genes at these loci are important in the gonadal differentiation cascade. In this regard, two genes, *DMRT-1* and *DMRT-2*, have been localized to the distal region of the short arm of chromosome 9 (Raymond et al., 1999). These genes are related to the sexual regulatory genes *Dsx* (double sex) in *D. melanogaster* and *MAB-3* in *Caenorhabditis elegans* (or double sex- and *MAB-3*-related transcription factor). Their evolutionary conservation, deletion from sex-reversed males with the 9p− syndrome, and male-specific expression in early human gonadogenesis suggest that one or both genes have a role in human sex determination (Calvari et al., 2000).

WNT-4, a vertebrate homologue of the *D. melanogaster* polarity gene ("wingless"), is involved in the regulation of steroid biosynthesis in the fetal gonad (Uusitalo et al., 1999). *Wnt-4* knockout female mice lack müllerian ducts and exhibit decreased levels of oocyte development and decreased rates of survival. *WNT-4* is downregulated in the fetal testis, presumably by *SRY*. Consequently, testosterone synthesis occurs in the XY individual. It has recently been demonstrated that *WNT-4* in humans is located on chromosome 1p35 and that duplication of *WNT-4* upregulates *DAX-1* expression and causes sex reversal in a 46,XY individual. 46,XX mice with homozygous disruption of the *Wnt-4* gene manifest testosterone synthesis in the fetal ovary and masculinization of the wolffian ducts. This observation suggests that *Wnt-4* expression in the fetal ovary inhibits gonadal androgen biosynthesis.

Organogenesis of the Testes

Until about the 12-millimeter stage (approximately 42 days of gestation), the embryonic gonads of males and females are indistinguishable. By 42 days, 300 to 1,300 primordial germ cells have reached the undifferentiated gonad from their extragonadal origin in the dorsal endoderm of the yolk sac. These large cells are the progenitors of oogonia and spermatogonia. In the absence of primordial germ cells, the gonadal ridges in the female remain undeveloped. Germ cells are not essential for differentiation of the testes (Grumbach and Conte, 1998).

There is a striking sexual dimorphism in the timing of gonadal differentiation under the influence of *SRY* and other testis-determining genes (Figures 3-2 and 3-3). Organization of the indifferent gonad is definitive by the 6th to 7th week of gestation; the testes develop more rapidly than the ovaries. The ovary does not emerge from the indifferent stage until 3 months of gestation, when the earliest sign of differentiation into ovaries appears: the beginning of meiosis, as evidenced by the maturation of oogonia into oocytes. The precursor of the Sertoli cell that arises from the coelomic epithelium expresses *SRY*, leading to differentiation of Sertoli cells, which marks testis differentiation (Capel, 2000). The Sertoli cell is the only cell in the testes in which *SRY* has a critical effect. Germ cells in the XY gonad are sequestrated inside the forming testis cords. Anti-müllerian hormone (AMH) (or müllerian-inhibiting factor or substance) is a member of the transforming growth factor beta family, one of the earliest known products of Sertoli cells. The organization of testicular cords regulates Leydig cells to the interstitial region between the primitive seminiferous tubules.

The early endocrine function of the fetal testis is the secretion by the Sertoli cells of anti-müllerian hormone (AMH), a homodimeric glycoprotein that functions as a paracrine secretion (Donahoe et al., 1987; Josso et al., 1993). It passes by diffusion to the paired müllerian ducts and induces their dissolution by apoptosis. The versatile Sertoli cell also secretes inhibin, nurtures the germ cells, expresses stem cell factor, synthesizes an androgen binding protein, and prevents meiosis. Leydig cells are first found at about 60 days of gestation. Leydig cells secrete testosterone, the regulator of male differentiation of the wolffian ducts, urogenital sinus, and external genitalia. After differentiation of the primitive testicular cords, they rapidly proliferate during the 3rd month and the first half of the 4th month. During this period the interstitial spaces between the seminiferous tubules are crowded with Leydig cells.

The onset of testosterone biosynthesis occurs at about the 9th week (Siiteri and Wilson, 1974). Human chorionic gonadotropin (hCG)-lutein-

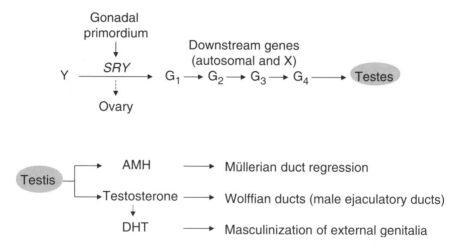

FIGURES 3-2 and 3-3 Hypothetical diagrammatic representations of the cascade of sex chromosomal and autosomal genes involved in testis determination (Figures 3-2 and 3-3A) and the hormones involved in male sex differentiation (Figures 3-2 and 3-3B). Genes indicated by italic capital letters have been shown to be involved in human sex determination and differentiation. *WT-1*, Wilm's tumor suppressor; *SF-1*, steroidogenic factor-1; *DAX-1*, dosage-sensitive sex reversal congenital adrenal hypoplasia congenital-critical region on the X chromosome, gene 1 (AHC, adrenal hypoplasia congenita, or hypogonadotropic hypogonadism; a double dose [2X DAX-1] of *DAX-1* [AHC] inhibits *SRY* and results in inhibition of testis determination; *SRY*, sex-determining region Y; *SOX-9*, SRY-

A

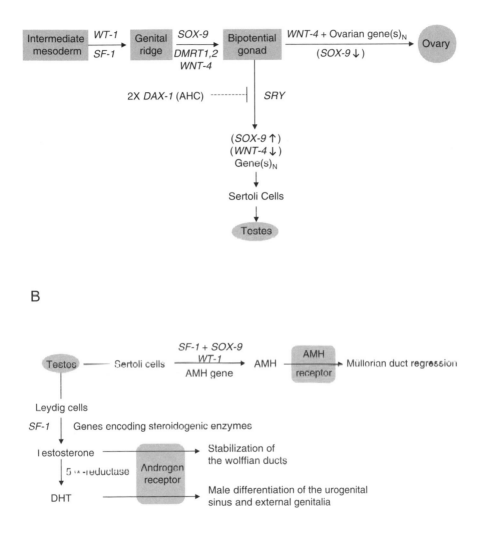

B

like HMG–box, gene 9; *WNT-4*, a member of the vertebrate homologue family of the *Drosophila* segment polarity gene("wingless"), a locally acting secreted growth factor (duplication of *WNT-4* in an XY individual led to a sex reversal with a female phenotype); *DMRT-1*, *DMRT-2*, *Dsx mob3*-related transcription factors 1 and 2; AMH, anti-müllerian hormone; DHT, dihydrotestosterone. Source: Grumbach and Conte (1998). Adapted, with permission, from M. M. Grumbach and F. A. Conte. 1998. *In: Williams Textbook of Endocrinology,* 9th ed. J. D. Wilson, D. W. Foster, H. M. Kronenberg, and P. R. Larsen, eds. Philadelphia: W. B. Saunders Co. Copyright by W. B. Saunders Company, Philadelphia.

izing hormone (LH) receptors are present in fetal Leydig cells by at least the 12th week of gestation, an observation that suggests that the initial secretion of testosterone at about 8 to 9 of weeks gestation is independent of hCG and fetal pituitary LH.

The concentration of testosterone in the plasma of the male fetus correlates with the biosynthetic activity of the fetal testis. Peak concentrations in the fetal circulation are 200 to 600 nanograms per deciliter (ng/dl), values comparable to those in the adult male, and are reached by about the 16th week of gestation (Grumbach and Conte, 1998; Grumbach and Gluckman, 1994). Between 16 and 20 weeks of gestation the testosterone levels fall to about 100 ng/dl; after 24 weeks the plasma testosterone level is in the range found in early puberty. Clinical as well as biochemical data indicate that the hCG secreted by the syncytiotrophoblast of the placenta stimulates testosterone secretion during the critical period of male sex differentiation. The number of Leydig cells decreases after week 18 of gestation, probably by dedifferentiation.

Fetal pituitary gonadotropins are essential for the continued growth and function of the fetal testis after the early period of sex differentiation. Fetal pituitary LH seems necessary in concert with hCG for the normal growth of the differentiated penis and scrotum during the latter half of gestation and for descent of the testes. Fetal Leydig cells differ from adult Leydig cells in their morphologies, their regulatory mechanisms, and their lack of desensitization to high doses of hCG and LH. Figure 3-4 correlates the pattern of testosterone, hCG, and fetal pituitary LH and follicle-stimulating hormone (FSH) concentrations during gestation with the histological changes in the fetal testis.

In sum, organogenesis of the testis involves successive differentiation of the Sertoli cell and the seminiferous tubules with envelopment of the extragonadally derived germ cells by Sertoli cells, development of the tunica albicans, appearance of Leydig cells, and differentiation of the mesonephric tubules into ductule efferentes, which connect the seminiferous tubules and network with the epididymis to provide the pathway for sperm transport at the ejaculatory duct system (Grumbach and Conte, 1998).

Organogenesis of the Ovaries

In the absence of testis-determining genes, the gonadal primordium has an inherent tendency to develop as an ovary, provided that germ cells are present and survive. The indifferent stage persists in the female fetus weeks after testis organogenesis begins. There is, however, continued proliferation of the coelomic epithelium and primordial germ cells, which gradually enlarge and become oogonia. Steroid biosynthesis by the fetal ovary is meager in early and midgestation and appears to arise from hilar

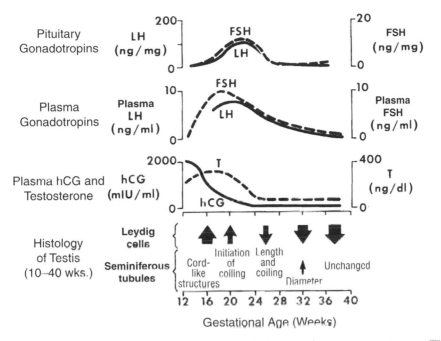

FIGURE 3-4 Comparison of the pattern of change of serum testosterone (T) levels and hCG and serum pituitary LH (LER-960) and FSH (LER-869) levels in the human male fetus during gestation with morphological changes in the fetal testis. Source: Grumbach and Conte (1998, Figure 29-18, p. 1321), adapted from Kaplan and Grumbach (1978). Adapted, with permission, from M. M. Grumbach and F.A. Conte. 1998. *In: Williams Textbook of Endocrinology*, 9th ed. J. D. Wilson, D. W. Foster, H. M. Kronenberg, and P. R. Larsen, eds. Philadelphia: W. B. Saunders Co. Copyright by W.B. Saunders Co., Philadelphia.

interstitial cells in the ovarian primordium at about the 12th week of gestation. Both female and male human fetuses are bathed in estrogens of placental origin. The fetal ovary does not contribute significantly to circulating estrogens, which in the fetus are almost exclusively of placental origin, nor does it secrete AMH. The ovary has no documented role in differentiation of the female genital tract (Grumbach and Auchus, 1999).

At about the 11th to 12th week of gestation, long after differentiation of the testis in the male fetus, germ cells in the ovary begin to enter the meiotic prophase, which characterizes the transition of oogonia to oocytes and marks the onset of ovarian differentiation. The *Wnt-4* gene, at least in the mouse, acts as a suppressor of the differentiation of steroidogenic cells in the fetal ovary.

Differentiation of the Genital Ducts

At the 7th week of intrauterine life, the fetus is equipped with both male and female genital ducts derived from the mesonephros. Müllerian ducts serve as the analog of the uterus and fallopian tubes, whereas the mesonephric or wolffian ducts have the potential to differentiate further into the epididymis, vas deferens (or ejaculatory ducts), and seminal vesicles. During the 3rd fetal month, either the müllerian or the wolffian ducts complete their development and involution occurs simultaneously in the opposite structure.

More than 50 years ago Alfred Jost, the French developmental endocrinologist, demonstrated that secretions from the fetal testis played a decisive role in determining the direction of genital duct development. In the presence of functional testes, the müllerian structures involute and undergo programmed cell death and the wolffian ducts complete their development; in the absence of testes, the wolffian ducts do not develop and müllerian structures differentiate. The regression of the müllerian ducts and the stabilization and differentiation of wolffian ducts are mediated by different secretions by the fetal testis: a glycoprotein, AMH, secreted by the fetal Sertoli cells and a sex steroid, testosterone, synthesized by fetal Leydig cells.

Female development is not contingent on the presence of an ovary because development of the uterus and tubes occurs if no gonad is present. However, the müllerian ducts fail to differentiate in the absence of the mesonephric ducts, which serve as the analog for both the male urogenital tract and the metanephros (primordial kidney). The influence of the fetal testis on duct development is exerted locally and unilaterally; if one testis is removed in an early stage of development, the oviduct develops normally on that side but müllerian duct regression occurs on the side of the intact testis. It is through the secretion of AMH by the fetal Sertoli cells that apoptosis of the müllerian ducts is induced, which leads to their degeneration.

Although müllerian duct involution is not androgen dependent, the differentiation of primitive wolffian ducts into the epididymis, vas deferens, and seminal vesicles requires testosterone and the androgen receptor. Differentiation of the wolffian ducts to form the epididymis, vas deferens, and seminal vesicles is testosterone dependent (the wolffian ducts lack the enzyme 5α-reductase type 2, which converts testosterone to a more potent androgen, dihydrotestosterone) (Wilson et al., 1981). Experimental data and studies with humans with steroid 5α-reductase type 2 deficiency provide additional evidence that testosterone, not dihydrotestosterone, mediates the differentiation of the wolffian ducts. This is in striking contrast to the dihydrotestosterone-dependent differentiation of the urogenital sinus and genital tubercles, which express steroid 5α-reductase 2 even before the testis has developed the capacity to synthe-size testosterone. Thus, testosterone leads to the development of the internal genitalia and dihydrotestosterone leads to the development of the external genitalia (see Figures 3-1, 3-2, and 3-3).

In patients with ambiguous genitalia, male genital ducts are well differentiated only in those who have testes. Females with congenital adrenal hyperplasia do not display wolffian duct differentiation, even though their external genitalia may be highly virilized in utero. It is the critical role of the testes in male duct development to provide high local concentrations of testosterone. Male duct development is therefore deficient, even though testes may be present, in patients with severe defects in steroid biosynthesis and in XY patients whose tissues are unresponsive to testosterone (Grumbach and Conte, 1998).

Differentiation of External Genital and Urogenital Sinus

At the 8th fetal week the external genitalia of both sexes are identical and have the capacity to differentiate in either direction. They consist of the urogenital slit bounded by periurethral folds and more laterally by labioscrotal swellings. The urogenital slit is surrounded by genital tubercles consisting of corpora cavernosa and glans. The mucosa-lined urethral folds may remain separate, in which case they are called labia minora, or they may fuse to form a corpus spongiosum enclosing a phallic urethra. The fleshy labioscrotal swellings may remain separate to form labia majora, or they may fuse in the midline to form the scrotum and the ventral epidermal covering of the penis. The distinction between the clitoris and penis is based primarily on size and whether or not the labia minora fuse to form a corpus spongiosum.

By the 50-mm crown-rump stage, male and female fetuses can be distinguished by inspection of the external genitalia; in the male, the urethral folds have fused completely in the midline to form the cavernous urethra and corpus spongiosa by the 12th to 14th weeks of gestation. Penile length in the male increases linearly at about 0.7 millimeter/week from the 10th week to normal term. A 12-fold increase occurs from 0.3 centimeter (cm) at 12 weeks to 3.5 cm at term, a rate of growth about 3.5 times that of the clitoris.

The urogenital sinus separates from a common cloaca in early fetal life. It is thought that the müllerian duct contributes to the upper part of the vagina. There is disagreement about the relative contribution of the müllerian ducts and the urogenital sinus to the vagina, but the contact and interaction of the fused müllerian ducts with the urogenital sinus are essential for normal development of the vagina. In female development, proliferation of the vesicovaginal septum pushes the vaginal orifice posteriorly so that it acquires a separate external opening; thus, no urogenital sinus as such is preserved. In male development, the vaginal pouch is usually obliterated when the müllerian ducts are reabsorbed, although a vestigial blind vaginal pouch known as the prostatic utricle can sometimes be demonstrated. The prostate gland and the urethral glands of Cowper in the male are outgrowths of the urogenital sinus, in which male differentiation is mediated by dihydrotestosterone and requires the presence of androgen receptors (Grumbach and Conte, 1998).

The induction of differentiation of the external genitalia and urogenital sinus in males is affected by dihydrotestosterone, the 5α-reductase-reduced metabolite of testosterone (Wilson, 1999). Testosterone is a prohormone, and it is delivered through the bloodstream to these target tissues, which are rich in the enzyme 5α-reductase type 2 and which can readily convert testosterone to dihydrotestosterone even before the fetal testes acquire the capacity to secrete testosterone. Dihydrotestosterone binds to the androgen receptor and initiates the events that lead to androgen action.

As in the case of genital ducts, there is an inherent tendency for the external genitalia and urogenital sinus to feminize in the absence of fetal gonadal secretions. Complete differentiation of the external genitalia and urogenital sinus in males occurs only if the androgen stimulus is received during the critical period of development. Dihydrotestosterone stimulates growth of the urogenital tubercle and induces fusion of the urethral folds and labial fold swelling during this critical period; it also induces differentiation of the prostate and inhibits growth of the vesicle vaginal septum, thereby preventing the development of the vagina (Griffin et al., 1995; Grumbach and Conte, 1998). Androgen stimulation however, can cause clitoral hypertrophy at any time during the fetal life or after birth in the female.

Table 3-2 provides some examples of variations in sexual differentiation.

PUBERTY

Puberty is the transitional period between the juvenile state and adulthood during which the adolescent growth spurt occurs, secondary sexual characteristics appear (resulting in the striking sexual dimorphism of mature individuals), fertility is achieved, and profound psychological changes take place. Puberty tends to be regarded as a set of physical changes arising from reactivation of the hypothalamic-pituitary-gonado-tropin-gonadal apparatus (the feedback system integrating nervous and hormonal signals in the hypothalamus). These changes can be timed and measured. On the other hand, adolescence is a more general and gradual coming of age that transpires during most of the second decade of life. Physiological and hormonal processes are involved in many aspects of

TABLE 3-2 Selected Examples of Variations in Sexual Differentiation

Condition	Karyotype	Effective Prenatal Hormones	External Genitalia	Usual Rearing Sex	Can Provide Information Regarding
Congenital adrenal hyperplasia	46,XX	↑ A levels, nl female E levels	Ambiguous	Female	Early A levels
Complete androgen insensitivity	46,XY	No A action	Female	Female	Early A levels, male-typical E levels, Y chromosome, rearing sex
Partial androgen insensitivity	46,XY	↓ A action, nl male E levels	Ambiguous	Varies	Early A levels, male-typical E levels
Cloacal exstrophy	46,XY	nl male A levels, nl male E levels	Absent penis	Female	Early A and E levels, Y chromosome, rearing sex
5-α-Reductase deficiency	46,XY	nl T levels, ↓ DHT, nl male E levels	Ambiguous, masculinized at puberty	Male	T versus DHT levels
Aromatase deficiency	46,XX	↑ A levels, ↓ E levels	Ambiguous, clitoral growth at puberty	Female	Early A levels
Turner syndrome	45,X	↓ E levels at puberty	Female	Female	

NOTE: Abbreviations and symbols: nl, normal; A, androgen; E, estrogen; T, testosterone; DHT, dihydrotestosterone; ↑, increase; ↓, decrease.

this growth and development, with the onset of puberty a benchmark of the passage from childhood to adolescence.

Puberty is not a de novo event but rather is a phase in the continuum of development of the hypothalamic-pituitary-gonadal function from fetal life through puberty to the attainment of full sexual maturation and fertility (Grumbach and Styne, 1998). Endocrine events recognized as adolescent puberty actually begin early in fetal life. The hypothalamic-pituitary-gonadotropin-gonadal system differentiates in function during fetal life and early infancy, is suppressed to a low level of activity during childhood (the juvenile pause), and is reactivated at puberty (Grumbach and Kaplan, 1990; Grumbach and Styne, 1998). As mentioned earlier, a significant sex difference in fetal pituitary gonadotropin levels and the high circulating testosterone levels in the male fetus through the 24th week of gestation are the most prominent features of the hypothalamic-pituitary-gonadotropin-gonadal system. There is no evidence that the concentrations of estradiol or other estrogens in serum differ in male and female fetuses.

Within a few minutes after birth, the concentration of LH in serum increases abruptly (about 10-fold) in the peripheral blood of the male newborn but not in that of the female newborn. This short-lived surge in LH release is followed by an increase in the serum testosterone level during the first 3 hours that persists for 12 hours or more. In the female neonate, LH levels do not increase, and FSH levels in both males and females are low in the first few days of neonatal life. After the fall in circulating placental steroid levels, especially estrogens, during the first few days after birth, serum FSH and LH levels increase and exhibit a pulsatile pattern with wide perturbations for several months. The FSH pulse amplitude is greater in female infants, and the FSH response to hypothalamic luteinizing hormone-releasing hormone (LHRH) or gonadotropin-releasing hormone is higher in females than males throughout childhood; LH pulses are higher in males. A sex difference in plasma FSA and LH values is also present in anorchid boys and agonadal girls less than three years old.

The high gonadotropin concentrations in infancy are associated with a transient second wave of differentiation of fetal-type Leydig cells and increased serum testosterone levels in male infants for the first 6 months or so and with elevated estradiol levels intermittently in the first 1 to 2 years of life in females. The mean FSH level is higher in females than males during the first few years of life. By approximately 6 to 8 months of age in the male and 2 to 3 years of age in the female, plasma gonadotropin levels decrease to low values until the onset of puberty. Thus, the restraint of the hypothalamic LHRH pulse generator and the suppression of pulsatile LHRH secretion (and thus FSH and LH release) attain the prepubertal level of quiescence in late infancy or early childhood and earlier in boys than in girls (for reviews see Grumbach and Styne [1998] and Grumbach and Gluckman [1994]).

The juvenile pause (that interval between early childhood and the peripuberty period when the LHRH pulse generator is at a low level of activity and circulating pituitary gonadotropin levels are low) is not associated with complete suppression of pituitary gonadotropin-gonadal function. Some studies have used highly sensitive immunoassays to show that both prepubertal boys and prepubertal girls have a pulsatile pattern of serum LH and FSH concentrations, with higher concentrations during the night than during the day (see Mitamura et al., 1999, 2000). The pulses are of very low amplitude compared with the increase in the pulse amplitude that occurs with the approach of puberty. There is apparently no change (or only a modest one) in pulse frequency with the onset of puberty (Mitamura et al., 1999, 2000).

A striking sex difference has been detected in prepubertal children by a highly sensitive immunoassay for estradiol in serum. Prepubertal girls have a mean estradiol concentration of 0.6 picograms per milliliter (pg/ml), whereas the mean value in prepubertal boys is 0.08 pg/ml (Klein et al., 1994). During prepuberty in both sexes, serum testosterone concentrations are detectable, but at a very low level. The higher concentration of estradiol in prepubertal girls is associated with about a 20 percent advancement in bone age and may be a factor in the earlier onset of puberty in girls. For example, a bone age of about 11 years in girls is the equivalent of a bone age of 13 years in boys.

In addition, striking sex differences exist in the gonadally synthesized glycoprotein hormone inhibins throughout development in boys and girls (Andersson et al., 1997; Sehested et al., 2000). Inhibin B concentrations are strikingly elevated in males for the first 2 years of life and show a striking increase from childhood levels to adult levels at the onset of puberty, whereas levels of inhibin B are low or undetectable in prepubertal girls, followed by a sharp increase through midpuberty and then a decline.

Data on the normal variations in pubertal development in the United States are becoming more plentiful but are still incomplete. In recent years striking ethnic differences in the time of onset of puberty have been detected for girls but not for boys (Biro et al., 1995; Herman-Giddens et al., 1997). In girls, two distinct phenomena occur in the development of secondary sex characteristics. The development of breasts is under the control of estrogen secreted by the ovaries; the growth of pubic and axillary hair is under the influence of androgen secreted by the adrenal cortex and the ovary. Most recent data suggest that the mean age of onset of breast development in Caucasian girls is 10.6 years, with limits between 7 and 13 years, and that in African-American girls is 9.5 years, with limits between 6 and 13 years. The onset of breast development in African-American girls is about 1 year earlier than that in Caucasian girls, even though the average age of menarche in a large cross-sectional study was different by only 0.7 year (12.2 years for African-American girls and 12.9 years for Caucasian girls) (Herman-Giddens et al., 1997).

A careful review of U.S. studies of the onset of puberty in girls in the past three decades suggests that any change in the mean age of onset of breast development in Caucasian American girls is probably no more than 1 year earlier, if in fact a decrease in the mean age has actually occurred (Grumbach and Styne, 1998; Herman-Giddens et al., 1997). The age of menarche, a well-recognized landmark of pubertal development in girls, has not changed over the past four decades (Eveleth and Tanner, 1990). In African-American girls the mean age of onset of breast development apparently is 1 year earlier; while ethnic differences in fat mass maybe a factor (Kumanyika, 1998), the nature of the discordance is uncertain. In girls (as will be discussed below) the onset of puberty, in retrospect, is marked by an increase in the growth rate even before breast development.

The beginning of pubertal onset in boys is marked by an increase in the size of the testes, which occurs in both white and African-American boys at a mean age of about 11 years (Biro et al., 1995), with the normal limits being between 9 and 13.5 years. It is well established that the changes in the levels of sex steroid and gonadotropin secretion may precede or anticipate for some years the onset of physical changes of puberty. The actual dimorphic physical changes of puberty are primarily the consequence of testosterone secretion by the Leydig cells in boys and of estrogen secretion by the granulosa cells in girls (Grumbach and Styne, 1998).

Leptin

Leptin, a hormone produced by adipose tissue, appears to have an important permissive action in the progression into puberty and the maintenance of normal secondary sex characteristics through its effect on hypothalamic-pituitary-gonadotropin-gonadal function (Clement et al., 1998; Farooqi et al., 1999; Strobel et al., 1998). The leptin concentration in serum correlates with body mass index or percent body fat and even more highly with the absolute amount of adipose tissue. There is a striking sexual dimorphism in the circulating concentration of leptin at birth, at which time females have higher levels than males, and again in late puberty and adulthood. A sexual dimorphism in circulating leptin concentrations has not been detected during childhood, however (Horlick et al., 2000), with the rise in leptin concentrations occurring 1 year earlier in girls than in boys. The levels in boys peaked at Tanner stage 2 and decreased by Tanner stage 5. In contrast, in girls, leptin levels increased in breast stage 2 and peaked at breast stage 5 (Blum et al., 1997; Clayton et al., 1997; Horlick et al., 2000). The decreased leptin levels in late puberty in boys have been attributed to the action of testosterone

Pubertal Growth Spurt

One of the most striking sex differences in puberty is the earlier age of onset of the pubertal growth spurt and the earlier attainment of peak height velocity in girls, in contrast to the later onset of the increased rate of growth and greater peak height velocity in boys. Prepubertal height and growth velocities are similar in boys and girls. Boys reach peak height velocity approximately 2 years later than girls and are taller at the beginning of the pubertal growth spurt.

In contrast to girls, in whom the increase in height velocity is probably the earliest sign of pubertal maturation, in boys, peak height velocity does not occur until genital stage 3 or 4 of puberty (Boxes 3-1 and 3-2). The mean height difference of 12.5 cm between adult men and women results partly from the greater pregrowth spurt growth in boys, partly from the height difference at the age of takeoff (boys being taller at their later age of the beginning of the pubertal growth spurt), and partly from the greater gain in height of boys during the pubertal growth spurt (Figure 3-5).

The hormonal control of the pubertal growth spurt is complex. Growth hormone, insulin-like growth factor 1, and triiodothyronine are the principal regulators of prepubertal growth and regulate about 50 percent of the growth during the pubertal period; superimposed on this growth is the linear growth induced by estradiol in both boys and girls. Although the role of estradiol in the pubertal growth spurt in girls has been appreciated for more than 20 years, only now do new observations indicate that estradiol is the major sex steroid responsible for the pubertal

---

BOX 3-1
Sex Differences in the Relationship of Onset of Pubertal Growth Spurt to Sexual Maturation in Girls and Boys

In Girls
The onset of the pubertal growth spurt precedes or is associated with the earliest signs of female secondary sexual maturation (e.g., pubic and axillary hair and breast development).

In Boys
The onset of sexual maturation including testicular enlargement and the development of male secondary sexual characteristics precedes the onset of the pubertal growth spurt. Peak height velocity is not achieved until late stage 3 to stage 4 of sexual maturation.

BOX 3-2
Sex Differences in the Timing of the Onset of Estrogen
Synthesis in Girls and Boys

In Girls
From late fetal life through puberty FSH stimulates aromatase and estrogen synthesis by the ovary.

In Boys
FSH leads to enlargement of the testes, the earliest sign of puberty in the male; spermarche occurs early in puberty, and spermaturia occurs at a mean age of 13.3 years before the sharp rise in testosterone levels and peak height velocity.
Estrogen synthesis is not detectable in fetal or prepubertal Leydig cells and is at a very low level until LH stimulates Leydig cell aromatase at late stage 2 to stage 3 of male secondary sexual maturation. Estradiol levels in males do not reach the levels found in early puberty in girls, who are exhibiting a pubertal growth spurt, until at least midpuberty.

---

growth spurt in boys as well as girls (reviewed in Grumbach [2000] and Grumbach and Auchus [1999]).

In boys, the estradiol is derived mainly from the extragonadal conversion of testosterone to estradiol in a wide variety of tissues, but there is also a small testicular contribution (Siiteri and MacDonald, 1973). Furthermore, estradiol, but not testosterone, appears to be the critical mediator of skeletal maturation and epiphyseal fusion and the major sex steroid in bone mineral accrual in boys as well as girls (Grumbach, 2000; and Grumbach and Auchus, 1999). This conceptual sea change has emanated from studies of men, women, and children with mutations in the gene encoding aromatase (Bilezikian et al., 1998; Grumbach and Auchus, 1999; Morishima et al., 1995) and from studies of one man with a null mutation in the gene encoding the estrogen receptor α (Smith et al., 1994).

There is a very striking and poorly understood difference in the prevalence of so-called idiopathic true or central precocious puberty in boys and girls. The idiopathic form is about 10 times more common in girls than in boys. In contrast to the striking sex difference in idiopathic true precocious puberty, constitutional delay in growth in adolescents (idiopathic delayed puberty) is more common in boys than in girls.

Adrenarche Versus Gonadarche

In both boys and girls, beginning before age 8 (skeletal age, 6 to 8 years), an increase in the levels of secretion of adrenal androgens and androgen precursors, called "adrenarche," occurs. It is marked biochemically by progressive increases in plasma dehydroepiandrosterone and

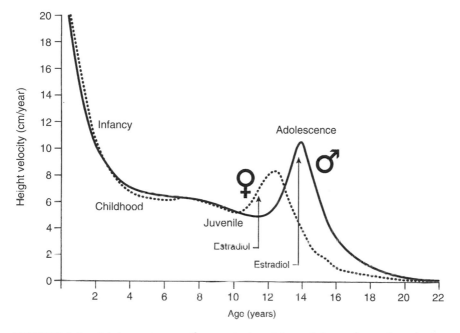

FIGURE 3-5 Adolescent growth spurts in girls and boys (growth velocity curves). Note the later onset of pubertal growth in boys than in girls, the approximately 2-year difference in peak height velocity between boys and girls, and the greater magnitude of peak height velocity in boys than in girls. The timing of the effects of estradiol is indicated, as is its important role in the growth spurt in both sexes. Progressive epiphyseal fusion terminates the growth spurt and leads to final or adult height. Source: Grumbach (2000). Reprinted, with permission, from M. M. Grumbach and D. M. Styne. 1998. *In. Williams Textbook of Endocrinology*, 9th ed. J. D. Wilson, D. W. Foster, H. M. Kronenberg, and P. R. Larsen, eds. Philadelphia: W. B. Saunders Co. Copyright by W. B. Saunders Company, Philadelphia.

dehydroepiandrosterone sulfate (DHEAS) concentrations. The mechanism of activation of adrenal androgen secretion or adrenarche is independent of the mechanisms that regulate the onset of sex steroid secretion by the gonads, which is called "gonadarche" (Grumbach and Styne, 1998).

Premature adrenarche, which is more common in girls than in boys, is characterized by the precocious appearance of pubic hair or axillary hair, less commonly an apocrine odor, and comedones and acne without other signs of puberty or virilization (Grumbach and Styne, 1998). Adrenarche is premature when it occurs in Caucasian girls before age 7 or African-American girls before age 5. In boys the diagnosis is limited to those who develop pubic hair or axillary hair before the age of 9. In contrast to boys, in whom premature adrenarche is usually a benign, self-limited normal variant of puberty, girls with premature adrenarche are at increased risk (about 10-fold) for the development of insulin resistance and ovarian hyperandrogenism, in particular, polycystic ovary syndrome (PCOS) (Dunaif et al., 1992; Ibáñez et al., 1996; Morales et al., 1996; Oppenheimer et al., 1995). PCOS affects about 5 to 10 percent of women of reproductive age and is the most common endocrine disorder in women. A proportion of girls with exaggerated adrenarche (Likitmaskul et al., 1995), which is marked by higher levels of circulating DHEAS, may exhibit insulin resistance and hyperinsulinism or dyslipidemia, and beginning in late adolescence they are at increased risk for the development of ovarian hyperandrogenism and anovulation (Ibáñez et al., 1998, 1999a). Affected girls, however, usually begin gonadarche within the normal range of time.

There is a correlation between the occurrence of exaggerated adrenarche in prepubertal girls and a higher risk for ovarian hyperandrogenism at puberty. The androgen excess is a consequence of PCOS and is associated with an increased risk of metabolic complications, including type II diabetes mellitus, hypertension, dyslipidemia, and possibly, cardiovascular disease. There is a tendency for familial aggregation of women with PCOS, and evidence suggests that this heterogeneous disorder represents a complex, multifactorial trait.

A promising area of research is the increasing body of evidence that supports an association of premature adrenarche, insulin resistance, and dyslipidemia in girls with intrauterine growth retardation (Francois and de Zegher, 1997; Ibáñez et al, 1999b). Recent studies (Ibáñez et al., 2000) suggest that girls with prenatal growth restriction have at birth a smaller complement of primordial follicles than infants of appropriate weight for gestational age and have at adolescence a small uterus and ovaries. After menarche these girls tend to show ovarian hyporesponsiveness to FSH.

In sum, the evidence suggests a link between intrauterine growth retardation and the increased risk of exaggerated adrenarche followed by PCOS, including hyperandrogenism, insulin resistance, dyslipidemia (with or without obesity), and cardiovascular disease (Barker, 1995, 1997; Cresswell et al., 1997). As first advanced by Barker (1995) from observational studies, the association of impaired or disproportionate fetal growth, related to fetal undernutrition, with premature adrenarche and PCOS is another example of disorders in adolescence and adulthood that may be programmed in fetal life. Many issues, however, remain unresolved (Jaquet et al., 1999).

Sex Differences in Behavior

The hormonal and physical changes at puberty described above have implications for sex differences in behavior in early adolescence. Some behavioral changes probably result from the direct effects of gonadal hormones acting directly on the brain. For example, in early adolescence, increasing testosterone levels in boys have been associated with increasing aggression and social dominance, and changes in estrogen levels in girls have been associated with mood changes (Brooks-Gunn et al., 1994; Buchanan et al., 1992; Finkelstein et al., 1997; Olweus et al., 1980; Schaal et al., 1996; Susman et al., 1987). Some behaviors appear to relate to the absolute level of the hormone, others appear to relate to the ratio of hormone levels (for example, the testosterone level/estradiol level ratio), and others appear to relate to hormonal variation. (These associations are not always noted and probably depend on the reliability of hormone level measurements, intersubject variation, and the specific behaviors measured.) It is important to note that hormone levels themselves can be changed by behavior. For example, winning an athletic event has been shown to increase testosterone levels in males (Booth et al., 1989).

As discussed later, the rise in estrogen levels at puberty may contribute to females' superior phonological skills and may allow females with dyslexia to compensate for their reading deficiencies. There is also some suggestion that other cognitive changes in adolescence are related to hormonally induced maturation of the frontal lobe (Spear, 2000). Given the sex difference in the timing of gonadarche, there may well be sex differences in the developmental timing of behaviors subserved by the frontal lobe (including planning and judgment), although probably not in the ultimate levels of those behaviors at maturity.

The hormonal and physical changes that occur during puberty also contribute in indirect ways to differences between adolescent boys and adolescent girls. For example, the development of secondary sex characteristics in girls creates social signals that result in different responses from peers, parents, and teachers. There is a substantial literature showing that girls who mature earlier than their peers are at greater risk than girls who mature on time or later than their peers for problems during the pubertal transition and continuing into adulthood. These problems include substance use, depression, and eating disorders (Caspi and Moffitt, 1991; Graber et al., 1997). Some of these effects are mediated by the fact that girls who mature early are more likely than others to associate with older adolescents and to be treated as if they are older (including increased responsibilities from parents and increased expectations of parents). Boys who mature earlier than their male peers do not have a similarly increased risk of problems compared with the risk for boys who mature on time or later, in part because the absolute age of boys who mature early is, on average, 2 years later than that of girls who mature early and because their physical maturation gives them status among adolescents, who value athleticism and physical skill in boys.

Adolescence is associated with changing social roles, and there is good reason to believe that gender socialization intensifies at that time of life (Crouter et al., 1995; Hill and Lynch, 1983; Stein, 1976). These changes in social roles will have wide-ranging effects, including, for example, variations in interpretations of harmful stimuli and responses to injury, as discussed below.

ADULTHOOD

During the long period of about 40 years of fertile adulthood, an individual's occupation(s), social roles, and lifestyle change episodically and develop slowly as experiences accumulate. Although societal norms are rapidly changing, in general it remains the case that women still predominate as caregivers and organizers with wide-ranging obligations and duties spanning the family, workplace, and leisure realms, whereas men still predominate in more focused aggressive and physically demanding activities with a relatively narrower range of social obligations. Accompanying these developing and highly individual psychosocial characteristics are the more consistent (but not constant) sex differences in anatomy, organ function (physiology), and endocrine function. Thus, on average, women, relative to men, have a higher percentage of body fat, smaller muscle mass, lower blood pressure, higher levels of estrogens and progestins, and lower levels of androgen. The challenge in understanding the significance of this vast array of sex differences for health and health care lies not so much in assessing the influence of each of these factors in isolation but, rather, in deciphering how the factors interact throughout the course of adulthood to affect each individual at any moment.

In addition, women, but not men, undergo fluctuations associated with the reproductive condition (such as the ovarian cycle and pregnancy) that influence numerous bodily functions (e.g., gastrointestinal transit time, urinary creatinine clearance, liver enzyme function, and thermoregulation), including brain function. (The effects of pregnancy, lactation, and parity are obviously important to the health of women later in their lives but are not addressed specifically in this report.)

Effects of Menopause on Women's Health

After the fertile years in women there is a 5- to 10-year period of menopause-related alterations in hormone patterns, terminating in the sharp decline in female hormone levels. As follicle depletion occurs in the ovaries, the rate of ovarian hormone production slows. The tissues most affected by reduced estrogen levels are the ovaries, uterus, vagina, breast, and urinary tract. However, other tissues such as the hypothalamus, skin, cardiovascular tissue, and bone are also substantially affected. A major challenge to the prevention of disease in older women lies in exploring the effects of both short-term and long-term reductions in ovarian hormone levels on the development of symptoms and disease.

The lack of ovarian estrogens appears to contribute significantly to the onset of several postmenopausal diseases, such as osteoporosis and cardiovascular disease, two leading causes of morbidity and mortality in older women. Much of the evidence to support the finding of a cardioprotective effect for estrogen has come from observational studies of women on estrogen replacement therapy, which has shown that estrogen users experience half as many cardiovascular events as nonusers, but numerous questions remain (also discussed in Chapter 5). An adverse influence of hormone therapy on cardiovascular risk in women with coronary heart disease has been shown during the initial year of use; however, few data are available on the effects of long-term hormone therapy (Grodstein et al., 2000). The protection conferred by estrogen has been shown to be mediated by mechanisms acting at different levels, including a beneficial effect of estrogen on plasma lipid concentrations (Lamon-Fava, 2000).

In addition, research has identified estrogen receptors in bone (reviewed in Grumbach and Auchus, 1999; Khosla et al., 1999; Prestwood et al., 2000). Declines in estrogen production correlate with rapid bone loss, which predisposes a woman to osteoporosis. Although age-related bone loss is a universal phenomenon shared by men and women, the effect of osteoporosis on women is much more profound and pervasive. Several reports have shown that combining high-calcium supplements with a regimen of hormone therapy increases the efficacy of estrogen in bone conservation. Hormone replacement by estrogen therapy or the newly developed therapy with selective estrogen receptor modulators may prevent the development of osteoporosis and its related fractures (Kamel et al., 2001).

In men, more inconsistent and complex changes in hormone metabolism, called "andropause" by some, occur over a longer period of time, on average, between the ages of 48 and 70 (Morales et al., 2000; Vermeulen, 2000). Currently, much more is known about the consequences of menopause than about those of andropause. Androgen deficiency has been shown to be associated with osteoporosis. Although testosterone replacement therapy in hypogonadal men decreases bone resorption and increases bone mass, placebo-controlled trials are needed to better define the effectiveness and risks of such therapy in older men. The effect of testosterone is, at least in part, related to its conversion in bone (Bilezikian et al., 1998; Grumbach, 2000; Khosla et al., 1998; Smith et al., 1994) to estradiol.

The Aging Human

The evolving effects of interactions between an individual's personal physiology and unique experiences make it difficult to assess how simply being female or male affects that individual's health as life progresses from birth through fertile adulthood into old age. Although the field of gerontology is growing rapidly, research from this perspective is meager. Most studies simply address the question of how elderly individuals differ from younger individuals, with little attention paid to how the differences might develop over time. Nevertheless, it is evident that the patterns of sex differences that exist during the long period of fertile adulthood change during old age in clinically relevant ways. For example, community prevalence estimates for chronic widespread pain and fibromyalgia show a general increase with age until about age 65, followed by a decrease, with the prevalence in women always being higher (LeResche, 1999). On the other hand, the prevalence of pain in the knee or finger joints shows a continual increase across the life span for both sexes, with no sex differences until age 50, after which the prevalence becomes higher in women (LeResche, 1999). A second example—in this case, one relevant to diagnosis—is that the symptom presentation of patients with confirmed acute myocardial infarction varies by sex, but, importantly, the pattern changes with age (Goldberg et al., 2000). Younger patients (less than age 55) were significantly more likely than older patients to complain of sweating and arm pain.

A third example—in this case, relevant to treatment—involves recent data showing sex- and age-related differences in the optimal effects of antihypertensive and antiplatelet therapies for the prevention of cardiovascular disease (Kjeldsen et al., 2000). For example, compared with treatment with a placebo, daily acetylsalicylic acid (ASA) treatment resulted in a significant reduction in the rate of occurrence of composite major cardiovascular events in younger patients (younger than age 65). Some reduction in the rate of occurrence of major cardiovascular events was also seen in ASA-treated older patients, but the reduction was not statistically significant.

From 1900 through about 1940, Americans who lived to age 65 had a life expectancy of another 11 or 12 years, regardless of sex. Since the 1940s differences in life expectancies between males and females after age 65 have emerged, and these differences favor females. Similarly, in 1900 individuals who reached the age of 85 had, on average, another 4 years of life, with very little difference between the sexes. Differences in survival began to appear in the 1960s, and these again favored females. Much of this difference can be attributed to differences in rates of death from cardiovascular disease. A breakdown by sex and age (65 to 74 years, 75 to 84 years, and 85 years and older) reveals that in each age group men have higher death rates from both heart disease and cancer than women (National Center for Health Statistics, 1999). Death rates from stroke, another leading cause of death, are more balanced between males and females.

Currently, life expectancy at birth is greater for females than males by ~6 years, but once old age has been attained, it becomes 2 to 3 years (Table 3-3). The actual life expectancy differs among ethnic groups and is, for example, notably shorter among African American than Caucasian Americans, but the consistency in the observation of an advantage for females across ethnic groups is striking (Figure 3-6). This consistent observation of greater life expectancy at birth for females has grown over time, from about 2 years in 1900 to 6 years in 1998 (Figure 3-7), with some fluctuations during the interim.

Although the mechanisms that underlie both the general increase in longevity and the increasing advantage for females are poorly understood, some components of the male longevity disadvantage can be identified. For example, rates of death from the major causes (both intentional and unintentional injuries and illnesses) are usually higher for males than for females at each stage of life (Leveille et al., 2000), although there are exceptions in which the rates are similar for the two sexes or are higher for females.

Stress and its hormonal consequences are complex factors that may contribute to longevity. A recent provocative suggestion is that the behavioral response to stress may differ between males and females (Taylor et al., 2000). According to this hypothesis males display the classic "fight-or-flight" response that in females is modulated to become a "tend-and-defend" response. On the basis of a meta-analysis (integrating the data from a number of independent studies), the female's response is apparently mediated by oxytocin, a hormone known to reduce stress and increase social affiliation in rodents (Carter et al., 1995; Witt et al., 1990). This proposed difference in response may have implications for the sex

TABLE 3-3 Life Expectancy at Birth, Age 65, and Age 75 Years, United States, All Races, 1998

| Age | Life Expectancy (years) | | Difference (Female minus Male) | Percent Difference[a] |
	Males	Females		
At birth	73.8	79.5	5.7	7
At age 65	16.0	19.2	3.2	17
At age 75	10.0	12.2	2.2	18

[a] Percent difference equals (life expectancy for females minus life expectancy for males) divided by life expectancy for females.
SOURCE: National Center for Health Statistics (2000a).

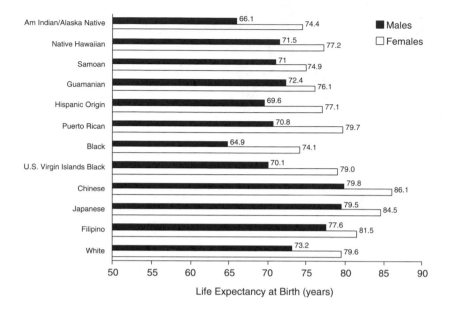

FIGURE 3-6 Life expectancy at birth for males and females in several U.S. ethnic groups (data are from 1989 to 1994). Source: National Center for Health Statistics (1996) and National Institutes of Health, Office of Research on Women's Health (1998).

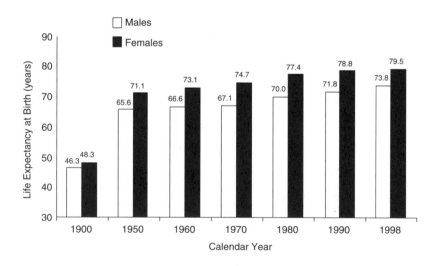

FIGURE 3-7 Life expectancy at birth for males and females, selected years between 1900 and 1998, United States, all races. Source: National Center for Health Statistics (2000a).

differences in stress-related disorders in human populations and may contribute to the longer life span of females.

The female longevity advantage, however, is not without cost. Although females live longer, those who do live longer experience more disabling health problems than males. Thus, a recent study of 10,263 older adults in three communities in the United States showed that the proportion of disabled women increased from 22 percent at age 70 to 81 percent at age 90, whereas the figures for men were 15 and 57 percent, respectively (Leveille et al., 2000). Similarly, another study showed that although the current life expectancy at age 32 is 39.45 years for men and 44.83 years for women, it becomes 31.8 years for men and 33.1 years for women when life expectancy is adjusted for "quality of life." In other words, a 5.38-year advantage for women is reduced to 1.3 years (Kaplan and Erickson, 2000).

Clearly, studies that address the mechanisms that underlie the development of these differences as individuals age could yield important information of benefit to both sexes.

FINDINGS AND RECOMMENDATIONS

Findings

Sex differences occur throughout the life span, although their specific expression varies at different at stages of life.

- *Intrauterine environment:* Some sex differences originate in events that begin in the womb, where developmental processes differentially organize tissues for later activation..
- *Early development:* During the prepubertal period there are behavioral as well as subtle hormonal sex differences.
- *Puberty:* During sexual maturation, hormones activate organ systems differently between males and females; these include brain anatomy and functions that were previously organized by hormones and modified by the environment.
- *Adulthood:* Throughout the life span, including midlife and old age, the brain, as well as many other organs, retain plasticity and continue to be modified by gene expression, hormones, and environmental factors. These factors act in an integrative manner but may be expressed differently in males and females.

To continue to advance human health and health care, research on sex differences in health and illness across the life span is essential. Such research can be aided by information obtained from the observation and study of other species. In this regard, the committee makes the following recommendations.

Recommendations

RECOMMENDATION 2: Study sex differences from womb to tomb.

The committee recommends that researchers and those who fund research focus on the following areas:

- **inclusion of sex as a variable in basic research designs,**
- **expansion of studies to reveal the mechanisms of intrauterine effects, and**
- **encouragement of studies at different stages of the life span to determine how sex differences influence health, illness, and longevity.**

Sex is an important marker of individual variability. Some of this sex-related variability results from events that occur in the intrauterine environment but that do not materialize until later in life. Current research varies in its level of attention to these matters.

The committee acknowledges that inclusion of people, animals, or cells and tissues of both sexes in all studies is not feasible or appropriate. Rather, the committee is urging researchers to regard sex, that is, being male or female, as an important basic human variable that should be considered when designing, analyzing, and reporting findings from studies in all areas and at all levels of biomedical research. Statistical methods can be used to evaluate the effect of sex without necessarily doubling the sample size of every study. In addition, it is particularly important that researchers revisit and revise approaches to studying whole-animal physiology in light of what has been learned in the past decade about major sex differences.

RECOMMENDATION 3: Mine cross-species information.

- **Researchers should choose models that mirror human sex differences and that are appropriate for the human conditions being addressed. Given the interspecies variation, the mechanisms of sex differences in nonhuman primates may be the best mimics for some mechanisms of sex differences in humans. Continued development of appropriate animal models, including those involving nonhuman primates, should be encouraged and supported under existing regulations and guidelines (see the *Guide for the Care and Use of Laboratory Animals* [National Research Council, 1996]).**
- **Researchers should be alert to unexpected phenotypic sex differences resulting from the production of genetically modified animals.**

Sex differences and their relevance to human health can be examined through the use of cross-species comparisons. The use of appropriate animal models can reveal underlying mechanisms of normal and pathogenic processes.

4
Sex Affects Behavior and Perception

ABSTRACT

Basic genetic and physiological differences, in combination with environmental factors, result in behavioral and cognitive differences between males and females. Sex differences in the brain, sex-typed behavior and gender identity, and sex differences in cognitive ability should be studied at all points in the life span. Hormones play a role in behavioral and cognitive sex differences but are not solely responsible for those differences. In addition, sex differences in perception of pain have important clinical implications. Research is needed on the natural variations between and within the sexes in behavior, cognition, and perception, with expanded investigation of sex differences in brain structure and function.

The purpose of this chapter is not to review all the evidence about the nature and determinants of sex differences in behavior or any other characteristic but to describe how basic genetic and physiological differences between males and females might produce phenotypic differences throughout the life span.

SEX DIFFERENCES IN BEHAVIOR AND COGNITIVE ABILITIES

Behavioral sex differences may originate in events that begin in the womb. The fetal environment, particularly hormones present during development, affects aspects of later behavioral and cognitive sex differences. Sex differences in behavior are important in their own right, but also suggest ways in which prenatal influences can contribute to sex differences in nonbehavioral traits, including those associated with health and illness. The information presented in this section should not be interpreted to mean that all behavioral sex differences are caused by hormones during prenatal development but, rather, should serve as an illustration of the potential role of prenatal hormones in producing phenotypic sex differences.

No single factor produces sex differences in any one behavioral or cognitive trait, let alone in all of them. Until recently, it has been popular to focus on cultural or experiential causes of these differences. Thus, for example, sex differences in the occurrence of depression have been considered to reflect women's greater social orientation (which is itself assumed to be cultural) or stresses associated with women's multiple social roles (as also mentioned in Chapter 3). In the past 10 years, however, there has been increasing appreciation of the fact that genetic and physiological differences between males and females might also influence behavioral sex differences. Although some might argue that the pendulum has swung too much in favor of genes and physiology (Fausto-Sterling, 2000), there is considerable interest in examining the joint effects of genes, physiology, and experiences. In particular, there is recognition that the environment is not independent of the individual (Scarr and McCartney, 1983). Individuals actively construct their environments and are responded to by others in their environments. The effects of imposed environments are not the same for everyone. When one considers sex differences, one must also remember that females and males "inhabit" different cultures and that some behavioral sex differences are more marked when people are in social groups than when they are alone. Thus, questions about sex differences concern not just differences between individual males and females but also differences between male and female cultures (Maccoby, 1998).

Psychosexual Differentiation

Studies with nonhuman vertebrate species suggest that the sexual role adopted at maturity is determined by the hormonal environment in early life. As for other aspects of sex differentiation, there appears to be a predisposition for individuals to develop female sexual postures. The development of male patterns of sexual behavior in nonhuman species is influenced to a large extent by exposure to androgens—in particular, testosterone—during the prenatal and perinatal periods. This organizing capacity of testosterone administered at a critical stage of development has been localized to specific areas of the brain. Sexually dimorphic organizations of target cell nuclei detected during behavior-related events in other species are the result of local aromatization (conversion) of testosterone to estradiol in the central nervous systems of these species. In humans, masculinization of the central nervous system does not appear to result from aromatized estradiol but appears to result from forms of testosterone (Grumbach and Auchus, 1999).

Sex Differences in the Central Nervous System and Brain

Sex differences in the central nervous system extend beyond functions and structures traditionally associated with reproduction. These differences might be better understood if they were studied in the context of new and exciting conceptualizations of how the brain works, which encompass notions of lifelong plasticity, ensemble processing and distributed networks, and the brain's role as an endocrine organ.

The classic examples of sex differences in the brain involve neuroanatomical differences that are developmentally programmed. In several species, sex differences in the patterns of synaptic innervation are observed in the preoptic area and are influenced by the perinatal hormone environment but not by hormonal conditions in the adult animal (Gorski et al., 1978; Nottebohm and Arnold, 1976; Raisman and Field, 1971). These early studies reveal the effects of castration of males and the administration of testosterone to females early in development and established the idea that differences in the wiring of the brain are programmed at birth. There are now many documented sex differences in a wide range of species, including primates (Forger, 1998). In canaries and zebra finches, for example, differences in singing behavior between males and females have been correlated with differences in the sizes of three vocal control areas in the brain (Nottebohm and Arnold, 1976), but, importantly, the young male bird must hear the adult male song to initiate its own repertoire.

There are also sex differences in the human brain, including the higher cognitive centers. These differences have been observed in adults, and the nature and origins of these differences are subjects of active investigation. Recent studies suggest sex differences in brain structure size as the brain develops in children (Giedd et al., 1987; Lange et al., 1997). It is important to remember that these differences are not absolute and that it is currently not possible, nor may it ever be, to look at a brain or a brain image and know the sex of its owner.

The principles that have emerged from studies with nonhuman species have generally been confirmed in humans, although differences in details exist. For example, androgens act as masculinizing agents in all species, but they appear to do so through different metabolites. Another important principle that has emerged from studies with animals and that has been confirmed in humans is that the central nervous system remains plastic throughout the life span. Finally, former notions that discrete brain regions have specific and static functions have been modified by work on ensemble neuronal activity (Laubach et al., 2000) and distributed networks (Sanes and Donoghue, 2000).

Areas that have not been traditionally thought to be sexually dimorphic may be involved in sexually dimorphic behavior. Some examples are (1) dopamine functions within the striatum and nucleus accumbens (Becker, 1999); (2) the responsiveness of neurons in the gracile nucleus to stimulation of skin and pelvic organs (Bradshaw and Berkley, 2000) (neuronal responsiveness and activity in the two regions vary with the estrous cycle and hormonal manipulation in a manner that correlates with lordosis and other reproductive behaviors; and (3) modulation of functions in the hippocampus, inferior olive, and cerebellum (Smith et al., 2000).

The Brain as an Endocrine Organ

A great deal of evidence indicates that the brain functions as an endocrine (hormone-secreting) organ. Throughout life, there are profound sex differences in the brain's responsiveness to sex hormones, some of which are established early in development and which have implications for later behavior, including cognitive function.

The brain is also involved in the regulation of other hormones that show sex differences and that are involved in both reproductive and nonreproductive behaviors. For example, aggression in male mice is considerably more intense than that in female mice, and this difference is known to be influenced by testosterone. Recent studies suggest that the story may be more complex. Nitric oxide, a compound that participates in cell-to-cell signaling, may be involved. The neural form of nitric oxide is measured by changes in nitric oxide synthase (nNOS) and plays an important role in the expression of aggressive behavior in males (Nelson, 1997). This was discovered when nNOS knockout mice were created, and informal observations indicated that nNOS −/− male mice (where −/− indicates the absence of the gene on both chromosomes) were hyperaggressive but that female nNOS knockout mice were not (Nelson et al., 1995). Inappropriate aggressiveness was never observed among the nNOS −/− female mice. When given an opportunity to defend their pups, nNOS −/− mice were very docile, unlike their wild-type sisters. These studies suggest that nitric oxide from neurons has important but opposite effects in the mediation of aggression in male and female mice (Nelson and Chiavegatto, 2000).

In the rat brain, the ventromedial hypothalamus is important in the regulation of reproductive behavior such as lordosis. The estrogen-inducible progesterone receptors in the ventromedial nucleus appear to play a role (Parsons et al., 1984; Schumacher et al., 1992). Estrogens have also been shown to induce receptors for oxytocin in the hypothalamus, and blockage of oxytocin receptors interferes with the expression of lordosis behavior. Estrogens also cause the formation of new synaptic connections between ventromedial hypothalamic neurons in the hypothalamus.

Rats display a characteristic set of motor behaviors following activation of serotonin receptors or elevation of synaptic serotonin levels after treatment with L-tryptophan. Both males and females exhibit this "serotonin behavioral syndrome," but females display signs of the syndrome at much lower doses than males. Fischette and colleagues (1984) have shown that androgens, via androgen receptors, modulate the reduced sensitivity of male rats to the tryptophan drug challenge.

Sex-Typed Behavior and Gender Identity

Discussions about the determinants of human sex-typed behavior, especially gender identity, have recently become highly visible because of scientific and popular accounts of a prominent case (Colapinto, 2000; Diamond and Sigmundson, 1997). The case challenged the established belief that individuals are born with the potential to develop male or female gender identity and that the specific gender identity can be determined exclusively by sex of rearing (Hampson and Hampson 1961; Money and Ehrhardt, 1996; Money et al., 1955; reviewed in Grumbach and Conte, 1998). For detailed reviews and discussions, see Bradley et al. (1998), Colapinto (2000), Diamond and Sigmundson (1997), Fausto-Sterling (2000), Kessler (1998), Wilson (1999), and Zucker (1999).

The case involved a boy (46,XY karyotype) with male-typical development whose penis was ablated after a mishandled circumcision and whose gender was subsequently reassigned and reared as a female. Contrary to early reports, the child never adjusted to the female assignment, despite having no knowledge of his early history. Sex reassignment was requested, and the individual is now reported to live successfully and happily as a man. Because this individual is a normal genetic male who was exposed to male-typical hormones in prenatal and early neonatal life, this case lends credence to the view that gender identity is determined by early hormones that act on the developing brain and argues against the view that rearing sex is the main determinant of gender identity (Diamond and Sigmundson, 1997; Grumbach and Conte, 1998).

The conclusion, however, must be considered in light of other details of this case and other cases. The individual described above (Diamond and Sigmundson, 1997) was reared unequivocally as a boy at least until age 7 months, when the accident occurred, and perhaps longer, because the final decision about female reassignment was not made until his second year and surgery was not completed until age 21 months. Furthermore, the outcome for another individual with an ablated penis was very different: after an accident at age 2 months, another child was reassigned as a female at age 7 months and has reportedly adapted well to this identity. As an adult, she shows no evidence of gender dysphoria, although she has a male-typical occupation and a bisexual orientation (Bradley et al., 1998).

Ongoing studies with boys with cloacal exstrophy (malformed or absent penis with normal testes) who are reared as girls should help to provide systematic evidence about the determinants and malleability of gender identity. These boys are usually reassigned as girls because of concerns about adjustment problems associated with inadequate male genitalia. Preliminary reports from an ongoing systematic study (Reiner, 2000) indicate that more than half of these female sex-assigned XY children identify as boys, consistent with their male-typical prenatal androgen exposure, and not with their female-typical rearing. Interestingly, however, some of these children continued to accept their female assigned sex, so it will be important to determine what differentiates children with male identity from those with female identity, despite their common 46,XY chromosome constitutions. This is clearly an area deserving of further investigation.

Other Sex Differences in Human Behavior

Although identification as male or female is the most obvious psychological sex difference, it is far from the only one. A variety of important human behaviors covering a range of domains are more common or occur at higher levels in one sex than in the other. The behaviors that have received the most attention include aspects of normal social behavior and cognition, such as childhood play behavior and related activities and interests, personality (such as aggression and interest in babies), nonverbal communication, sexuality, and cognitive abilities (Hall and Carter, 1999; Halpern, 2000; Maccoby, 1998; Ruble and Martin, 1998). Activities related to these behaviors are performed at different frequencies by males and females in most cultures studied (Daly and Wilson, 1990). Again, the goal of this chapter is not to provide an exhaustive review of behavioral sex differences but to illustrate some of the differences and to indicate how they might be influenced in part by sex hormones.

There are also sex differences in health-related behaviors, such as frequency of visits to health professionals and use of complementary medicine, but these have not been well studied. There are also sex differences in the incidence and course of some mental disorders and substance abuse (National Institutes of Health, Office of Research on Women's Health, 1999b). These differences in mental health may also produce differences in physical health.

Cognitive Function

A large body of research has now converged to indicate that there are sex differences in specific areas of cognitive function. Although there has been some controversy over the proverbial question of which sex is the smarter one, a reasonable conclusion reached by many scientists is that there are no meaningful differences in intelligence between males and females (Halpern, 2000). A more probing question asks if there are particular areas of thinking or problem solving in which males and females differ; such cognitive abilities are referred to as "sexually dimorphic behaviors."

Before reviewing the research findings, it is important to bear in mind several factors. (1) In general, there is a marked overlap in the abilities of males and females. In some cases, the sex differences are most marked at the extreme ends of a particular ability, for example, among those who are the most skilled (Figure 4-1) (Hampson, in press; Hampson and

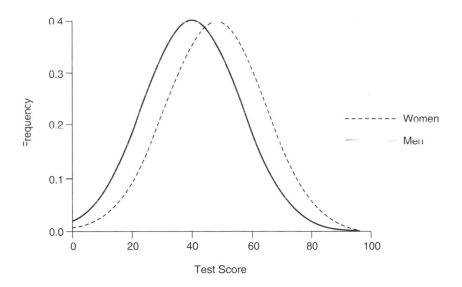

FIGURE 4-1 Frequency distribution of scores on a hypothetical cognitive test plotted separately by sex. As a consequence of the differences in the means, the number of individuals scoring above a given point will differ for the two sexes; for example, the mean for women is higher than the mean for men such that only 25 to 30 percent of males score above the mean score for females. Source: Hampson and Kimura (1992, Figure 12-1) Reprinted, with permission, from J. B. Becker, S. M. Breedlove, and D. Crews, *Behavioral Endocrinology*, Cambridge, MA: The MIT Press, 1992, p. 359.

Kimura, 1992). Although there may be slight but significant differences between the mean scores for males and females on some tests, they are invariably smaller than the differences between the highest- and lowest-scoring males (or females) on the same tests. (2) When differences are noted, they may apply only to individuals at a specific age or stage of life. (3) Finally, how an ability is measured may affect the results, for example, whether the response is multiple choice, fill in the blank, short essay, or oral.

Cognitive abilities can be subdivided and considered in any number of ways. Maccoby and Jacklin (1974) prepared a useful classification in which they delineated three general cognitive domains demonstrating sex differences: verbal, quantitative, and visuospatial abilities. Although for ease of presentation the report refers to these three main groups of cognitive abilities, these encompass heterogeneous areas of function, with each one representing several different functions. Furthermore, the specific cognitive processes of interest may be assessed quite differently, often leading to conflicting results.

Despite these caveats, it should be noted that a reasonable consensus has emerged relating sex differences to specific patterns of cognitive function: in general, women most often demonstrate an advantage in verbal abilities—particularly verbal fluency, speech production, the ability to decode a language, and spelling; perceptual speed and accuracy; and fine motor skills—whereas men frequently show an advantage on tests of spatial abilities, quantitative abilities, and gross motor strength (Hampson, in press; Hampson and Kimura, 1992). The following sections summarize data that support this general statement.

Verbal Abilities

Although it is often stated that females demonstrate better verbal abilities than males, it is important to note, as Halpern (2000) has, that "the term verbal abilities is not a unitary concept. The term applies to all components of language usage: word fluency, which is the ability to generate words (both in isolation and in a meaningful context), grammar, spelling, reading, writing, verbal analogies, vocabulary, and oral comprehension. The size and reliability of the sex differences depends on which of these aspects of language is being assessed" (pp. 93–94). Sex differences have been demonstrated for some but not all of these verbal abilities; however, when there is a difference, it invariably favors females.

Two aspects of language showing perhaps the most consistent sex differences are verbal fluency and speech production, both of which share the need to have the ability to quickly access and to produce speech sounds and words. Verbal fluency (Hampson and Kimura, 1992; Hines, 1990; Hyde and Linn, 1988) is tested by having a subject name as many words as rapidly as possible according to either a phonological or sound-based cue (words that begin with a particular letter) or rhyming with a specific sound or by having the subject name words that belong to a certain category such as food or plants. In studies investigating sex differences in verbal abilities, the largest difference (effect size $[D] = 0.33$) is typically found for speech production (Hyde and Linn, 1988), a measure, as discussed later, that is closely related to both reading and reading disability. Reliable sex differences have also been reported for spelling, another verbal ability closely related to reading; however, reports of sex differences in other areas of verbal ability such as vocabulary or reading comprehension have been inconsistent and are not considered reliable (Hampson and Kimura, 1992).

Sex differences have also been noted in tests of memory, particularly in tests of working memory (the ability to hold in memory information intended for temporary use). This is a particularly important ability because it affects many aspects of a person's everyday life, for example, remembering a phone number given by the information operator, where the keys were just put down, or a message on the answering machine. Females have an advantage over males in remembering both verbal and nonverbal information. Females' superiority in verbal memory has received much attention, although their skill in remembering visual details, for example, spatial locations, has often been overlooked. As summarized below, males outperform females in visuospatial abilities when the task requires the manipulation of the spatial information; females, however, remember visual information better (Halpern, 2000; Hampson and Kimura, 1992).

Articulatory Skills, Manual Fine Motor Skills, and Perceptual Speed and Accuracy

Females generally perform articulatory tasks or fine motor tasks more quickly and more adroitly than males. These skills all depend on the coordination of a sequence of movements. Articulatory skills are assessed by having the subject quickly repeat several syllables, for example, "puh tah kuh, puh tah kuh, puh tah kuh," for 1 minute or try to say a tongue twister such as "sweet Susie swept sea shells" as rapidly as possible. Females also outperform males in carrying out fine hand movements such as rapidly placing pegs in small holes or in carrying out a simple sequence of hand movements (Hampson and Kimura, 1992). In addition, females tend to perform better than males on tasks requiring perceptual speed and accuracy. This ability is assessed by asking subjects to quickly scan an array of symbols or figures and to indicate which one matches a previously indicated stimulus; for example, in the "random A's test," the subject rapidly scans letters scattered over a page and is asked to cross out only the letter "A."

Spatial and Quantitative Abilities

Males demonstrate an advantage on tests of visuospatial ability (as reviewed by Maccoby and Jacklin [1974] and more recently by Halpern [2000]). According to Halpern (2000), this refers to the ability "to imagine what an irregular figure would look like if it were rotated in space or the ability to discern the relationship between shapes and objects" (p. 98). Kerns and Berenbaum (1991) noted that a major issue is how to define and measure spatial ability. In a comprehensive meta-analysis, Linn and Petersen (1985) focused on three categories of spatial ability: spatial perception, mental rotation, and spatial visualization. The most consistent sex differences occur with measures of skills referred to as "spatial perception" and "mental rotation" (Linn and Petersen, 1985). In particular, the mental rotation task has demonstrated the most sensitivity at detecting sex differences in spatial ability (Sanders et al., 1982); here, a subject is asked to imagine how a figure would appear if it were rotated in a two- or three-dimensional space.

Sex differences in quantitative abilities have also been reported. Here, it is important to ask "what" particular abilities and in "which people." Quantitative abilities refer to a heterogeneous group of abilities; depending on the specific ability tested, males or females will have an advantage. For example, males seem to outperform females on tests of geometry, measurement, probability, and statistics as well as on tests of spatial and mechanical reasoning (Stones et al., 1982; Stumpf and Stanley, 1998). Some have suggested that the male advantage in quantitative abilities reflects the male's use of visuospatial approaches for problem solving. In contrast, females perform better on measures of calculation and also on tests in which the problem requires much reading.

Perhaps the most important finding from the various research studies is that differences in math ability are much smaller toward the middle of the distribution, where most males and females are represented, and are most pronounced at the upper end of the distribution. Males consistently outperform females on tests of quantitative ability, for example, the mathematics portion of the Scholastic Aptitude Test (SAT). Competitions among seventh and eighth grade boys and girls held to identify mathematically precocious youth on the basis of scores on the mathematics portion of the SAT greatly favor boys. A consistent finding on these tests is that differences between boys and girls tend to increase at the higher levels of performance. Thus, boys outscore girls 2:1 at scores of 500 and above, 5:1 at scores of 600 and above, and 17:1 at the highest scores, 700 and above (Benbow, 1988, Stanley and Benbow, 1982). One problem in interpreting such results is that the best predictor of performance on such standardized mathematics tests is experience. That is, most of the students who score the highest are enrolled in high-level mathematics courses. The data also indicate that many more males than females are enrolled in these high-level mathematics courses (Jones, 1984). However, even when one controls for the number of advanced mathematics courses, males continue to have an advantage, albeit a much smaller one (Meece et al., 1982).

Newer studies are shedding light on the nature of sex differences in quantitative abilities. A recent analysis (Gallagher et al., 2000) indicated that males performed better on various types of mathematics questions that had in common a dependence on a strategy to "construct and mentally transform a mental representation" (Halpern, 2000, p. 117). This suggests that it is not the type of mathematics problem that is important in evaluating sex differences but the kind of strategy required to solve it that is critical in determining whether males or females have ability. Reviews of the relationship between quantitative skills and spatial ability find that spatial ability is an important factor in predicting performance on advanced mathematics tests and that this relationship is especially strong at the highest levels of mathematics performance (Halpern, 2000).

EFFECTS OF HORMONES ON BEHAVIOR AND COGNITION

Prenatal Androgens and Sex Differentiation of Human Behavior

There is now good evidence that human behavioral sex differences are influenced by sex hormones present during prenatal development, confirming findings from studies with other mammalian species (described in Chapter 3). These hormones act by "organizing" neural systems that mediate behavior later in life. Much of the evidence about the behavioral effects of prenatal sex hormones comes from individuals with clinical conditions that alter these hormones (so-called experiments of nature), although in recent years there has been confirming evidence from studies with individuals with circulating concentrations of hormones in the normal range. The following section provides an illustration of work done in this area; for detailed reviews of hormonal influences on human behavior, see Berenbaum (1998), Collaer and Hines (1995), Hampson and Kimura (1992), and Wilson (1999).

Prenatal androgens alone do not determine behavioral sex differences. Social and environmental factors undoubtedly contribute to differences between males and females, but the focus of this section is on genetic and physiological factors. Rather than considering physiological-hormonal and social explanations as being mutually exclusive, however, it is important to think about how they might operate in concert to produce behavioral sex differences. For example, biologically influenced traits may affect an individual's response to the environment or the way that the individual is treated by others; such effects have been demonstrated in other species (Clark and Galef, 1998; Fitch and Denenberg, 1998).

Studies of Females with Congenital Adrenal Hyperplasia

The evidence for hormonal influences on human behavior is illustrated with findings from studies of females with congenital adrenal hyperplasia (CAH), a genetic disease in which the fetus is exposed to high levels of androgens beginning early in gestation (Grumbach and Conte, 1998; Miller, 1996; White et al., 1987). If sex differences in human behavior are affected by the levels of androgens that are present during early development, then females with CAH should be behaviorally more masculine and less feminine[1] than a comparison group of females without CAH (the best comparison group consists of the unaffected sisters of females with CAH because they provide a control for general genetic and environmental backgrounds). Indeed, females with CAH do differ from their sisters in sex-typed behavior (for a detailed description, see Berenbaum [2000]).

One of the largest differences between females with CAH and their unaffected sisters is in their activities: it is characteristic of girls with CAH to play with boys' toys in childhood and to be interested in boys' activities in adolescence (Berenbaum, 2000; Berenbaum and Snyder, 1995; Ehrhardt and Baker, 1974). For a variety of other behaviors, the differences between females with CAH and their unaffected sisters are almost as large as the differences between typical males and typical females. This includes interest in babies (Leveroni and Berenbaum, 1998), reported likelihood of using aggression in conflict situations (Berenbaum and Resnick, 1997), and spatial ability (Hampson et al., 1998; Resnick et al., 1986). Other differences between females with CAH and unaffected females are smaller relative to the difference between typical males and typical females. For example, most girls with CAH prefer girls as playmates (Berenbaum and Snyder, 1995), and most women with CAH are exclusively heterosexual in terms of their sexual fantasy and arousal characteristics (Zucker et al., 1996), although some do prefer boy playmates and some have bisexual fantasy and arousal characteristics. The differences are even smaller for gender identity: only a very small minority of females with CAH have male-typical gender identity or are gender dysphoric (Ehrhardt and Baker,

---

[1] Masculine and feminine are empirically defined and refer to a person's relative position on traits that show sex differences.

1974; Meyer-Bahlburg et al., 1996; Zucker et al., 1996). This is consistent with the idea that male-typical gender identity requires a higher level or different timing of exposure to androgen than is characteristic of that for females with CAH, rearing as a male, or exposure to other genetic or hormonal factors unique to or more common in males, for example, the *SRY* gene.

Limitations of Studies of Females with CAH

Females with CAH do not provide a perfect test of the behavioral effects of exposure to androgens early in gestation because they differ from their unaffected sisters in a number of ways that might affect behavior. Of particular importance from a social perspective is the fact that females with CAH have masculinized genitalia, and it is possible that their masculinized behavior results from the treatment of these girls by their parents in response to their physical appearance (Quadagno et al., 1977). Recent evidence, however, renders this explanation unlikely: the amount of time that girls with CAH spend playing with boys' toys is linearly related to their degree of prenatal androgen excess, as inferred from the degree of genetic mutation, and it decreases (rather than increases) when a parent is present (Nordenstrom et al., 1999; Servin, 1999).

Convergence of Evidence

Given the limitations of studies of females with CAH, it is important to seek a convergence of evidence across methods for the behavioral effects of hormones. Findings from studies of females with CAH have been confirmed from other "experiments of nature" and from studies of samples of typical (non-CAH) individuals. For example, girls who were exposed to masculinizing hormones because their mothers took medication (androgenizing progestins) during pregnancy are more likely than their unexposed sisters to report that they would use aggression in conflict situations (Reinisch, 1981). Males with reduced androgen levels because of an endocrine condition called idiopathic hypogonadotropic hypogonadism (IHH) have lower levels of spatial ability than controls; within the group of men with IHH, spatial ability correlated with testicular volume and did not improve with androgen replacement therapy (indications that the low level of spatial ability was associated with low levels of androgen early in development and not at the time of testing) (Hier and Crowley, 1982).

Converging evidence for these special cases has come from studies of normal individuals with typical variations in prenatal hormone levels. For example, 7-year-old girls who had high levels of testosterone in utero (determined from measurements of the concentrations in amniotic fluid at 14 to 16 weeks of gestation) had faster mental rotation (an aspect of spatial ability) capabilities than girls who had low levels of prenatal testosterone (Grimshaw et al., 1995), and females with a male twin appear to be more masculine than females with a female twin on several traits, including sensation seeking (Resnick et al., 1993), spatial ability (Cole-Harding et al., 1988), and auditory characteristics (McFadden, 1993). Gender-specific behavior in young adult women has been suggested to be related to their exposure to sex hormones during the second trimester of fetal development (Udry et al., 1995). Although some of these studies are imperfect, the limitations are different from those of studies of individuals with CAH.

Understanding How Prenatal Androgens Might Affect Behavior (and Other Traits)

The evidence presented above suggests that androgens present early in life do affect a variety of sex-typed behaviors and that the effects are complex (Wilson, 1999). It is unclear what might account for variations in a given behavior and among different behaviors among individuals. For example, it is not yet known what accounts for the fact that most girls with CAH play with boys' toys but that the majority of women with CAH are heterosexual. Investigators do not know the genetic, physiological, or stochastic factors that differentiate women with CAH who are aroused by members of the same sex from those who are not. It is not yet known why some individuals with male-typical prenatal hormone levels develop female-typical gender identity when they are reared as females but others develop male-typical gender identity in that environment. The developmental course of the behavioral effects of prenatal androgens is also not known. Finding the answers to these questions provides an opportunity to integrate hormonal explanations for behavioral sex differences with other explanations and to arrive at a more complete understanding of why males and females differ in their behavioral characteristics.

What Accounts for Variations?

Evidence from studies of other species indicates that differences in the nature or extent of hormone exposure can have implications for behavior. First, the timing of hormone exposure is important. The early prenatal period has generally been thought to be the crucial time for the organizational effects of hormones on mammalian brain development and later behavior, but other periods may be important, too. In primates, for example, there appear to be several distinct periods during which behavior is sensitive to the effects of androgen, with different behaviors masculinized by exposure early versus late in gestation (Goy et al., 1988):

female rhesus macaques exposed to androgen early in gestation (and thus with virilized genitalia) show increased mounting behavior, whereas those exposed late in gestation (with no genital virilization) show increased rough play.

Second, different aspects of physical and behavioral sexual differentiation may be affected by different forms of masculinizing hormones. For example, dihydrotestosterone is responsible for differentiation of the external genitalia (Siiteri and Wilson, 1974); in monkeys, dihydrotestosterone and testosterone propionate have different effects on learning (Bachevalier and Hagger, 1991). In some species, male-typical development results from estradiol metabolized from androgen in the brain, although aromatized estrogens do not appear to play a role in masculinizing the human brain or behavior (Grumbach and Auchus, 1999).

Third, the effects of specific hormones may be modified by other hormones (Goy and McEwen, 1980). There is increasing recognition of the importance of ovarian estrogens for both physical and behavioral sexual differentiation, and it seems likely that androgens are modified by the effects of ovarian estrogens.

Fourth, the behavioral effects of hormones may be modified by individual differences in hormone receptor sensitivity.

In both human and nonhuman species, sex differences and the effects of hormones on behavior are influenced by the social environment, with hormones having their greatest effects on behaviors that show consistent sex differences among affected individuals (Wallen, 1996). The theories and evidence regarding the role of cognitive and social factors in producing sex differences have recently been reviewed by others (e.g., Bussey and Bandura [1999], Lytton and Romney [1991], Maccoby [1998], and Ruble and Martin [1998]).

It seems likely that although prenatal hormones contribute to some behavioral sex differences, they do not act alone and do not produce all sex differences. For all behaviors studied, the differences between females with CAH and unaffected females are less than the differences between typical males and typical females. Although rearing as a female is not always sufficient to produce female gender identity (Diamond and Sigmundson, 1997; Wilson, 1999), in some cases it may be (Bradley et al., 1998). It is unclear how much these results can be explained by sex-related socialization and how much may ultimately be explained by hormonal factors that have not been delineated, such as ovarian estrogens.

Mechanisms by Which Androgens Affect Behavior

Although there is good evidence that at least some of the sex differences in behavior are influenced by the prenatal androgens operating on the developing brain, it is not at all clear how that happens. For example, it is not known what parts of the brain are particularly susceptible to organizational changes induced by high levels of androgen or what basic behavioral mechanisms cause someone who is exposed to high prenatal levels of androgen to play with boys' toys.

Hormone exposure might also affect behavior through the selection and interpretation of the social environment, particularly those aspects related to sex. Recent studies of gender development in typical children suggest that the social environment is actively constructed and interpreted in ways that reinforce sex differences through the use of gender identity and gender labels (for a review, see Ruble and Martin [1998]). Similar studies with children with variations in sexual differentiation (Table 3-2) have the potential to provide information about factors that affect gender cognition and interpretation of the social environment. Such studies should also help provide an understanding of the development of behavioral sex differences, that is, how differences between boys and girls arise as a result of maturation and transactions with the physical and social environments.

A Counterview:
The Artificial Separation of Biology from Environment

The concept that physiological and behavioral characteristics are prenatally organized by hormones, as first proposed by Phoenix et al. (1959), has been fundamental to understanding the development of sex differences in mammals. As is true for many overarching theoretical constructs, it has been significantly modified (Arnold and Breedlove, 1985) and has recently been reviewed critically (Fausto-Sterling, 2000; Wilson, 1999). Some of the anatomical, physiological, and biochemical changes resulting from the early organizational effects of hormones have been revealed, particularly in the central nervous system (Breedlove, 1994; Gorski et al., 1978). The effects of certain genes, such as the gene coding for the classic estrogen receptor alpha, on body and brain development depend on the sex of the individual in which it is expressed.

McCarthy and colleagues (1993) have been able to explain some of the organizational effects at the molecular level by showing that neural estrogen receptors are essential during the prenatal period for masculinization and defeminization of rats. Using estrogen receptor knockout (ERKO) mice, Simerly and colleagues (1997) have also demonstrated estrogen receptor-dependent sexual differentiation.

Such research is just beginning to reveal the mechanisms by which the effects of hormones early in gestation have long-term consequences. Among the mechanisms underlying the organizational concept are that the development of particular behaviors can be mediated and affected by a number of postnatal environmental experiences (Moore and Rogers,

1984; reviewed by Fausto-Sterling [2000]). The "organizational effect hypothesis" thus serves as a useful framework on which to attach facts as they become available and to stimulate additional research on the complex array of factors that produce sex and gender differences.

Two members of the committee, however, raised concerns about the use of the term *organizational effect*. Although is clear that the organizational effects of prenatal hormones on the later development of particular behaviors is mediated and affected by a large number of organismal factors and postnatal effects, it is often not clear what such an effect is or might mean at the cellular level. Two members of the committee argued that continuing to use the phrase *organizational effect* as an explanation could preclude experiments that might reveal the actual mechanisms by which hormones, genes, and a variety of postnatal experiences produce the sex and gender differences of interest.

Two members of the committee believed that reliance on analyses that divide variance into main effects and smaller contributing effects sidetracks other biologically appropriate analysis, such as pursuing developmental understanding of the emergence of cognitive skills. It also does not enable researchers to see how experience and biology work together to produce difference. What is called for here, argued the two committee members, is an approach that examines the mutual construction of cognition by physiology and by experience during key periods of development.

There are animal models that successfully integrate the study of hormones and experience as they contribute to cognitive and spatial abilities. For example, variations in maternal care in rats (specifically, the amount of licking and grooming) contribute to the development of spatial memory and learning. The effect is mediated by synaptogenesis in the hippocampus (Liu et al., 2000). Maternal licking can, in turn, be affected by a variety of factors, including an odor developed in the pup in response to an individual pup's testosterone levels (Moore, 1990; Moore and Rogers, 1984, Moore et al., 1992). This example illustrates part of a process by which a particular capacity emerges. Nature is not distinct from nurture, since maternal behavior responds to both pup odor and other inputs and directly influences pup brain development and, hence, the pup's behavior as an adult. Such effects are transmitted across generations.

There are other examples of this sort in the literature on studies with animals (Crews, 2000; Gottlieb, 1997). A variety of studies have shown postnatal effects on the development of hormonally influenced behaviors (summarized schematically in Figure 4-2). For further discussion see Fausto-Sterling (2000) and Tobet and Fox (1992).

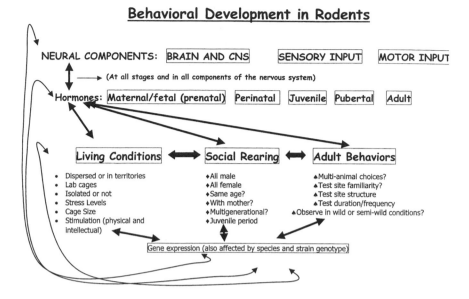

FIGURE 4-2   Behavioral development in rodents. Source: Fausto-Sterling (2000, p. 228). Reprinted, with permission, from A. Fausto-Sterling. 2000. *Sexing the Body: Gender Politics and the Construction of Sexuality.* New York: Basic Books. Copyright 2000 by Basic Books, a Member of the Perseus Books Group.

An Approach to Studying Multicausal Development

Two members of the committee supported a new approach to studying multicausal development that has emerged in recent years. The general claims of developmental systems theory are as follows.

1. Some aspects of development are self-organizing, but these self-organizing aspects are rarely sufficient for the emergence of a trait or a behavior. For example, early in the embryogenesis of retina-brain nerve connections, nerve cells begin to fire spontaneously. This spontaneous nervous activity is, in turn, required for an initial "rough targeting" of cells between the thalamus and the cortex (Catalano and Shatz, 1998). However, the rough embryonic connections still require postnatal visual experience for fully functional visual circuits to develop (Katz and Shatz, 1996).

2. The initial spontaneous and apparently random activities of cells, such as nerve or muscle cells, eventually stabilize (via self-organizing properties and because of feedback from outside the body), leading to periods of great stability or stasis. Thus, certain features of development emerge as apparently fixed. Some features of development are more stable

than others, but as researchers come to understand the systems that generate and maintain them, they will come to understand both stasis and its loss. By overly focusing on the "main effect" rather than examining a developmental system out of which differences emerge and are maintained, important data may be missed.

3. The emergence of sex and gender differences, then, "can be seen in dynamic terms as a series of states of stability, instability and phase shifts"(Thelen, 1995. p. 84) These ideas have been applied at length to cognitive development in general in a National Research Council and Institute of Medicine report entitled *From Neurons to Neighborhoods* (2000). What remains is serious thought about how these ideas should be applied to the development of sex and gender.

Cognitive Effects of Sex Hormones on Adults

Sex hormones not only act in prenatal life, to organize the brain for later behavior, but also continue to exert effects later in life. This is clearly seen with respect to cognitive abilities. One of the areas most carefully studied has been the relationship between sex hormones in females and cognitive abilities, especially verbal skills. Studies of this relationship have found that performance on particular cognitive tests varies with changing hormone levels, demonstrating, too, that even mature neural systems in adult brains are responsive to the influence of sex hormones. Thus, in addition to their early influences on brain development, sex hormones may also exert influences later on. In addition, as noted below, sex hormones affect neural systems in adult women during their active reproductive years and postmenopausal years.

During adult life, women's hormone levels fluctuate monthly with the menstrual cycle, and some studies have shown that these variations to some degree affect performance on certain tests of cognitive abilities (although the sizes of the effects were quite small). In three studies, Hampson (1990a,b) and Hampson and Kimura (1988) tested women during their menses and during the preovulatory phase of their menstrual cycles to specifically compare states of minimal and maximal estrogen secretion, respectively. As hypothesized, the preovulatory phase, a time of relatively high estrogen levels, was found to be associated with modest decreases in spatial ability and improved ability on tests of manual coordination and articulatory skills.

These findings have been confirmed by subsequent researchers (e.g., McCourt et al. [1997], Moody [1997], Phillips and Silverman [1997], and Silverman and Phillips [1993]). A few studies, however, failed to detect any menstrual cycle effects (Gordon and Lee, 1993; Peters et al., 1995), although methodological differences could account for the different findings. For example, in the study by Peters and colleagues (1995), data on the menstrual cycle were not carefully verified, and verbal self-reports can be very inaccurate.

Epting and Overman (1998) also failed to replicate the performance fluctuations across the menstrual cycle. However, the women in the study of Epting and Overman (1998) were younger than women typically used for menstrual cycle studies. For example, in contrast, Hampson (1990a,b) and Hampson and Kimura (1988) excluded women younger than age 21 years. Even though menstrual cycles can seem to be regular in young women, young women have higher incidences of anovulatory cycles and lower levels of ovarian output than women in their 20s and beyond. Thus, it is possible that the cognitive effects of menstrual cycle changes are genuinely weaker in women in their teens than in women over the age of 21 years.

A particularly intriguing bit of evidence supporting the role of female sex hormones on language-related behaviors comes from studies of Koko, a female gorilla that has been trained to communicate using American Sign Language (Patterson et al., 1991). Both the number of discrete signs used and the total number of signs per day rose in the follicular phase of her reproductive cycle, when Koko's estrogen concentrations were raised. The investigators speculate that the increase in manual and verbal output at midcycle could serve to enhance the possibility of conception through more effective signaling to the male as a part of the proceptive behavior complex.

Taken together, these studies indicate that female sex hormones appear to enhance performance of those skills usually performed better by females, whereas they cause a decrement in performance of those skills usually performed better by males.

Hormonal levels in women also change during menopause, when the levels of the hormone estrogen undergo dramatic declines after the cessation of cyclic ovarian function. Given the demonstrated sex differences in cognitive function that favor verbal abilities in females and the association of better performance of these skills during phases of the menstrual cycle when estrogen levels are high, there has been great interest in the effects of hormone replacement therapy (exogenous estrogen) on these cognitive abilities. Although evidence suggests that estrogen positively affects basic neural processes and cognitive function in animals (McEwen and Alves, 1999), the influence of estrogen on cognitive function in humans, especially postmenopausal women, has been much more difficult to establish. Results to date from observational studies and clinical trials with women receiving hormone replacement therapy are far from consistent (Barrett-Connor, 1998b; Haskell et al., 1997; Rice et al., 1997; Sherwin, 1997; Yaffe et al., 1998).

Such inconsistency may reflect differences in the ages of the women studied. For example, at midlife, estrogens tend to have a positive effect on cognitive function (Shaywitz et al., 1999; Sherwin, 1997). Studies with older populations have more varied results, with some indicating a positive influence of estrogen on cognitive function (Jacobs et al., 1998; Resnick et al., 1997; Steffens et al., 1999) but others failing to show such an effect (Barrett-Connor and Kritz-Silverstein, 1993; Matthews et al., 1999). Furthermore, it may be that the effects of estrogen on cognitive function are observed most strongly when the agent is first used, an effect noted in studies with animals (Miranda et al., 1999). Nevertheless, when effects are observed they invariably tend to be positive influences on verbal function, particularly verbal memory and verbal fluency.

Most recently, estrogen has been found to improve the oral reading ability of postmenopausal women (S. E. Shaywitz et al., submitted for publication). The notion that estrogen has a positive influence on cognitive function received further support from another recent study in which postmenopausal women were monitored for a 6-year period, with their cognitive function measured initially and after 6 years. The amount of free circulating estrogen was also measured. The investigators found that women with the highest levels of hormone were those least likely to show signs of cognitive decline on testing (Yaffe et al., 1998).

Possible Mechanisms Influencing Effects of Estrogen on Cognitive Functions

Is it reasonable to suppose that estrogen may have salutary effects on certain cognitive abilities? A large body of evidence supports the notion that estrogen has significant effects on neuronal function and affects a range of neural activities in mature animals (McEwen and Alves, 1999). Thus, it is logical to suggest that estrogen has potent effects on central nervous system functioning, including cognitive functions. The next question relates to how estrogen may affect the specific cognitive functions demonstrated to be sensitive to its actions. To address this question, some investigators have turned to another large body of evidence, but in this instance the studies related to the process of reading (Shaywitz et al., 1998; Shaywitz et al., submitted.)

Reading and Language Processes

This discussion should be appreciated in the context that reading is related to language (as determined from a newer understanding of the reading process) and that within language the reading process is related to phonological processing. Interestingly, the key cognitive functions affected by estrogen (verbal fluency, verbal memory, and articulation) are the same cognitive processes that are deficient in individuals who have difficulty reading. These processes share a dependence on the need to access the basic sound structure of words, that is, phonological process-ing. Synthesis of the findings from the literature on hormonal influences on cognitive function and from the literature on reading has led to the novel hypothesis that hormones, specifically estrogen, influence phono-logical processing, which in turn influences the development of verbal fluency, speech production, and reading skills.

Current theory supported by substantial empirical data supports the belief that the same processes that serve language also serve reading. Although speaking is a universal behavior, not everyone learns to read; speaking is automatic, whereas reading must be learned. These observa-tions have led to the belief, from an evolutionary perspective, that the biological systems that serve reading are not newly developed but, rather, represent a modification of those biological processes already in place to serve language. One hypothesis suggests that the language apparatus forms a distinct biological system or module (Fodor, 1983) that is served by specific brain mechanisms and structures (Liberman and Mattingly, 1989; Liberman, 1989). In this view, the same processes and processors that serve language also serve reading, the major difference being that speaking is automatic but reading must be learned. Much has been learned about the nature of the reading process and the component skills neces-sary for the acquisition of reading skills, particularly the importance of phonological processes (Catts, 1986; Shaywitz, 1996).

The Phoneme

Reading and language share the same basic elemental unit, the pho-neme, the smallest unit of sound that gives meaning to a word. The pho-neme represents the sound structure that underlies all words, written or spoken. For words to be understood, spoken, read, stored, or retrieved, they must first be segmented into phonemes. Deficits in phonological processing have been intimately related to reading disability, and a large body of literature now indicates that a phonological core deficit is respon-sible for the difficulties that dyslexic children have in learning to read.

Areas of impaired phonological processing consistently related to reading disability represent the same areas of language most sensitive to the actions of estrogen, that is, word fluency (e.g., naming) and speech production (e.g., speed of articulation). For example, deficits in naming colors, common objects, and numbers consistently characterize reading disability (Denckla and Rudel, 1976; Wolf, 1984; Wolf and Goodglass, 1986). Problems with naming are conceptualized as reflecting problems with registering, storing, or retrieving phonemes (Catts, 1986). Similarly, children with reading disabilities have difficulties with speech produc-tion (Catts, 1986, 1989); in this case, poor readers have difficulty either selecting, ordering, or articulating phonemes during speech (Catts, 1986).

Reading and the Actions of Estrogen

This very brief summary has reviewed information that supports the well-accepted belief that reading and reading disability are related to language and, in particular, to phonological processing. Disruptions in phonological processing predict, characterize, and explain many of the difficulties experienced by poor readers. These data relating phonological processing to reading and reading disability converge with the consistent findings that within the domain of verbal ability, the specific measures that are sensitive to the positive effects of estrogen are those very same tasks that tap specific components of phonological processing disrupted in those with reading disabilities.

Such converging findings from two different areas of investigation have important implications: they suggest that there may be commonalities to the mechanisms of reading and reading disability and to the actions of the female sex hormone, estrogen. Both reading and reading disability reflect language, and estrogen's strongest influence is on verbal abilities. Within the language system, phonological processing has been identified as the critical component relating to reading and reading disabilities; and among the actions of estrogen on language, the areas most sensitive to hormonal effects are verbal fluency, naming, and speech production-speed of articulation, those areas most related to phonological processing.

Together, these findings suggest that the deficit in reading ability and the action of estrogen on specific verbal skills may have a common base: phonological processing. These findings are exciting because they represent a link between studies of the influence of sex hormones on cognitive function and studies relating specific cognitive subskills to the reading process. They indicate that the notion that reading may be influenced by female sex hormone is consonant with current theories of reading. Furthermore, it is of particular interest that Hampson (1990a,b) reported that a surge in estradiol levels enhanced performance on tests of specific verbal skills, including color naming and syllable repetition. Similar results have also been found with exogenously administered hormones in studies of the effects of estrogen replacement therapy in postmenopausal women; for example, Kimura (1995) reported that another measure of phonological processing, speeded articulation, was performed better by postmenopausal women in the on phase of their estrogen replacement therapy. Thus, the specific verbal abilities that are sensitive to change in estradiol levels are those verbal skills that also reflect phonological processing and that have been implicated in the reading process.

Evidence relating sex hormones to reading comes from epidemiological and developmental studies suggesting that hormonal changes during puberty in females may influence phonological processing skills and read-

ing. These data suggest that although sex ratios for dyslexia are comparable during childhood (Shaywitz et al., 1990), these ratios may change as
children mature into adults. Thus, studies of adults in the same family
have consistently indicated sex ratios for dyslexia of 1:1.5 to 1:1.8 in favor
of males (DeFries et al., 1991), whereas investigations of compensated
dyslexics (adults who were dyslexic as children but who are able to read
with some degree of accuracy as adults) report that preponderance (72
percent) are females (Lefly and Pennington, 1991). Thus, reports of equal
sex ratios for children with dyslexia, in contrast to a sex ratio favoring
males in studies of adults in the same family, may reflect hormonal influences associated with puberty.

Similarly, reports of an increased prevalence of females in the group
of dyslexic readers who have become more accurate readers but who are
not automatic readers may reflect the positive effects of female sex hormones on dyslexic readers. Such findings could be interpreted to suggest
that as young women progress through puberty they improve their linguistic skills and that these improved linguistic skills allow them to compensate, to some degree, for their reading disability. This explanation is
appealing because it is parsimonious, accounting both for the observed
difference in prevalence ratios for children compared with those for adults
and for the known positive effects of female sex hormones on the cognitive and linguistic skills that underlie reading.

More recent studies, using sophisticated imaging technology, demonstrate sex differences for language, specifically for phonological processing, and add further evidence that supports the notion that estrogen may
exert its effects on cognitive function through its actions on phonological
processing (Shaywitz et al., 1995). Thus, researchers interested in localiz-
ing the neural systems used for reading, particularly those engaged by
phonological processing, studied a group of 19 men and 19 women using
functional magnetic resonance imaging (fMRI). fMRI captures changes in
blood flow associated with cerebral activity and acts to identify those
regions of the brain used to perform a cognitive task. The men and women
in that study were asked to sound out nonsense words, for example,
"lete" and "jeat," and to indicate if the pairs of words rhymed or not. To
carry out this task, the subject must sound out the words, that is, rely on
phonological processing. The results of the study were remarkable: they
indicated that men and women carry out phonological processing using
different neural systems; that is, men rely on the left inferior frontal gyrus
(Broca's area), whereas women use both the left and the right inferior
frontal gyri (Figure 4-3) (Shaywitz et al., 1995).

These findings of a sex difference in brain systems underlying phonological processing stimulated efforts to understand the origins of these
differences, including the possible influence of female sex hormones. In
one investigation, Shaywitz and colleagues (1998) studied a group of post-

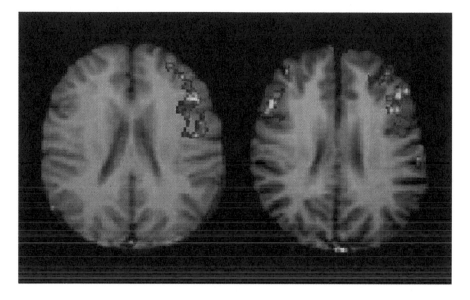

FIGURE 4-3 Composite images of the distribution of activations upon performance of rhyme-case tasks (phonological processing) for 19 males (left image) and 19 females (right image). Males show unilateral activation, primarily in the left inferior frontal gyrus. In females, phonological processing activates both the left and right inferior frontal gyri. (Color dots represent pixels for which the mean value for the split *t* statistic from the average for the 19 subjects was greater than 0.4. Dark red dots represent mean values close to 0.4; yellow dots represent mean values that approach 1.0) Source: Shaywitz et al. (1995) Reprinted, with permission, from B. A. Shaywitz, S. E. Shaywitz, K. Pugh, R. T. Constable, P. Skudlarski, R. K. Fulbright, R. A. Bronan, J. M. Fletcher, D. P. Shankweiler, L. Katz, and J. C. Gore. 1995. Sex differences in the functional organization of the brain for language. *Nature* 373:607–609. Copyright 1995 by *Nature.*

menopausal women (mean age, 50 years) while they were on and off estrogen replacement therapy. Each woman's brain was imaged as she was given a series of tasks that tested her verbal and nonverbal working memory. Examination of the fMRI scans of the women on and off estrogen replacement therapy showed a significant influence of estrogen on the neural systems for memory. Overall, these results demonstrated that brain plasticity continues into midlife and that "functional brain organization in women (and, we assume, men) is neither fixed nor immutable" (Shaywitz et al., 1998, p. 1201). More specifically, prior studies had indicated different patterns of neural organization for memory in older men and women compared with those in younger men and women. Shaywitz and colleagues (1999) found that estrogen usage in older individuals was associated with brain activation patterns different from those in younger individuals. Interestingly, the inferior parietal lobule, a region of the brain known to be engaged by phonological processing, was activated while a woman was on estrogen, supporting the notion that estrogen influences phonological processing.

To this large body of evidence linking estrogen to phonological processing is a new report indicating that estrogen improves the reading ability in postmenopausal women (Shaywitz et al., submitted). Thus, a range of evidence taken together indicates that estrogen may exert its actions through its influence on a fundamental component of the language system, phonological processing, which is critical for speaking, remembering, and reading. This hypothesis brings together seemingly disparate data and provides a reasonable explanation for at least one group of sex differences in cognitive function that have been observed.

Future Work

Future studies are needed to focus on the possible relationship between male sex hormones and reported male advantages in spatial and quantitative functions. A good beginning has been made in a recent investigation that used fMRI to study brain organization during the performance of navigational skills (Gron et al., 2000). In that study, a group of males and females were imaged as they searched their way out of a three-dimensional, virtual-reality maze. The investigators noted sex differences in the regions of the brain activated; males activated the left hippocampus but females activated the right parietal cortex and right prefrontal cortex during the same navigational task. Similar to the findings of sex differences in brain organization for observed differences in language skills, specifically, phonological processing, these findings now provide a neural basis for observed sex differences in spatial performance. One interpretation of these findings is that females rely mostly on landmark cues (Sandstrom et al., 1998) and that activation of the prefrontal region reflects efforts to hold these cues in working memory. On the other hand, males depend on both landmark and geometric cues so that they activate the hippocampus, which allows them to process geometric cues.

The advent of newer brain imaging technologies should now provide more information on the underlying neural substrate of a range of observed sex differences in cognitive function. It is hoped that, with time, new hypotheses will also emerge that offer possible explanations of the mechanisms that underlie the observed sex differences in spatial performance and other areas of cognition and the observed sex differences in brain organization.

SEX DIFFERENCES IN PERCEPTION OF PAIN

The issue of sex differences in pain during adulthood has been the subject of considerable research and meta-analysis, much of which has recently been reviewed (Berkley, 1997a,b; Berkley and Holdcroft, 1999; Derbyshire, 1997; Fillingim, 2000; Fillingim and Maixner, 1996; Riley et al., 1998; Unruh, 1996). In general, the data consistently show that females are more sensitive than males to nociceptive (potentially or frankly damaging) stimuli, including those that occur in internal organs (Giamberardino, 2000). Added to this greater sensitivity of females is the higher prevalence of many painful disorders in females (Table 4-1). On the other hand, perhaps because there is a more permissive atmosphere for women to acknowledge the threat of injury (i.e., pain) and perceive dysfunction (Taylor et al., 2000), women seek more and more varied forms of health care than men, making use of it in a more positive, multidimensional manner, thereby deriving more relief than men (Affleck et al., 1999; Robinson et al., 2000; Unruh et al., 1999).

Also evident in all of the reviews, however, is frustration with applying to individuals the generality that females are more sensitive to pain because exceptions abound. Whether it be humans or nonhuman animals, the existence or even the direction of sex-related differences in pain have been shown to vary with different situations, for example, as one ages, by testing paradigm or setting, by type or location of pain, by subject demographics, by reproductive status, by genetic profile, by treatment utilization behavior, by the way in which pain is measured (and by whom), by analgesic, and by responses to different treatments. Thus, one is faced with what may be two separate problems: determining what factors underlie what appears to be a general greater female vulnerability to pain over the female's lifetime versus understanding how being female or male contributes to individual and circumstantial variations in pain and responses to treatment. Some constructive answers with potential application to human health are beginning to emerge from the latter approach as a result of research with both laboratory animals (mostly rodents) and humans, with implications for either sex. Two examples follow.

Genes, Nociception, and Sensitivity to Analgesics

Neuroscientist Mogil (2000) has recently published an elegant series of studies on the responses of different strains of rodents to noxious stimulation and to analgesics. He summarizes this work as follows: "Recent findings in my laboratory strongly suggest that the modulatory effect of either of these organismic variables (genetic variation, sex) on pain-re-

TABLE 4-1 Sex Prevalences of Some Common Painful Syndromes and
Potential Contributing Causes

Female Prevalence	Male Prevalence
Head and Neck	
Migraine headache with aura	Migraine without aura
Chronic tension headache	Cluster headache
Postdural puncture headache	Posttraumatic headache
Cervicogenic headache	Paratrigeminal syndrome[a]
Tic douloureux	
Temporomandibular disorder	
Occipital neuralgia	
Atypical odontalgia	
Burning tongue	
Carotodynia	
Temporal arteritis	
Chronic paroxysmal hemicrania	
Limbs	
Carpal tunnel syndrome	Thromboangiitis obliterans[b]
Raynaud's disease	Hemophilic arthropathy[c]
Chilblains	Brachial plexus neuropathy
Reflex sympathetic dystrophy	
Chronic venous insufficiency	
Piriformis syndrome	
Peroneal muscular atrophy[c, d]	
Internal Organs	
Esophagitis	Pancoast tumor[e, f]
Gallbladder disease[f]	Pancreatic disease
Irritable bowel syndrome	Duodenal ulcer
Interstitial cystitis	
Proctalgia fugax	
Chronic constipation	
General	
Fibromyalgia syndrome	Postherpetic neuralgia
Multiple sclerosis,T[g]	
Rheumatoid arthritis, T	
Acute intermittent porphyria[c]	
Lupus erythematosus, T	

[a] Raeder's syndrome.
[b] Buerger's disease.
[c] Sex-linked inheritance is a potential contributory cause.
[d] Charcot-Marie-Tooth disease.
[e] Bronchogenic carcinoma.
[f] Lifestyle is a potential contributory cause.
[g] T, autoimmune.
SOURCE: Berkley and Holdcroft (1999). Sex prevalence information is mainly from Merskey
and Bogduk (1994) and was cross-checked by using MedLine and other search sources.

lated traits can only be understood in the context of the other. That is, sex differences vary with, and are specific to, the particular genetic background in question, and genetic differences (between strains) can sometimes only be observed in one sex but not the other" (Mogil, 2000, p. 26). It is important to understand that in these studies the effects were revealed by using a specific set of experimental tests of nociception (tail withdrawal from a 49°C hot plate) and antinociception (reduction in nociception with systemic morphine or a κ-opioid or cannabinoid receptor agonist). As Mogil readily admits, the results of such tests can be influenced by many factors, such as time of day, the type of stimulus (mechanical versus thermal), diet, pre- and postnatal stress, housing (in a group versus in isolation), current or prior injury, reproductive status of the comparison females, and more (Berkley, 2000). Thus, Mogil's observations herald a huge potential for the emergence of individual differences in phenotype as genotypic influences are further affected by life's accumulating circumstances.

Mechanisms of Analgesia, Sex Steroid Hormones, and Central Sensitization

An exciting series of findings from research with rodents is that sex differences emerge from complex interactions between stress and endogenous analgesia. In other words, it may be that there are more potent sex differences in mechanisms of pain and analgesia than in measured pain behaviors. The differences seem to lie in how sex steroid hormones exert their effects (Aloisi, 2000; Gintzler and Liu, 2000; Sternberg and Wachterman, 2000). Thus, stress gives rise to an analgesia mediated by a nonopioid, N-methyl D-aspartate (NMDA), that is present primarily in males but that is also present in some females: those who have been ovariectomized or who were neonatally exposed to testosterone. Stress also gives rise to an estrogen-dependent, nonopioid, non-NMDA-mediated analgesia present only in intact females, the mechanisms of which are unknown. Furthermore, the hormonal milieu of pregnancy creates an antinociception involving δ- and κ-opioid systems but not μ-opioid systems.

When such an analgesia is created artificially by hormone treatments in gonadectomized rats, in females the analgesia results from a synergistic combination of spinal κ-opioid, δ-opioid, and α_2-noradrenergic pathways but not μ-opioid pathways, whereas in males the analgesia results from independent additive contributions of spinal κ- and μ-opioid pathways but neither the δ-opioid nor the α_2-noradrenergic pathway.

Finally, estrogen can influence cardiovascular responses (e.g., promotion of vasodilatory or spasmodic effects) and neuronal responses (e.g., expression of the *trkA* gene) to injury, thereby influencing nociception differently in females and males. Some of these findings may relate to recent studies with humans showing that κ-opioids are more effective analgesics in young adult women than in young adult men who have undergone molar tooth extraction (Gear et al., 1996, 1999).

Significance for Human Health

Assuming that the two sets of observations just described are applicable to humans, what might their significance be for health? One obvious area is in the development of analgesic medications. Is it possible that at some time in the foreseeable future analgesics will be prescribed on the basis of an individual's genotype, sex, and reproductive status? Given the first discussion on genotype, such a strategy would likely be pursued only with great care and only in special circumstances (Mogil et al., 2000). For example, individuals with mutations that lead to altered functioning of the cytochrome P450 2D6 enzyme are likely to be prescribed some analgesic other than codeine because they are unable to transform codeine into morphine (Sindrup and Brosen, 1995). Drug development must take into consideration both the sex and the reproductive status of the research subjects not only during all phases of clinical trials but also during the drug development stages of basic research with animals.

On the other hand, before concluding that a specific drug may eventually be prescribed on the basis of the sex of the individual or the reproductive or hormonal status of the patient, it also seems important to consider how stress exerts its cumulative effects over the life span of an individual. Of relevance here is the plasticity of neural function: the ability of neural elements to change their phenotype, to "learn." Considerable research on these changes in the context of pain has led to the discovery of what is called "central sensitization," which is an enhanced responsiveness of central nervous system neurons induced by intense stimulation or injury or by a stressor that, importantly, continues long after the initial noxious event has resolved (Dubner and Ruda, 1992; McMahon et al., 1993). Thus, if the different complex modulatory mechanisms of endogenous sex steroids discovered in female and male rats also exist in human females and males, it is likely that how they influence pain behaviors and the effects of analgesics will change in an ever more complicated manner as the different sociocultural stressors in human females and males exert themselves across their life spans. It may therefore be that one of the most important clinical insights from these two disparate areas of research (mechanisms of endogenous analgesia and central sensitization) is realization of the importance of understanding the chronology and sociocultural context of stressor events for each individual, with that individual's being female or male forming only one of many components considered for drug prescription and therapeutic strategies. Two examples follow.

Sex Differences in Efficacy of μ-Opioids in Clinical Setting

Miaskowski and colleagues (2000) have carried out an extensive review of the clinical literature and have concluded that μ-opioid analgesics are more effective in human females than in human males. Verification of such a conclusion might lead toward research on the development of different analgesics or combinations of analgesics for use as treatments for males. However, it is important to consider the basis for this conclusion. As pointed out by those investigators, the effects have been measured mainly by determination of the amount of μ-opioid medication that females and males consume postsurgically. In most studies males consume more medication than females (when the levels are measured) to achieve comparable levels of pain reduction. The question of whether the consumption of larger amounts of μ-opioids postsurgically by males indicates that they have lower levels of efficacy in males then arises.

One possible way to interpret the finding of greater μ-opioid usage by males is to consider the results of other studies demonstrating that females and males make use of different strategies to reduce pain. As recently reviewed by Robinson and colleagues (2000), females bring a greater variety of coping strategies to bear on their pains than males; that is, females make greater use of what might be called self-polytherapy than males (Berkley and Holdcroft, 1999) (Table 4-2). It is therefore possible that females use smaller amounts of μ-opioids because they are able to engage other forms of positive coping strategies, thereby reducing their need for opioids, and that males use more μ-opioids because that is the only relief they can find. Thus, efficacy depends not simply on whether the drug user is female or male but, rather, depends on sociocultural factors. Such an hypothesis can be tested. Is it in fact the case that in the postoperative setting females engage more coping mechanisms than males? On the other hand, do individuals who have learned to engage multiple coping measures, regardless of their sex, use smaller amounts of opioid medication than others? If so, could opioid usage be reduced overall if individuals were encouraged and educated on how to engage additional constructive coping mechanisms?

Impact of Menstrual Cycle on Pain

Along with genetic and developmentally programmed sex differences in neural organization and physiology, the entire nervous system is potently influenced by the hormonal milieu of the individual (McEwen, 1999; McEwen and Alves, 1999). One arena in which this influence becomes evident is the ovarian cycle (one should keep in mind, however, that the basis for ovarian cyclicity in any realm of physiology or behavior may not necessarily be entirely due to the hormonal milieu). Several stud-

TABLE 4-2　Growing List of Therapies for Pain

Drugs	Somatic Interventions	Situational Approaches
Primary analgesics	**Simple**	**Clinician**
Nonsteroidal anti-	Heat or cold	Education
inflammatory agents	Exercise	Attitude
Acetaminophen	Massage	Clinical setting and
Opioids	Vibration	arrangement
	Relaxation	
Other analgesics		**Self**
α_2 Agonists	**Minimally invasive**	Education
β-Adrenergic antagonists	Physical therapy	Meditation
Antidepressants	Traction	Diet
Anticonvulsants	Manipulation	Art, music, poetry,
Antiarrhythmics	Ultrasound	performing arts
Calcium channel blockers	Transcutaneous electrical	Sports, gardening,
Cannabinoids	nerve stimulation	hobbies
Corticosteroids	Acupuncture	Humor
Cox-2 inhibitors	Local anesthetics	Aroma therapy
γ-Aminobutyric acid		Religion
type B agonists	**Invasive**	Pets
Serotonin agonists	Radiation therapy	
	Dorsal column stimulation	**Interactive**
Adjuvants	Nerve blocks	Hypnosis
Antihistamines	Neurectomy	Biofeedback
Laxatives	Local ganglion blocks	Support groups
Neuroleptics	Sympathectomy	Advocacy groups
Phenothiazines	Rhizotomy	Networking
	Dorsal root entry	Self-help groups
Routes	zone lesions	
Topical, transdermal, oral	Punctate midline	**Structured settings**
Buccal, sublingual,	myelotomy	Group therapy
intranasal	Limited myelotomy	Family counseling
Vaginal, rectal	Commissural myelotomy	Job counseling
Inhalation	Cordotomy	Cognitive therapy
Intramuscular,	Brain stimulation	Behavioral therapy
intraperitoneal	Brain lesions	Psychotherapy
Intravenous		Multidisciplinary clinic
Epidural, intrathecal		Hospice
Intraventricular		

SOURCE: Berkley (2000).
NOTE: Women are more likely than men to take advantage of most of the therapies listed in the "simple" and "minimally invasive" sections of the middle column and nearly all of the therapies listed in the "situational approaches" column (Berkley and Holdcroft, 1999).

ies with rodents have shown the powerful impact of the ovarian (estrous) cycle on the functioning not only of the parts of the brain associated with reproductive functions but on other regions of the brain as well, such as (so far) the hippocampus, striatum, inferior olive, cerebellum, and dorsal column nucleus (Becker, 1999; Bradshaw and Berkley, 2000; Smith and Chapin, 1996a,b; 1998; Woolley and McEwen, 1993; Xiao and Becker, 1994). Importantly, these changes are not always predictable according to the hormonal milieu (Bradshaw and Berkley, 2000).

Given that brain imaging studies show that many parts of the brain are engaged when the subject is in pain (Ingvar and Hsieh, 1999), it is not surprising that numerous studies have found that pain can vary with the menstrual cycle, especially pain that occurs when noxious stimuli are delivered to healthy individuals under certain tightly controlled experimental conditions (Riley et al., 1999). One consequence of this situation is that results of studies comparing pain in young adult females and young adult males may depend on the time of the menstrual cycle in which the women's pain was assessed.

The clinical significance of these findings, however, is unclear because the existence and pattern of the menstrual effects that have been reported are not consistent, especially for painful clinical conditions (Berkley, 1997a,b; Fillingim and Ness, 2000). Part of the inconsistency across studies may be due to technical factors, such as how different parts of the menstrual cycle are classified and the manner in which the analysis has been made. Given that brain imaging studies, however, are beginning to show that the brain regions engaged while an individual is under painful conditions vary with the individual (Davis et al., 1998; Gelnar et al., 1999), it is relevant to consider other factors. For example, a recent study compared skin and muscle pain thresholds in the lower abdomen and limbs across the menstrual cycle in women with severe menstrual pain (dysmenorrhea) and women without dysmenorrhea and across the month in similarly aged young men (Giamberardino et al., 1997). For the men, limb pain threshold did not vary across the month, but abdominal thresholds could not be measured because of the men's extremely high sensitivity (all refused further testing of this region after the first set of trials). For women, the presence of dysmenorrhea gave rise to a generalized muscle (but not skin) hyperalgesia and a significant enhancement of the different patterns for skin and muscle across the menstrual cycle. Comparison of the limb pain thresholds in men and women showed no differences between the men and nondysmenorrheic women, regardless of the time of the month, but did show a higher threshold for both groups compared with that for the dysmenorrheic women.

Although these results highlight the complexity of the issue of differences in pain by sex and time of the menstrual cycle, they point to several potentially important clinical issues. First, the results suggest that dysmenorrhea might enhance the severity and cyclicity of other visceral conditions ("viscero-visceral interactions"). This hypothesis is being tested in parallel studies with animals with endometriosis and ureteral stones and with humans with dysmenorrhea and ureteral stones. So far the results show significant interactions between the two conditions that have implications for diagnosis and treatment in both females and males (Giamberardino, 2000; Giamberardino et al., 1999).

Second, a number of painful clinical disorders vary significantly with the menstrual cycle in some women but not others, such as certain types of headache, irritable bowel syndrome, interstitial cystitis, temporomandibular disorder, and fibromyalgia (Bradley and Alarcón, 2000; Fillingim and Maixner, 2000; Holroyd and Lipchik, 2000; Mayer et al., 1999; Naliboff et al., 2000). It is possible that the women with cyclical pains also suffer from dysmenorrhea, a possibility that can be tested experimentally. If so, it is also possible that treatment directed at the dysmenorrhea might alleviate those women's other pains, and this is also testable. Furthermore, an analysis of what factors reduce the pains during certain phases of the menstrual cycle might yield clues about the mechanism of the pain and treatments that could be applied to men with similar conditions.

Third, what might be the basis for the surprising extreme abdominal sensitivity exhibited by the men, and what implications does this sensitivity have for symptom reporting and clinical testing?

Summary

Overall, the results from research on sex differences in pain mechanisms and responses to treatment provide good examples of a constructive approach toward understanding the mechanisms of other sex differences. This approach highlights the importance of considering how sex differences in genetic, hormonal, psychosocial, and stressful environmental circumstances interact and evolve across the life span to give rise to an individual's ever-changeable "pain phenotype" at any particular time of her or his life (Berkley and Holdcroft, 1999; LeResche, 1999).

ANIMAL MODELS OF CEREBROVASCULAR AND CARDIOVASCULAR DISEASES

Sex-specific responses to experimental traumatic or ischemic brain injury have been reported and are summarized in Table 4-3.

The role of sex in behavioral outcomes after traumatic brain injury has also been studied. Clinical studies report improved outcomes for female patients with head injuries compared with those for male patients with head injuries, as determined by the ability of patients with head injuries to return to their preinjury work levels (Groswasser et al., 1998).

TABLE 4-3 Sex-Specific Responses to an Experimental Traumatic or Ischemic Cerebral Insult

Animal	Model	Results
Gerbil	3-h carotid occlusion	M have more CA1 hippocampal and cortical neuronal loss (Hall et al., 1991)
	Permanent carotid occlusion	M have more strokes (Berry et al., 1975)
Rat	Permanent bilateral carotid occlusion	M have higher rates of mortality and larger numbers of brain lesions (Sadoshima et al., 1988)
	2-h MCAO	M have larger infarcts (Alkayed et al., 1998; Belayev et al., 1996; Zea-Longa et al., 1989)
	Impact/acceleration closed-head injury	M have worse rates of survival (Roof and Hall, 2000a)
	Traumatic brain injury	M have more cerebral edema (Roof et al., 1993a)
	Progesterone after traumatic injury	Equally beneficial effect on edema in both M and F (Roof et al., 1993a)
	Entorhinal cortex injury	M perform worse in maze test (Roof et al., 1993b)
	Ovariectomy, global ischemic insult	Ovariectomized F have greater neurological dysfunction than intact F (Wang et al., 1999)
	Post menopausal, MCAO	M and F similar in infarct size (Alkayed et al., 2000)
	Estradiol pretreatment of ovariectomized F, temporary MCAO	Increased survival and decreased ischemic area in treated versus nontreated F (Simpkins et al., 1997)
	MCAO, estrogen treatment of M	Prognosis improves in estrogen-treated M (Toung et al., 1998)
	MCAO, estrogen receptor antagonist	Ischemia increases in F but not in M (Sawada et al., 2000)
Mice	Unilateral carotid occlusion	Larger lesion in M (Roof and Hall, 2000b)
	Unilateral carotid occlusion in SOD overexpressers	M protected by overexpression of SOD (Roof and Hall, 2000b)

NOTE: MCAO, middle cerebral artery occlusion; M, male; F, female; SOD, superoxide dismutase.

In studies with rats, sex-specific neuroprotection was lost when female rats were ovariectomized, suggesting that circulating gonadal hormones are responsible for the sex differences (Simpkins et al., 1997). Several reports demonstrate that estrogen and progesterone treatment has a neuroprotective effect. This area of research has recently been reviewed (Roof and Hall, 2000b). Results of experiments with rats suggest that estrogenic neuroprotection is not sex specific and is not affected by testosterone.

The mechanisms by which female sex or by which estrogen or progesterone attenuates brain damage are complex. Estrogen could preserve autoregulation or antioxidant activity, affect leukocyte adhesion, or upregulate nitric oxide synthase. Estrogen modulates leukocyte adhesion in the cerebral circulation during resting conditions as well as after transient forebrain ischemia. Leukocyte adhesion and infiltration have been linked to the neuropathology in the brain; estrogen's neuroprotective effects may be due to modulation of this inflammatory pathway (Santizo et al., 2000).

In a model of the rate of progression of atherosclerosis in rabbits fed a high-cholesterol diet, the concentrations of lipids (total cholesterol, high-density lipoprotein cholesterol, and triglycerides) in serum were the same in males and females; however, the rate of progression of disease as determined by histological examination of the thoracic aorta differed (greater in males than in females). Estrogen administration to oophorectomized rabbits fed high levels of cholesterol resulted in a reduced degree of atherosclerosis (Haarbo et al., 1991). The inflammatory response that occurs during atherogenesis involves adhesion of monocytes to endothelial cells and migration across endothelial cells (Nathan et al., 1999). Adhesion of monocytes to endothelial cells is slower in females. In addition, the level of VCAM-1 protein expression in aortas from oophorectomized rabbits fed an diet enriched in cholesterol was increased and was attenuated by the ischemia. These sex differences in VCAM-1 expression in this model suggest an estrogen-mediated anti-inflammatory mechanism.

Transgenic (TNF1.6) mice with cardiac-specific overexpression of tumor necrosis factor alpha (TNF-α) develop ventricular hypertrophy, cardiac dilatation, interstitial infiltrates, massive pleural effusion, and fibrosis and die from congestive heart failure (Kubota et al., 1997). The 6-month survival rate was significantly better in females. The marked sex differences in survival cannot be the result of differences in the levels of expression of TNF-α since at both the transcript and the protein levels the levels of expression of TNF-α was the same in males and females. Rather, male TNF1.6 mice had higher steady-state levels of messenger RNAs encoding both TNF-α and -β receptors. The investigators (Kubota et al., 1997) demonstrated the physiological relevance of this increased level of expression of TNF receptors in male mice by looking at ceramide production, a TNF-dependent process, from myocardial tissue (male transgenic mice produced more ceramide than females). These results suggest that enhanced survival in female mice in the presence of TNF overexpression may be attributable to sex-related differences in TNF receptor levels. The etiology of this differential regulation of TNF receptors remains unknown. In human patients with heart failure, women live significantly longer than men (Becker et al., 1994; Greenland et al., 1991; Steingart et al., 1991).

Animal models provide an important research tool for the study of pathophysiological mechanisms of disease and therapeutic approaches. Male animals have predominantly been used in such animal models, however, on the basis of the assumption that the results obtained from studies conducted with male animals could be extrapolated to female animals. Furthermore, the inclusion of female animals in preclinical studies increases the complexity of a study because of the female estrous cycle and the need to control for the associated hormonal fluctuations (Panetta and Srinivasan, 1998). Thus, the roles of sex and sex hormones in mechanisms of disease outcome have not been routinely studied in animal models. It is not clear whether estrogen's effects are mediated via receptor-based or nongenomic mechanisms. However, continuing efforts to tease apart the mechanisms of sex-based differential vulnerability to traumatic and ischemic brain injuries and cardiovascular diseases could lead to improved understanding of the pathophysiologies of these injuries and diseases and may suggest new mechanistic approaches to their treatment.

FINDINGS AND RECOMMENDATIONS

Findings

Sex hormones do not act alone. No one factor is responsible for sex differences; rather, a number of genetic, hormonal, physiological, and experiential factors operating at different times during development result in the phenotype called an individual. To better understand the influences and roles of factors that may lead to sex differences, the committee makes the following recommendations.

Recommendations

RECOMMENDATION 4: Investigate natural variations.

• **Examine genetic variability, disorders of sex differentiation, reproductive status, and environmental influences to better understand human health.**
• **Naturally occurring variations provide useful models that can be used to study the influences and origins of a range of factors that influence sex differences.**

RECOMMENDATION 5: Expand research on sex differences in brain organization and function.

New technologies make it possible to study sex-differential environmental and behavioral influences on brain organization and function and to recognize modulators of brain organization and function. Explore innovative ways to expand the availability of and reduce the cost of new technologies.

Also see Recommendation 3 (Chapter 3) for a discussion of the need to mine cross-species information.

5

Sex Affects Health

ABSTRACT

Males and females have different patterns of illness and different life spans, raising questions about the relative roles of biology and environment in these disparities. Dissimilar exposures, susceptibilities, and responses to initiating agents and differences in energy storage and metabolism result in variable responses to pharmacological agents and the initiation and manifestation of diseases such as obesity, autoimmune disorders, and coronary heart disease, to name a few. Understanding the bases of these sex based differences is important to developing new approaches to prevention, diagnosis, and treatment. Sex should be considered as a variable in all biomedical and health-related research. Studies should be designed to control for exposure, susceptibility, metabolism, physiology (cycles), and immune response variables.

Males and females have different patterns of illness and different life spans, which leads to important questions about how these differences might be biologically determined. Diseases other than those of the reproductive system affect both sexes, often with different frequencies or presentations, or they may require different treatments. This chapter explores how these differences result from differences in exposures, susceptibilities, and responses to disease-initiating agents, differences in energy storage and metabolism, and disparate diagnostic and therapeutic interventions.

Because it is not possible to explore all diseases, disorders, and conditions with sex differences, the committee chose several illustrative examples. The committee first briefly describes the complexities of sex differences in response to therapeutic agents and energy metabolism. The subsequent section focuses on differences in energy metabolism, obesity, and physical performance and then uses two illustrations—melanoma and osteoporosis—to describe sex differences. The chapter then focuses on the complexities of a normal immune response that has gone awry or that has spontaneously lost its normal immune regulation system (autoimmune diseases). These diseases in particular demonstrate variable susceptibilities between human males and human females, as well as differential exposures to environmental factors. The chapter concludes by describing a disease whose etiology occurs from conception to the grave but that affects both sexes differently, coronary heart disease.

SEX DIFFERENCES IN RESPONSE TO THERAPEUTIC AGENTS: DIAGNOSTIC AND THERAPEUTIC INTERVENTIONS

Background

Pharmacological agents can be used as probes to diagnose, prevent, and treat human illnesses. How much of an agent one encounters depends on the route of entry into the body (see Figure 5-7), absorption, distribution, metabolism, and excretion and is a major factor in the body's response, whether it is a therapeutic or an adverse response. The following discussion uses the definitions provided in Box 5-1 and the schema presented in Figure 5-1.

BOX 5-1
Definitions

Bioavailability: fraction of the dose that is absorbed and that reaches the systemic circulation unaltered by biotransformation.

Biotransformation: enzymatic conversion of the compound, usually to a more water-soluble form of the compound.

Dose-response: relationship between the dose of a drug and the magnitude or intensity of the response.

Pharmacodynamics: the body's response to a drug.

Pharmacokinetics: the time course of the drug's absorption, distribution, metabolism (biotransformation), and excretion (see Figure 5-1).

Therapeutic index: relationship between the desired and undesired effect(s) of a drug, that is, the benefit/risk ratio.

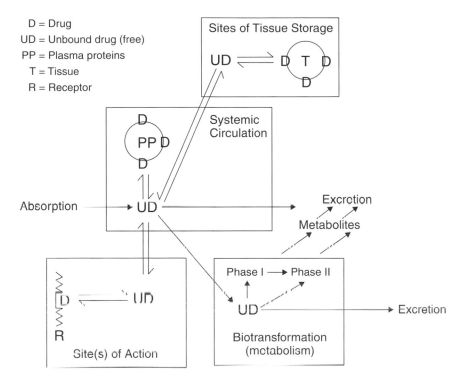

FIGURE 5-1 Schematic representation of the absorption, distribution, metabolism, and excretion of drugs.

Pharmacokinetic and pharmacodynamic variables can be measured and can demonstrate differences between males and females. Pharmacokinetic and pharmacodynamic differences between males and females exposed to the same compound and dose do not necessarily result in different health outcomes. Outcome data that can be used, however, to establish whether differences between the sexes are clinically meaningful are sparse.

The methods used to study sex differences in the effects of drugs can serve as a template for the study of the relative effects of any foreign chemical, including volatile organic chemicals. For example, most standards for the human carcinogen benzene have been based on studies involving males, even though physiologically based pharmacokinetic modeling shows that females have higher levels of metabolism of benzene (Brown et al., 1998). Greater appreciation of these methods will yield significant clinical data regarding the importance of sex both in drug development, prescription, and dosing and in assessments of environmental exposures.

In reviewing the examples described below, the committee was cognizant of the small numbers of subjects involved in some of the studies, the sometimes conflicting results of studies, and the significant variations observed in the results of many of the studies that purport to evaluate sex and age differences. It will be essential in future studies to define the stages of a woman's menstrual cycle, use protocols with sufficient power to detect statistically significant differences, and determine whether demonstrated differences deemed to be sex relevant affect clinical outcomes. Although many studies are designed to demonstrate sex differences in pharmacokinetics, few look at pharmacodynamics, and even fewer determine clinical outcomes.

Processes of Drug Absorption and Metabolism

Absorption of Pharmacological Agents Through Different Routes of Entry

Absorption of small organic molecules is usually passive, but it may involve a facilitated process or an active process that requires energy. The factors that affect the absorption of chemicals from the gastrointestinal tract are listed in Table 5-1.

TABLE 5-1 Factors Affecting Absorption of Chemicals

Physical characteristics	pK_a
	Aqueous solubility
	Lipid solubility
Dosage form	Disintegration
	Dissolution
	Enteric coating
	Controlled-release properties
Gastrointestinal characteristics	Presence of food and type of food in the gastrointestinal tract
	Rate of gastric emptying
	pH of the different segments of the gastrointestinal tract
	Intestinal microorganisms
	Intestinal transit time
	Gastrointestinal blood flow
	Gastrointestinal enzymes
	Alcohol dehydrogenase
	Cytochrome P450
	Glucuronosyltransferase
	Sulfotransferase
	Gastrointestinal transport systems
	P glycoprotein
	Effects of other drugs

The venous blood supply of the entire gastrointestinal tract except the rectum goes directly to the liver, where absorbed compounds may be metabolized (first-pass metabolism). This observation may be explained by the high prevalence of CYP3A4 in the upper part of the intestine and its absence from the colon and rectum. Drugs given through the rectum (suppositories) and urinary bladder do not go through significant first-pass metabolism (Buyse et al., 1998). Interestingly, drugs applied to the vagina accumulate to a greater extent in the uterus than when administered by other routes; that is, they have a "first-uterine-pass effect" (Bulletti et al., 1997; Mizutam et al., 1995).

Gastrointestinal Tract Absorption of drugs from the stomach is affected by a variety of factors (Table 5-1). (For a general review of the effect of gastrointestinal motility on the absorption of drugs, see Hebbard et al. [1995].) Gastric emptying (Malagelada et al., 1993) can be measured by several techniques, of which transit times determined with a radiolabeled liquid or solid meals provide the best-validated and clinically meaningful measurements (Camilleri et al., 1998).

Differences in age, sex, body mass index, phase of menstrual cycle, and type of meal consumed lead to large inter- and intrasubject variabilities. The preponderance of evidence (Bennink et al., 1999; Datz et al., 1987; Gryback et al., 1996; Hermansson and Silvertsson, 1996; Hutson et al., 1989; Knight et al., 1997; Tucci et al., 1992) supports the conclusion that females empty solids more slowly than men; however, others have found that all transit variables are unaffected by sex (Madsen, 1992). The gastric emptying of liquids has also been reported to be slower in women than men (Datz et al., 1987; Mohiuddin et al., 1999); however, others have found no differences (Bennink et al., 1998). In addition, young people empty their stomachs faster than elderly people do (Jann et al., 1998; Moore et al., 1983; Teff et al., 1999). The small-bowel transit time of solids and liquids do not differ between the sexes (Horowitz et al., 1984; Madsen, 1992), but differences are seen between old and young subjects (Bennink et al., 1999; Madsen, 1992).

Slower gastric emptying in females does not likely affect the absorption of most solid drugs since most absorption takes place in the small intestine. The rate of absorption of enteric coated forms is delayed (Mojaverian et al., 1987). Drugs with narrow therapeutic indices are most likely to be harmful (Greiff and Rowbotham, 1994) or lack efficacy in persons with slow rates of gastric emptying. A slow rate of gastric emptying also decreases the level of absorption of alcohol.

Progesterone may be responsible for the slower rate of gastric emptying in women (Gill et al., 1985, 1987; Hutson et al., 1989; Mathias and Clench, 1998; Riezzo et al., 1998). Females are less sensitive than males to muscarinic blockade of stomach motility, possibly because of differences in autonomic tone (Teff et al., 1999). It is of interest that 80 to 90 percent of diabetic patients with gastroparesis (paralysis of the stomach) are females (Bennink et al., 1998).

Basal acid output, pH, and gastrin secretion are independent of sex (Bernardi et al., 1990; Dressman et al., 1990; Straus and Raufman, 1989) and age (Russell et al., 1993). In patients with gastroesophageal reflux, however, the mean basal level of acid output is greater in males than females (Collen et al., 1994).

Transport systems within the gastrointestinal tract may have significant effects on drug absorption. For example, a component of the intestine and liver, P glycoprotein (Pgp), is a transmembrane efflux protein that actively transports many compounds including drugs out of cells. The livers of males express twofold larger amounts of Pgp than the livers of females (Schuetz et al., 1995). This suggests that males transport drugs out of hepatocytes more rapidly than females, decreasing the time for biotransformation, although further studies are needed. The absorption of many drugs might be affected if a sex difference in intestinal Pgp activity also exists, and it is important to determine whether such a sex difference exists. Drug absorption rates from the rectum may also be sex dependent. Females absorbed one of the two specially prepared ondansetron suppositories (an antiemetic) differently than males (Jann et al., 1998), although this could be attributed to normal variability.

The menstrual cycle has no effect on motility in the esophagus (Mohiuddin et al., 1999) or on whole-gut transport (Kamm et al., 1989). However, evidence for a menstrual cycle effect on gastric emptying is conflicting (Gill et al., 1987; Horowitz et al., 1985; Mones et al., 1993; Parkman et al., 1996; Petring and Flachs, 1990).

Skin   Gels, ointments, creams, or patches deliver small organic compounds through the skin (Brown and Langer, 1988; Xu and Chien, 1991). Transit through the stratum corneum (outer skin) barrier often requires the use of absorption enhancers (Kanikkannan et al., 2000).

The level of transepidermal water loss, a measure of epidermal barrier permeability following injury to and recovery of the stratum corneum, does not differ between males and females or between Caucasians and Asians (Reed et al., 1995). Dark skin recovers from an injury more quickly than lightly pigmented skin. In a clinical trial of transdermal clonidine for the treatment of hypertension, blood pressure reduction was independent of race, ethnicity, sex, and age (Dias et al., 1999). In vitro, transdermal absorption of fentanyl and sufentanil (analgesics) was neither age nor sex dependent (Roy and Flynn, 1990).

Pulmonary tract   Absorption of drugs via the pulmonary tract varies with breathing rate and depth (ventilation) (Gonda, 2000). Progesterone may be a ventilatory stimulant. Females have greater minute ventilations and lower tidal volumes than males, and the ventilatory response to high carbon dioxide levels is greater in males (White et al., 1983). A drug, ethionamide, given orally to healthy and ill men and women appeared in equal concentrations in alveolar cells of both sexes (Conte et al., 2000). Women have higher ventilatory responses in the luteal phase than in the follicular phase of the menstrual cycle.

Protein Binding

Most small organic compounds bind to albumin or α_1-acid glycoprotein (AAG) and less frequently to alpha, beta, and gamma globulins, lipoproteins, or erythrocytes. AAG binds with a high affinity to basic drugs. Albumin binds to acidic drugs in a complex in which the drug readily dissociates to maintain an equilibrium between the bound and unbound (free) fractions. The unbound fraction is in equilibrium with the receptor (Anton, 1960; Shoeman and Azarnoff, 1975). Thus, the degree of binding of drugs to plasma proteins can influence their dispositions (Gillette, 1973).

The plasma protein binding of enantiomers (mirror-image compounds) in racemic mixtures (containing both enantiomers) may differ, and selective binding of the enantiomers does occur (Gross et al., 1988; Walle et al., 1983).

The level of AGG, an acute-phase reactant, increases in patients with infections, cancer, and rheumatoid arthritis. Decreased albumin levels or increased AAG levels occur in patients with renal, liver, and thyroid Crohn's disease, myocardial infarction, cancer, and burns (Reidenberg and Affrime, 1973). Increased levels of unbound drug occur in patients with uremia (Garland, 1998; Reidenberg and Affrime, 1973) and cirrhosis (Goldstein et al., 1969). It is not known whether sex differences exist in these circumstances.

In a very small study (nine women each examined through one menstrual cycle), the concentration of AGG was higher on day 4 of the menstrual cycle than on days 12, 20, and 28 (Parish and Spivey, 1991), but the study had very significant inter- and intrapatient variabilities. The level of sex hormone binding globulin has also been found to increase during the luteal phase of the menstrual cycle (Plymate et al., 1985).

The concentration of a drug in the fetus is a function of the concentration in the mother, placental permeability, fetal drug clearance, and differences in the levels of protein binding between maternal and fetal plasma (Boulos et al., 1971). The placental transfer of lipophilic drugs is good, but the transfer of hydrophilic drugs is slow.

The concentration of protein is significantly lower in the fetal circula-

TABLE 5-2 Differences in Drug Concentrations Between the Mother and Fetus and Between Males and Females

Mother-fetus comparisons	Binding of propranolol and verapamil is lower in fetal serum
	Propranolol *R/S* enantiomer ratio is larger in maternal serum
	Verapamil *R/S* enantiomer ratio is similar in maternal and fetal serum
	AAG levels are higher in maternal serum
	Albumin levels are slightly lower in maternal serum (Belpaire et al., 1995; Notarianni, 1990)
Male-female comparisons	Unbound concentrations of chlordiazepoxide, diazepam, imipramine, and nitrazepam are higher in women (MacKichan, 1992)
	The level of the unbound fraction of *S*-propranolol but not *R*-propranolol is decreased in older women (Walle et al., 1983)

tion than in the maternal circulation during early pregnancy, but the concentration in the fetus exceeds that in the mother at term. The maternal AAG level is very low before 16 weeks of gestation and thereafter increases at a constant rate to a fetal concentration-maternal concentration ratio of 0.37 near term (Perucca and Crema, 1982). Examples of circumstances in which plasma protein variables affect drug concentrations are shown in Table 5-2.

Body Composition

Male-female differences in body fatness may account for the increased volumes of distribution for lipophilic drugs (such as benzodiazepines) in females (Parker, 1984; Sciore et al., 1998) and for alcohol in males (Loebstein et al., 1997; Parker, 1984; Petring and Flachs, 1990).

The level of total body water decreases with age because of a disproportionate decrease in intracellular water levels (Kashuba and Nafziger, 1998; Phipps et al., 1998). It is important to adjust body composition models not only for sex but also for age and body size (Kasuba and Nafziger 1998; Phipps et al., 1998). (It is important to note, however, that some sex differences in pharmacokinetics reported in the literature are a result of differences in weights between males and females receiving the same fixed dose of the drug. Thus, pharmacokinetic parameters should be corrected by weight before concluding that a sex difference exists. The effects of differences in body fat, as noted above, can confound weight issues and should also be considered.)

Biotransformation

Sex has a complex effect on the pharmacokinetics of drugs metabolized in the liver (Harris et al., 1995; Yonkers et al., 1992). Temazepam and oxazepam, benzodiazepines that are metabolized through conjugation, are cleared faster by males (Divoll et al., 1981; Greenblatt et al., 1980; Smith et al., 1983). Alprazolam (Kristjansson and Thorsteinsson, 1991) and diazepam (Greenblatt et al., 1980) are metabolized via an oxidative mechanism and are cleared faster by females. Nitrazepam (Jochemsen et al., 1982) is metabolized via reduction of its nitro group, and its metabolism shows no sex differences. Thus, sex affects differently even drugs within the same pharmacological class and drugs with the same structures.

Cytochromes P450   The cytochromes P450 (CYPs) are a superfamily of at least 17 isozymes that modulate the oxidative metabolism of drugs in the liver (Wrighton and Stevens, 1992). CYP1, CYP2, and CYP3 are thought to be responsible for most hepatic metabolism of drugs. The CYP3A4 subfamily is the most abundant of the CYPs in the human liver and is responsible for the metabolism of cyclosporine, quinidine, erythromycin, dapsone, and lidocaine (Harris et al., 1995; Wing et al., 1984). The major CYP isoform found in the human embryonic, fetal, and newborn liver is CYP3A7. The activity of CYP3A4 is very low before birth but increases rapidly at birth and reaches 50 percent of the level in adults between 6 and 12 months of age. This maturation of drug-metabolizing enzymes is the main factor for age-associated changes in nonrenal drug clearance (de Wildt et al., 1999).

Studies with tirilazad (an antioxidant) (Hulst et al., 1994), erythromycin (Watkins et al., 1985), and diazepam (Greenblatt et al., 1980) suggest that females have greater CYP3A4 activity, but studies with other probe drugs yield conflicting results. Drugs metabolized by CYP3A4 are extensively cleared by females, whereas drugs cleared by other isozymes are usually cleared faster by males (Harris et al., 1995). The sex-specific differences in CYP3A4 activity are related to estrogen and progesterone, which regulate the activity of CYP3A4 at the gene level (Harris et al., 1995). However, the metabolism of ranitidine, also metabolized by CYPs, shows no sex difference (Abad-Santos et al., 1996). The metabolism of some drugs eliminated through conjugation shows sex differences (Divoll et al., 1981; Greenblatt et al., 1980, 1984; Macdonald et al., 1990; Miners et al., 1983, 1984).

Excretion

The kidney is the major organ of drug excretion. Drugs diffuse in their un-ionized form across the kidney glomeruli and tubules or are secreted and reabsorbed by active tubular transport systems. Drugs are also excreted in the feces if either the drug has not been absorbed from the gastrointestinal tract or it is excreted from the liver into the bile in the intestinal tract. Reabsorption (enterohepatic circulation) may occur as the excreted drug travels through the intestines.

Males have higher levels of creatinine in serum and urine and higher rates of creatinine clearance (CL_{CR}) than females. The difference is related to the greater lean body mass of males (James et al., 1988). In a three-way crossover study with young and elderly men and women, the renal clearance of amantadine was significantly inhibited by quinine and quinidine only in the male subjects. There were no age-related effects (Gaudry et al., 1993). The mechanism of this interaction is probably related to the differential effects of quinine and quinidine on the tubular excretion rate of cations (Charney et al., 1992). A physician would not need to consider this interaction when treating an elderly woman with quinidine for muscle cramps who developed influenza and was prescribed amantadine; a lack of attention to this drug-drug interaction in a male, however, could lead to a significant adverse reaction.

CL_{CR} is lower during the first week of menses and increases by week 4 by 20 percent. Overnight CL_{CR} measured three times a week during 11 menstrual cycles found the median CL_{CR} to be 7.3 percent higher during the luteal phase than during the follicular phase. Similar changes were found when intravenous chromium 51-labeled EDTA was used, a more accurate measure of the glomerular filtration rate (Paaby et al., 1987a,b). Estradiol and estriol do not affect the glomerular filtration rate, urine flow, renal plasma flow, or tubular reabsorption in humans (Christy and Shaver, 1974; Davison, 1987). CL_{CR} was found to be slightly increased only in the midluteal phase in another study (Phipps et al., 1998). However, the changes were attributable to changes in creatinine excretion and are not considered clinically important. It is surprising that investigators are still attempting to determine the effect of the menstrual cycle on CL_{CR}.

The renal clearance of the aminoglycoside antibiotics tobramycin (Nafziger et al., 1989) and amikacin (Matsuki et al., 1999) are not significantly altered during the menstrual cycle. In a recent review, Kashuba and Nafziger (1998) reported that most published studies have been conducted with small numbers of women and limited numbers of menstrual cycle phases within one menstrual cycle. In addition, studies of the effects of estrogen or progesterone on renal clearance are limited and their results are contradictory. They further conclude, "there are no demonstrated clinically significant changes that occur in the absorption, distribution or elimination of drugs" during a normal menstrual cycle (Kashuba and Nafziger, 1998, p. 204). Beierle et al. (1999) concluded that sex-related differences in the renal clearance of drugs is generally only of minor importance. However, a meta-analysis of 10 studies with 172 healthy volunteers administered an oral therapeutic dose of the antibiotic fleroxacin provided evidence that the volume of distribution/systemic availability ratio (V/F) is 20.4 liters greater in males than females and that the clearance/systemic availability ratio is 10.8 milliliters per minute (ml/min) greater in males than females (Reigner and Welker, 1996).

Pharmacodynamics

Receptors are macromolecules on or in cells to which a drug binds to initiate its effect. Continued stimulation of a receptor may lead to its downregulation or desensitization (refractoriness). Hyperreactivity may also occur and may result from long-term administration of antagonists or the synthesis of additional receptors. Drugs may also act as substrates for enzymes or may inhibit enzymes competitively or noncompetitively.

Although there is marked interindividual variation (Levy, 1998), pharmacodynamic differences between the sexes do occur. Several examples are shown in Table 5-3. (For additional examples, see Table B-1 in Appendix B.)

Clinical Implications

Some pharmacokinetic and pharmacodynamic sex differences may affect drug efficacy or make serious adverse events more likely. A sex difference will more likely affect drugs with narrow therapeutic indices than those with wide therapeutic indices. Adjustment of the dose or dosing interval of the drug may be sufficient to correct the difference, or it may be necessary to use a different drug or treatment modality.

Given the amount of resources being dedicated to drug development worldwide, it is especially important to consider sex-specific issues relating to clinical trials research, the effects of drugs on receptors (or sexual dimorphisms of receptors and neurotransmitters), and the sexual dimorphism of treatment responses. Sex-related variables should be specifically and comprehensively included in all diagnostic, longitudinal, and treatment research studies (i.e., all clinical studies involving humans) whenever feasible. Studies should be designed to determine the relative effects of covariables to clearly establish the contributions of sex to outcome data.

Analyses should be planned a priori (even if they are secondary or exploratory analyses) that address sex-related hypotheses (i.e., they should not rely primarily on post hoc analyses). In addition, at least some diagnostic, longitudinal, and treatment studies should be powered specifically to permit the appropriate analysis of sex-related variables (post hoc analyses are usually conducted with sample sizes that are too small, making it likely that type II errors [the assumption that no relationship exists when in, fact, it does] will occur). The Office of Research on

TABLE 5-3   Receptor, Enzyme, and Structural Differences Between Males and Females

Sex Difference	Clinical Relevance
Intra-arial α_1-adrenoceptor agonist phenylephrine induces greater vasoconstriction during the luteal phase than during the follicular phase of the menstrual cycle in African-American and white females. The α_2-adrenoceptor agonist clonidine induces greater vasoconstriction in the follicular phase than in the luteal phase in white females but not African-American females (Freedman and Girgis, 2000). Men show a significant dose-response to vasodilatation to isoproterenol; females do not.	Blood pressure regulation.
Correlation curves of blood alcohol levels and sedation; the slope of the curve is steeper in females (Ammon et al., 1996).	The sedative effects of ethanol are greater in women.
Angiotensin I and II infusion; negative relationship between change in heart rate and mean arterial pressure during infusion in females only. The renal vasoconstrictor response is increased in females (Gandhi et al., 1998).	Sex differences in cardiorenal fluid balance at the pharmacodynamic level.
The rise of D1 and D2 striatal dopamine receptors in males but not females parallels the early developmental appearance of motor symptoms of attention deficit hyperactivity disorder (Andersen and Teicher, 2000).	Possible explanation for higher attention deficit hyperactivity disorder incidence in males.

NOTE: See also Appendix B.

Women's Health of the National Institutes of Health (1999a,b) has made numerous recommendations in this regard.

Sex Differences in Adverse Events

Drugs from classes as diverse as antihistamines (terfenadine), antibiotics (erythromycin) (Makkar et al., 1993), and antiarrhythmic drugs (*d,l*-sotalol) (Kuhlkamp et al., 1997; Lehmann et al., 1996) can induce a potentially lethal cardiac rhythm called torsades de pointes. The risk of having this drug-induced complication is far greater in females than in males. Hypokalemia, hypomagnesemia, bradycardia, and the baseline QT[1] inter-

---

[1] The QT interval on an electrocardiogram is the duration of activation and recovery of the ventricular muscle. Because QT interval varies inversely with heart rate the corrected QT, or QT_c, is often used.

val and the degree of QT prolongation (electrocardiographic variables) increase ones susceptibility to this event (Napolitano et al., 1994). As females possess a longer average electrocardiographic QT interval-corrected heart rate (QT_c) than males, a difference not found in the newborn (Stramba-Badiale et al., 1995), sex differences in cardiac ion channel function account for the increased incidence in females (Rautaharju et al., 1992). In clinical studies it was found that quinidine, a drug that induces QT_c interval prolongation, also induces a greater prolongation of the QT_c interval in females (Benton et al., 2000). Furthermore, in animal models, estrogen has been found to prolong the QT_c interval, affecting cardiac repolarization (Drici et al., 1996). Recent studies with women suggest that drug-induced QT interval prolongation may be affected by the phase of the menstrual cycle (Rodriguez et al., 2001).

Studies of isolated ventricular myocytes indicate that active drugs block the delayed rectifier potassium channel (I_k) (Wesche et al., 2000). Adjustment of dosage for body weight or surface area does not ameliorate this problem. Recently, the U.S. Food and Drug Administration (FDA) has required label warnings for drugs that prolong the QT_c interval. One drug with this effect, cisapride, was removed from the market.

Although the prolongation of the QT_c interval by the d-sotalol enantiomer is said to be independent of dose and sex (Salazar et al., 1997), the small population size of the study (four males and four females, which is not sufficient to be able to draw general conclusions) exemplifies the inadequacy of the available literature on this topic.

Genes associated with the long QT syndrome and sudden death have mutations that affect ionic currents involved in the control of ventricular rhythm. Only those subjects with a mutation affecting the sodium-channel ionic current have sufficient prolongation of the nighttime QT interval to increase arrhythmic risk (Stramba-Badiale et al., 2000). The sex difference in QT_c interval observed in adults is not seen on the 4th day of life (Stramba-Badiale et al., 1995).

Other sex-related differences in side effects have also been noted. For example, females are twice as likely as males to develop a cough while taking angiotensin-converting enzyme inhibitors (Kubota et al., 1996; Strocchi et al., 1992).

Sex Differences in Effectiveness

Sex differences in the therapeutic response to the 5HT3 antagonist alosetron have been reported. FDA has recently approved alosetron for the treatment of nonconstipated irritable bowel syndrome in females. It is ineffective in males, but the reasons for this are unknown (Bardhan et al., 2000; Camilleri et al., 2000). Another example of sex differences in the therapeutic response to a compound that acts by a serotonergic mechanism is sertraline. FDA recently approved sertraline for the treatment of posttraumatic stress disorder in women. Two multicenter, placebo-controlled trials for the treatment of posttraumatic stress disorder demonstrated its effectiveness in females but not in males (Henney, 2000).

Differences in the rates of serotonin synthesis in the brains of female and male volunteers have been measured by positron emission tomography. This technique allows a direct measurement of the rate of serotonin synthesis in the living brain. The rate of brain serotonin synthesis was found to be 52 percent greater in male subjects than female subjects. The researchers suggest that this marked difference in rates of serotonin synthesis could contribute to the higher incidence in women of major unipolar depression and other psychopharmacologies in which serotonergic mechanisms are implicated in the pathophysiology of the disease. However, a few postmortem studies found no significant sex differences in serotonin levels (Arato et al., 1991; Dean et al., 1995; Nishizawa et al., 1997).

METABOLISM, LIFESTYLE, AND PHYSICAL PERFORMANCE

Male-female differences are very striking in terms of body size and composition (Björntorp, 1989; Legato, 1997; National Center for Health Statistics, 1987). These sex differences are closely linked to reproductive variables (Björntorp, 1989; Legato, 1997).

In addition, these differences can result from a combination of biological and social (lifestyle) differences, which are then manifest in variable rates of illness, for example, obesity and osteoporosis between males and females. The relative influence of biological factors on the development and prognosis for some diseases, such as melanoma, are sometimes difficult to sort out because of the different social practices of men and women, for example, in regard to styles of clothing, levels of sun exposure, and use of sunscreens.

As another example, the reduced rates of osteoporosis in males are likely a combination of basic molecular and hormonal differences combined with a greater tendency for men to engage in physical activity and weight-bearing exercise (Damien et al., 2000).

Nevertheless, there is a limited understanding of the underlying mechanisms of these apparently fundamental sex differences and their influence on aspects of health and functioning other than reproduction (Legato, 1997). A better understanding of how sex differences relate to physical performance variables such as strength, endurance, and overall work capacity is needed to address the question of when differential treatment by sex is justified.

Differences in Body Composition

Differences in body composition are mediated by sex hormones and sex differences in behavior and tend to diminish after the fertile adult years. It is thought that these differences emerge around puberty; however, sex differences in body composition have also been observed well before the onset of puberty (Taylor et al., 1997). Body fat is an important component of energy balance, and there is clearly a relationship between systems of energy regulation and reproduction (including puberty and menarche) in various animal species and humans, but this relationship is not as simplistic as was once thought (Caprio et al., 2001; Schneider et al., 2000; also discussed in Chapter 3). Mammary fat and gluteal-femoral fat are preserved in females under conditions of starvation and are preferentially mobilized during lactation. Food intake varies during the menstrual cycle, and hormonal changes during pregnancy may increase a female's appetite. Pregnancy causes weight gain over and above that from the fetus and placenta, and a return to the prepartum weight requires weight loss. Menopause is associated with a shift toward relatively more fat as well as toward the deposition of more fat in the abdominal region (Poehlman and Tchernof, 1998).

Adult males are, on average, taller than adult females and generally have a greater proportion of muscle and a lower percentage of body fat than females of the same weight and height. The greater muscle mass of males is associated with greater physical strength. Males also typically have relatively more abdominal fat and less gluteal-femoral fat than females.

Energy Metabolism and Body Composition

Foods and beverages contain substances that can be oxidized to energy (heat, measured in calories) as fuel for vital processes and physical work; these substances include fat (~9 kilocalories per gram), carbohydrate (~4 kilocalories per gram), and protein (~4 kilocalories per gram) (Goran, 2000). The ethanol in alcoholic beverages provides calories (~7 kilocalories per gram) but is also a toxin. Individual variation in the efficiency of energy utilization (the amount of heat produced per unit of food energy consumed) is in part genetically determined but can be influenced by behavioral factors such as physical training, cigarette smoking, and alcohol use (Collins et al., 1994; Goran, 2000; Suter et al., 1994).

Body weight reflects the weights of bone, visceral organs, skeletal muscle, adipose tissue (fat, both intra-abdominal and subcutaneous), blood, and other body fluids (Heymsfield et al., 1997). The adipose tissue component has the greatest variability. Daily energy requirements depend primarily on basal metabolic needs, that is, the amount of energy needed to support basic functions, such as during sleep or at rest. The basal or resting energy expenditure is determined primarily by body size and body composition (i.e., the proportions of fat and lean tissue). Energy expenditure during energy utilization is higher in muscle than in fat tissue. Thus, at the same weight and height, a fatter individual expends less energy than one with relatively more lean tissue. Other contributors to total energy expenditure include the small amount of energy needed to metabolize food and the variable amount of energy expended during physical activity. Energy intake in excess of energy requirements is stored preferentially and primarily as fat (Figure 5-2).

Sex differences in energy requirements derive from sex differences in body size, body composition, and activity levels (Goran, 2000). Larger individuals (e.g., males) have higher energy needs. Estimated energy requirements for males and females are similar before puberty (i.e., before the occurrence of sex hormone-driven changes in body size and fatness) (National Research Council, 1989). After puberty, energy requirements are higher for males. Compared with a man of the same weight and height, a woman has less lean tissue and, therefore, a lower basal metabolism and lower energy expenditure per unit of work.

Obesity

The interest in obesity has increased in recent years because of an alarming increase in the prevalence of obesity in both adults and children (Flegal et al., 1998; Mokdad et al., 1999; Troiano and Flegal, 1998) and because type II diabetes (adult-onset, non-insulin-dependent diabetes

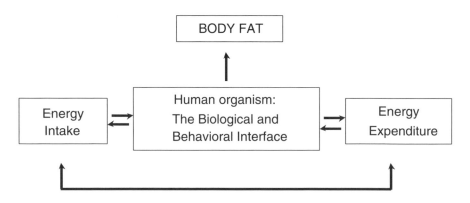

FIGURE 5-2 The major affectors of body fat. Source: Bouchard (1992). Reprinted, with permission, from C. Bouchard. 1992. Genetic aspects of human obesity. *In: Obesity.* P. Björntorp and B. N. Brodoff, eds. Philadelphia: J. B. Lippincott Company. Copyright 1992 by J. B. Lippincott Company).

mellitus), as one clear manifestation of the associated metabolic aberrations, is also increasing in parallel in both adults and children (Mokdad et al., 2000; Rosenbloom et al., 1999). Simultaneously, advances in genetics and molecular biology have begun to provide new insights into mechanisms of appetite regulation, energy metabolism, and obesity causation, with the promise of effective pharmacological approaches to the treatment of obesity in the foreseeable future. Taken together, these developments increase both the urgency of and the potential for the identification of the biological factors that underlie obesity and that interact with the plethora of identified sociocultural and behavioral contributors to obesity (World Health Organization, 1998a).

The following questions remain unresolved, however.

- Does the biological predisposition of women to develop fat stores also predispose women to become obese under conditions of high levels of food availability?
- Are sex-specific approaches needed in obesity treatment?
- Are the systems of energy regulation in females more primed for weight gain or weight retention relative to those in males? If so, under what circumstances is this tendency expressed or suppressed?
- Given that many obesity-related health risks are specifically linked to abdominal fat, is a given level of overall obesity less problematic for females than for males?
- Can the study of sex differences in energy balance facilitate understanding of the etiology of obesity?

These questions become particularly pressing in light of the current epidemic of obesity within both the United States and worldwide (Mokdad et al., 1999; World Health Organization, 1998a).

The development of obesity probably reflects a natural response to an overabundance of food energy and limitations of requirements for physical activity (Hill and Peters, 1998; James, 1995), conditions that overwhelm the physiological capability to maintain energy balance. There are, nevertheless, numerous scientific questions related to variations in individual susceptibility to these conditions, physiological aberrations that may result from a chronic overabundance of food and physical activity limitations (e.g., changes in set points for energy regulation), and ways to leverage compensatory responses through genetic or drug therapy. Sex differences in obesity, along with age and ethnic variations in overall levels of obesity and in the sex ratio of obesity, provide interesting leads that can be used to address these questions.

Commonly used definitions of obesity are based on relative weight for height but do not account for either fatness or fat patterning. These definitions may therefore overestimate fatness in males relative to that in females. To the extent that obesity-related health risks are tied to abdominal obesity (Björntorp, 1996), definitions of obesity based only on body size will overestimate the health risks associated with obesity in females (who have relatively less abdominal fat) in comparison the health risks associated with obesity in males (Laws et al., 1997). Obesity prevalence data also indicate that the tendency of females to be more obese than males differs according to ethnic, socioeconomic, and environmental circumstances (Table 5-4). This makes the question of sex differences in obesity more complicated; that is, what is the underlying predisposition to obesity in females, and under what circumstances is it expressed or not expressed?

Possible explanations for a greater prevalence of obesity in females include the following: (1) overconsumption, that is, eating behaviors that predispose females to consume too much food in relation to energy needs, possibly including physiologically determined disorders of appetite regulation; (2) metabolic efficiency, for example, physiological factors that predispose females to store relatively more consumed energy at any given level of intake; (3) low energy expenditure, that is, possible behavioral sex differences in the ability to offset energy intake through routine or leisure time physical activity; and (4) less success in voluntary weight control because of either behavioral of physiological factors.

These explanations are complementary and may combine to increase the predisposition of females to a positive energy balance. From an epidemiological perspective, exploration of these possibilities might include comparisons by ethnicity and socioeconomic status to determine whether one or more are particularly applicable or inapplicable to subgroups of females. For example, assuming that the underlying biological sex differences in obesity determinants are relatively similar, the higher level of obesity in non-Hispanic African-American females compared with that in non-Hispanic white females might be due to higher levels of occurrence of the behavioral risk factors implied above in the African-American female population (overeating, low levels of activity, less effective weight control) (Kumanyika, 1998).

Sex differences in energy metabolism are not observed in all species, but when differences are observed, females are more obese (Hoyenga and Hoyenga, 1982). A convincing scenario can be constructed in which differential evolutionary pressures on males and females would lead females to be smaller (i.e., shorter) than males and females to have less muscle but to be more efficient users of energy (Hoyenga and Hoyenga, 1982), as follows. In mammals, sex differences in body size appear to occur in relation to the degree of differentiation in reproductive roles. Larger size confers a greater advantage with respect to the reproductive roles usually held by males (e.g., competition for territory, defense of the group, and competition for females). The greater muscle mass in human

TABLE 5-4 Obesity Prevalence Data for Selected U.S. Adults, by Sex

Group	Percent Males	Females	Female:Male
Non-Hispanic whites, 1988–94, age ≥20[a]	20	23	1.2
Non-Hispanic whites, 1988–91, age ≥25, <grade 12 education[b]	39	39	1.0
Non-Hispanic whites, 1988–91, age ≥25, grade 12 education[b]	36	38	1.1
Non-Hispanic whites, 1988–91, age ≥25, >grade 12 education[b]	30	30	1.0
Non-Hispanic African Americans, 1988–94, age ≥20[a]	21	37	1.8
Non-Hispanic African Americans, 1988–91, age >25, <grade 12 education[b]	29	55	1.8
Non-Hispanic African Americans, 1988–91, age ≥25, grade 12 education[b]	29	51	1.8
Non-Hispanic African Americans, 1988–91, age ≥25, >grade 12 education[b]	36	49	1.4
Mexican Americans, 1988–94, age ≥20 [b]	21	33	1.6
Mexican Americans, 1988–91, age ≥25, <grade 12 education[b]	39	53	1.4
Mexican Americans, 1988–91, age ≥25, grade 12 education[b]	43	40	0.9
Mexican Americans, 1988–91, age ≥25, >12 grade education [b]	40	47	1.2
Puerto Ricans, 1982–84, age 20–74[b]	25	37	1.5
Cuban Americans 1982–84, age 20–74[b]	29	34	1.2
American Indians in OK, 1994–96[b] (questionnaire)	38	36	0.9
American Indians in NM and AZ, 1994–96[b] (questionnaire)	33	34	1.0
American Indians in WA and OR, 1994–96[b] (questionnaire)	33	43	1.3
American Indians in ND and SD, 1994–96[b] (questionnaire)	46	47	1.0
Alaska Natives, 1996[b] (questionnaire)	41	30	1.0
Asian Americans, ages 18–59[c] (questionnaire)	57	38	0.7
Samoans in Manu'a[b]	56	77	1.4
Samoans in Oahu[b]	75	80	1.1

[a] Obesity was defined as a body mass index of ≥30 kilograms per square meter.

[b] Obesity was defined as a body mass index of >27.8 kilograms per square meter for males and a body mass index of ≥ 27.3 kilograms per square meter for females.

[c] Obesity was defined as a body mass index of ≥25 kilograms per square meter.
SOURCES: Lauderdale and Rathouz (2000); National Heart, Lung, and Blood Institute, National Institutes of Health (1998); and Will et al. (1999).

males would be consistent with this. Greater metabolic efficiency would confer resistance to starvation in times of limited food supplies or of cycles of feast and famine. This would be more advantageous for the females of species in which the main role of females is not only to bear the offspring but also to rear them until they are independent and would particularly apply in cases of a long period of dependency of the offspring. Low levels of heat production per calorie consumed would promote starvation resistance but would predispose an individual to store fat during periods with increased food supplies. The link between reproductive function and energy balance implies that progesterone and possibly estrogen affect processes related to food intake, weight gain, heat production, and heat loss. Some such effects can apparently be identified in the perinatal period (Hoyenga and Hoyenga, 1982).

Current approaches to the study of sex differences in energy metabolism and obesity are compatible with the general view that there are physiologically mediated differences in energy regulation, storage, and utilization. Many differences appear to be mediated by male-female differences in fat patterning, for example, the amounts, types, and metabolic characteristics of fat in the abdominal and gluteal-femoral regions (Björntorp, 1989). Mechanisms under study include hormonal influences on appetite regulation (Hassink et al., 1996; Kennedy et al., 1997; Roca et al., 1999), energy expenditure (Nicklas et al., 1997), gastric emptying time (Gryback et al., 1996), resting metabolic rate (Carpenter et al., 1998; Weyer et al., 1999), use of fatty acids as energy sources and rate of mobilization of fatty acids (Fletchner-Mors et al., 1999; Laws et al., 1997; Lonnqvist et al., 1997; Sumner et al., 1999), and changes in body composition and energy metabolism associated with menopause (Poelhman and Tchernof, 1998) or puberty (Molnár and Schutz, 1997).

Females are less likely to mobilize fat from certain adipose tissue stores (Laws et al., 1997; Lonnqvist et al., 1997; Sumner et al., 1999), although this varies with age and ethnicity. The gluteal-femoral fat depots in females are much larger than those in males and have higher lipoprotein lipase activity, which promotes the uptake of lipid and greater α-adrenergic activity than β-adrenergic activity, which promotes the retention of fat in the cells. Changes in the lipid-accumulating patterns of cells in this fat depot are observed with pregnancy (increased) or menopause (decreased), consistent with the theory that this aspect of female fat accumulation and fat metabolism has a reproduction-related function (Björntorp, 1989). In addition, within the abdominal area, females demonstrate more lipolytic activity in subcutaneous fat, whereas visceral fat is more active in males. These differences do not apply after menopause.

The finding that age- and sex-related differences are mediated primarily by changes in the energy density rather than the volume of foods consumed (Marti-Henneberg et al., 1999) implies sex differences in appetite regulation. Studies of sex differences in levels of circulating leptin—a hormone involved in appetite regulation—also suggest sex differences in appetite regulation. Higher leptin levels occur in females at all levels of body weight, with a steeper gradient of increase in leptin levels occurring with obesity in females. However, an increase in abdominal fat levels and insulin resistance associated with leptin levels was observed only in males. Leptin levels were always higher in obese girls than in obese boys. These studies suggest that girls are relatively resistant to the appetite-suppressing effects of leptin. The appetite-regulating effects of serotonin (5-OH-tryptophan) may also differ between the sexes (Roca et al., 1999).

Physical Performance

Studies of physical performance and energy metabolism during exercise and physical work suggest intriguing sex differences that may be qualitatively different from the sex differences in energy regulation that are observed under resting conditions (Björntorp, 1989). From an evolutionary perspective, in keeping with sex role differentiation, males may be more adapted than females for brief spurts of intense energy expenditure, whereas females may be more adapted than males for sustained but less intense energy expenditure (Hoyenga and Hoyenga, 1982). For example, under conditions of moderate exercise, females preferentially utilize fatty acids, sparing muscle glycogen reserves and permitting sustained performance (Björntorp, 1989; Tate and Holtz, 1998). This difference could, however, be related to physical training rather than underlying sex differences. In the same vein, sex differences in the ratios of different types of muscle fiber are consistent with a greater potential for oxidative metabolism in the muscles of females. Again, however, these differences may reflect sex differences in muscle morphology that are influenced by behavior (through differences in activity and exercise habits) instead of intrinsic differences. In addition, some part of the sexual dimorphism in muscle fiber composition appears to be mediated by sex hormones; for example, it is not observed after menopause (Björntorp, 1989).

The Institute of Medicine Committee on Military Nutrition Research (1992, 1998) described some major policy implications potentially associated with sex differences in body weight and composition and their relationship to physical performance. With respect to the armed services, a conflict was identified between the standards of body composition required for women to achieve an appearance goal and those necessary for performance of many types of military tasks (Institute of Medicine, 1992). Specifically, among heavy women, greater lean body mass and upper body strength confer advantages for physical fitness and endurance, but higher weights are considered a disadvantage with respect to appearance (that is, the proper "military bearing," which is associated with leanness).

The Committee on Military Nutrition Research observed that both the standards for percent body fat used for eligibility and the methods used for assessment of body composition and evaluation of physical performance varied considerably among the different branches of the military, suggesting a need for evidence on which to base a sound consensus. The 1998 Committee on Military Nutrition Research (Institute of Medicine, 1998) cited the earlier recommendation of the 1992 Committee (Institute of Medicine, 1992) that "body composition standards be based on considerations of task performance and health and be validated with regard to the ethnic diversity of the military" (Institute of Medicine, 1998, p. 2).

The need to improve the scientific basis for sex-specific criteria for body size and composition for military performance is evident (Institute of Medicine, 1998). The fundamental questions are whether and under what circumstances men and women can be held to similar performance standards and what health or reproductive benefits or risks accrue to women under these circumstances.

Bone Metabolism and Osteoporosis

Osteoporosis is a disorder of low bone mass, microarchitectural degeneration, and bone weakness that leads to fracture. The most common sites of osteoporotic fracture are the thoracic vertebrae and femoral neck (hip). Fifteen percent of all Caucasian women in the United States and 35 percent of women in the United States over age 65 have osteoporosis; one of every two Caucasian women will suffer an osteoporotic fracture in her lifetime (*American Journal of Medicine*, 1993), a lifetime risk similar to the combined risk of developing breast, endometrial, and ovarian cancer (Holbrook et al., 1985). The rate of mortality within the first year after fracture is 15 to 20 percent; less than one-third of fracture patients return to their prior functional status.

The bones of humans reach their peak mass in the third or fourth decade of life. Thereafter, men lose bone density at a slow, steady pace (0.3 to 0.5 percent per year). Women lose bone density at this same pace until menopause, at which time they lose 2 to 3 percent per year for approximately 10 years and then resume a rate of loss comparable to that in men (Khosla et al., 1999). Osteoporosis results when the rate of bone resorption by osteoclasts outstrips the rate of bone formation by osteoblasts (Manolagas, 2000).

Bone is composed of a honeycomb-like structure (trabecular bone in vertebral bodies and the femoral neck) and dense bone (cortical bone in the outside tube-like structures of long bones). Trabecular bone has a greater surface area per gram of mineral and is more likely to be subjected to osteoclastic degradation than cortical bone. Trabecular struts, like the architectural cross-struts that support bridges, give strength to bone. In osteoporosis, these struts erode through, weakening bone strength disproportionately to the amount of calcium loss.

Many factors contribute to bone health. Regarding the whole organism, both body size and frailty are important factors in clinical osteoporosis: large people have large bones and are less likely than small people to suffer a fracture. Heavy people have subcutaneous fat to absorb trauma in falls and are therefore less likely than thin people to suffer a fracture if they fall. Old people have relatively slow reflexes and frequent gait disturbances and are thus more likely than young people to fall.

Behavioral habits contribute to bone strength: weight-bearing exercise creates strong bone structure; loss of weight bearing, for example, during space travel or bed rest, weakens bone (Turner, 1999). Extreme exercise resulting in amenorrhea causes bone loss (Drinkwater et al., 1984; Hobart and Smucker, 2000). Caloric repletion, however, restores the menses and protects the bones (Warren and Stiehl, 1999). Smokers are at high risk for the development of osteoporosis (Kato et al., 2000).

Hormones are also important to bones. Both estrogen and testosterone are critical for achievement and maintenance of peak bone mass. A deficiency of either hormone in both men and women or a deficiency of growth hormone reduces bone mass (Braidman et al., 2000). Rapid bone turnover can result in osteoporosis (Garnero et al., 1996; Ross and Knowlton, 1998). Bone resorption follows a circadian cycle, being maximal at night.

Among the various life events that affect bones, pregnancy and lactation divert calcium from the mother's bones to the baby; if the mother does not replete her calcium, she will suffer a net bone loss (Black et al., 2000; Horst et al., 1997).

Genetic factors also affect bones. In controversial studies, different alleles of the vitamin D receptor make individuals' susceptibilities to osteoporosis different. Mutations of the collagen I gene, as in osteogenesis imperfecta, lead to extremely weak bones (Heegaard et al., 2000; McGuigan et al., 2000).

Various environmental factors affect bones. Dietary calcium and vitamin D (from diet or sun exposure) are required for bone formation, and calcium and vitamin D deficiencies during childhood cause rickets. Calcium requirements differ by age and sex: infants should obtain 400 to 600 mg of calcium per day, children should obtain 800 mg per day, adolescents should obtain 1,200 to 1,500 mg per day, premenopausal women should obtain 1,000 mg per day, and postmenopausal women should obtain 1,000 to 1,500 mg per day. Men under age 65 should obtain 1,000 mg of calcium per day, and men over age 65 should obtain 1,500 mg per day.

Many pharmaceutical agents cause bone loss. Corticosteroids, for instance, hinder the actions of osteoblasts, promote renal calcium loss, and inhibit the absorption of dietary calcium. Other drugs that cause bone loss are heparin, thyroxin, and several anticonvulsants, while diuretics prevent calcium loss.

The major risk factors for osteoporosis are positive family history, weight less than 127 pounds and current tobacco use. Lesser risk factors are white race, female sex, age more than 65 years, postmenopausal status, low levels of calcium intake, alcoholism, sedentary life style, and chronic illness (Huopio et al., 2000). Bone strength thus has genetic, hormonal, life stage, life event, behavioral, and environmental components. Those factors that contribute most to the predominance of osteoporosis among women are estrogen loss at menopause, lower levels of exercise among women, lower levels of sun exposure among women, and pregnancy.

Exposures and Different Patterns of Melanoma Occurrence and Survival

The different rates of melanoma between men and women serve as an example of the complex interaction of biology, exposures, and social factors in the manifestation and progression of disease.

Melanoma, a malignancy of melanocytes (pigment cells), which are primarily found in the skin, is a public health concern for several reasons:

- It is largely preventable; two-thirds of cases are attributable to sun exposure (Gilchrest et al., 1999).
- Most deaths should be avoidable, as most lesions are easily recognized early on, when excision is still curative (Piepkorn, 2000).
- The incidence of melanoma and the rate of mortality from melanoma are increasing more rapidly than those for almost any other malignancy (Koh et al., 1995; National Cancer Institute, 1986; Piepkorn, 2000).
- It is the most common fatal malignancy in young adults (Kosary et al., 1996).

The incidence of melanoma is slightly higher among women than men, but the rate of mortality from melanoma is higher among men (Stidham et al., 1994; Tsao et al., 1998). Both sex and gender differences appear to play important roles in the risk for melanoma.

Most melanomas can be attributed to ultraviolet (UV) light-induced mutations in key regulatory genes in melanocytes; UV light-induced cutaneous immune suppression may also contribute to melanoma (Piepkorn, 2000). Risk factors include fair skin, red or blonde hair, easy sunburning (specifically, a history of sunburns during childhood), a large number of nevi (benign proliferations of pigment cells, commonly called "moles"), and a family history of melanoma (Piepkorn, 2000). Melanomas are statistically associated with intermittent sun exposure and occur on body sites intermittently exposed to the sun (Bentham and Aase, 1996; Nelemans et al., 1993). In men the midback is the most common site, and in women the posterior calves are the most common site (Piepkorn, 2000). Because melanocytes are present in approximately equal numbers and have the same distribution over the body in both sexes, it is difficult to invoke a biological explanation for these differences in the locations of occurrence of melanoma; instead, the differences are attributed to clothing styles. The startling increase in the incidence of melanoma over the past 70 years, from a 1 in 1,500 to a 1 in 75 lifetime risk for Americans (Koh et al., 1995; Piepkorn, 2000), may reflect the increasing popularity of revealing bathing suits and other casual attire.

The possibility that hormones influence melanoma has long been a subject of debate. The darkness of skin pigmentation at some body sites is affected by estrogenic hormones (Abdel-Malek, 1998). For example, pregnancy is associated with melasma (a reticulated facial pigmentation also known as the "mask of pregnancy"), the linea nigra (hyperpigmentation extending from the umbilicus to the pubic area along the midline), and darkening of the areolae (Abdel-Malek, 1998). Several studies suggest an adverse effect of pregnancy on the prognosis of melanoma (Piepkorn, 2000), and melanoma cells have been reported to express estrogen receptors (Piepkorn, 2000). Melanoma is also influenced by immune factors. For example, melanoma is responsive to adjuvant immunotherapy (Piepkorn, 2000). Altered immune status during pregnancy may contribute to the spread of melanoma.

Men age 50 or older have a striking excess rate of mortality due to melanoma compared with that for women (Tsao et al., 1998). It is unclear whether this reflects biological or behavioral differences. It is known, however, that most melanomas are first suspected by women, whether the lesions are on themselves or on their spouses, and that women then arrange for physician examination (Koh et al., 1992).

Such observations suggest ways in which both sex and gender figure in the incidence and prognosis of melanoma. Sun exposure histories between men and women differ because of occupational and recreational sun exposures, clothing styles, and willingness to apply sunscreens. These gender-specific issues may influence who develops melanoma and at what site. Gender-specific influences can then be compounded by sex- and gender-neutral biological factors. For example, midback lesions (most common in men) carry a worse prognosis than lesions on other body sites (Piepkorn, 2000). Once a melanoma has developed, hormonal differences may influence the probability of disease spread; and differences in body awareness and social priorities may influence how quickly medical attention is sought, with a large consequent influence on the prognosis. Thus, a better understanding of the contributions of sex and gender differences to melanoma may have an enormous effect on the incidence and prognosis of this devastating malignancy.

SEX DIFFERENCES IN AUTOIMMUNE CONDITIONS

Because certain rheumatic, hepatic, and thyroid autoimmune diseases are predominant in females but other autoimmune diseases are not, the fact of autoimmunity alone does not explain the sex differences in autoimmune disease incidence. In humans, exposure and other extrinsic factors explain most sex differences in the incidence of infectious diseases. If infections induce autoimmune diseases, differences in exposure may likely explain the sex differences.

Background

Most mammals respond to infections with a combination of innate (inflammatory) and adaptive (immune responses (Medzhitov and Janeway, 2000). Infectious agents include viruses, prions, bacteria, mycobacteria, fungi, and parasites. The innate response engulfs, walls off, and, when appropriate, kills the invader with toxic cell products. The innate immune response recruits and in part directs the cells of the adaptive immune response. Adaptive immunity recruits and engages memory cells and their products to assist inflammatory cells. Autoimmunity occurs when the adaptive immune system attacks normal tissue. Autoimmunity may result from a normal immune response to an invading organism gone awry or from the loss of normal immune regulation.

The levels and types of models used to study infection and inflammation are listed in Box 5-2. Each can be tested by use of various challenges: spontaneous or induced infection, vaccination, and response to common environmental stimuli. Spontaneous illness constitutes another form of test.

Sex Differences in Types of Exposure and Portals of Entry

Portals of entry into the intact body include the skin; eyes; mouth, gastrointestinal tract, and rectum; nasal passages and lungs; and, in females, the vagina. The urethra is less commonly an entry point, but it may be important in venereal diseases. Exposure may occur through direct penetration, as from a knife wound or transmission of a parasite through an insect bite; indirect penetration, such as by radiation; inhalation of a gas, aerosol, or organism; percutaneous absorption (through the skin); ingestion; or absorption from a mucosal surface.

Sex differences in types of exposure and portals of entry are rarely

---

BOX 5-2
Levels and Types of Models for Study of
Infection and Inflammation

Whole organism (in its environment). This level describes the interaction of an animal or person with its society or with its environment, for instance, the response to a living or inanimate agent.

Whole organism (independent of its environment). This level considers hormones, chronobiology (menstrual cycling), and life events (pregnancy).

Organ models. This model considers sex differences in organs or organ systems, for instance, cellular elements of the immune system.

Cell model. This model considers individual cells, such as lymphocytes and vascular endothelial cells, which may differ intrinsically.

Molecular and genetic models. These models consider cell phenotypes, which reflect sex-specific genetic coding or responsiveness to single protein signals or sex differences at the chromosome and gene levels.

---

studied. Hypothetically, for behavioral and social reasons, males may experience more penetrating trauma and may inhale higher levels of toxic (industrial) materials. In general, a male's skin may be exposed to more (industrial) toxins, and female's skin may be exposed to more toxins in detergents and cosmetics. In the course of work or relaxation, males may be more likely to place more unusual materials (building nails, tobacco pipes) in their mouths. In addition, males and females may have different diets. Females have a mucosal surface (vagina) absent from males and encounter products and agents (tampons, semen, medical instruments, douches) through vaginal insertion that males do not. Furthermore, in females the cervical barrier between the internal and the external environments is transiently broken during menstruation. Finally, sexual practices present different types of exposure for males and females.

Normal Processes

Innate and Adaptive Immunities

This section reviews differences in innate and adaptive immunities between females and males. Gonadal hormones partly control these normal defense systems. The literature on the nonhormonal effects of sex on mechanisms of innate and adaptive immunities is sparse, however.

Adaptive immunity varies markedly by sex; innate immunity varies less. Mature young females mount more vigorous immune responses than others. Whole-organism elements of inflammation and immunity include cycling, hormones, growth and nutrition, life stages, and life events (discussed below). Of these, only hormones have been extensively studied.

Chronobiological events occur over short intervals (e.g., brain waves and heart beat), days (sleep cycle), weeks (menstrual cycle), or years (seasonal cycles) (Young, 2000). Male and female chronobiologies, that is, menstrual or estrous cycles, should thus be considered separately from the associated hormonal changes. Both sleep deprivation and jet lag, examples of chronobiological events, are immunosuppressive (Ishida et al., 1999). Hypothetically, a chronobiological effect on immunity may occur in menstruating females or may render a fertile female vulnerable at certain times of the month. Studies that have compared exogenously cycled and noncycled castrated animals have not been done.

Leukocytes and their products constitute the innate immune system. Leukocyte function, which is assessed by cellular synthesis of degradative enzymes (Kuslys et al., 1996), oxidative metabolism (Garcia-Duran et al., 1999), and adherence and phagocytosis (Ito et al., 1995; Josefsson et al., 1992; Miller, 1999; Mondal and Rai, 1999; Spitzer, 1999; Spitzer and Zhang, 1996a,b; St. Pierre Schneider et al., 1999), is modulated by estrogen. Some estrogen-induced changes increase the levels of functioning of leukocytes in females; others decrease their level of functioning. Overall changes are small, and sex differences in levels of leukocyte functioning probably do not affect human illness.

The adaptive immune response includes activation and suppression of T and B lymphocytes, macrophages, and dendritic cells; secretion of their cytokine products; production of immunoglobulin antibodies; and activation of the complement and coagulation systems.

The adaptive immune response of females, as measured by determination of the level of cell proliferation or immunoglobulin levels, is more vigorous than that of males. The sex differences are relatively small. Comparable differences are seen between Caucasians and African Americans and between young and old individuals. Persons with chronic inflammatory illnesses have activated immune systems. The implication of the differences between males and females is unknown.

As a rule, estrogenic hormones upregulate and androgenic hormones downregulate the cellular effectors of human adaptive immunity: lymphocytes, macrophages, and dendritic cells (Ahmed and Talal, 1999; Kanda et al., 1999). The adaptive immune response varies during the menstrual cycle. However, most experiments on immune cells examine specific questions (e.g., does estradiol upregulate expression of a certain substance without considering physiological age, menstrual cycle, or other

TABLE 5-5   Sex Differences in Immunocytes as Determined in Representative Recent Studies

Human

Estrogen stimulates mononuclear cell nitric oxide synthase (Stefano et al., 1999)

Estrogen stimulates macrophage inflammatory mediators (D'Agostino et al., 1999)

Lymphocyte glutathione S-transferases are not correlated with sex (Van Lieshout et al., 1998)

Stress and depression downregulate hypopituitary-pituitary-adrenal axis (Olff, 1999)

CD4/CD8 ratios are higher in Guinean girls (Lisse et al., 1997)

Estrogen decreases apoptosis of mononuclear cells of menstruating women (Evans et al., 1997)

Estrogen inhibits monocyte interleukin 1 production (Morishita et al., 1999)

Animal

Estrogen downregulates monocyte adhesion and migration in females (rabbits) (Nathan et al., 1999)

Estrogen receptor is nonfunctional in male thymocytes (mice) (Kohen et al., 1998)

Lymph nodes from myelin basic protein-immunized male mice are less encephalitogenic than those from female mice (Kim and Voskuhl, 1999)

Intracerebroventricular interleukin 1 beta upregulates progesterone and prolactin in females but not males (rats) (Turnbull and Rivier, 1995)

Mononuclear cell binding to atheromas is lower in hypercholesterolemic females (rabbits) (Holm et al., 1998)

Estrogen upregulates Bcl-2 and blocks tolerance (mice) (Bynoe et al., 2000)

variables (Lockshin, 1999). Reviews are readily available (Cannon and St. Pierre, 1997; Cutolo et al., 1995; Draca, 1995; Gaillard and Spinedi, 1998; Kammer and Tsokos, 1998; Marchetti et al., 1998; Wilder, 1995). Representative recent data are displayed in Table 5-5.

The hypothalamic-pituitary-adrenal-gonadal axis, which exerts important control on the adaptive immune system, differs between males and females. Exercise, stress, and depression all downregulate immune function (Irwin, 1999; Nehlsen-Cannarella et al., 1997). Since each of these differs between the sexes, sex differences in the resultant illness may occur.

Immunization

Sex-specific studies of responses to immunizations with vaccines show intriguing serological differences (differences in circulating antibody levels) but few clinical differences between females and males (Table 5-6). Sex differences in serological response are not generalizable among organisms. Adverse systemic reactions to immunization, particularly arthritis, are more common in females.

TABLE 5-6 Sex Differences in Immunization

Reference	Disease	Finding
Trollfors (1997)	Pertussis	No sex difference
Singh and Datta (1997)	Measles	No sex difference in antibody response
Singh et al. (1999)	Measles	Girls have higher case fatality rates (because of a lack of immunization)
Atabani et al. (2000), Forthal et al. (1995)	Measles	Antibody-dependent cellular cytotoxicity is lower in females, but neutralizing antibody levels are equal in both sexes
Sankilampi et al. (1997)	Pneumococcal infection	Elderly women have lower antibody levels
Nichol et al. (1996)	Influenza	More systemic adverse reactions in females
Govaert et al. (1993)	Influenza	More local adverse reactions in females
Cardell et al. (1999), Havlichek et al. (1997)	Hepatitis B	Seroconversion rates are equivalent in males and females
Chiaramonte et al. (1996)	Hepatitis B	Antibody titers are higher in young women
Chen et al. (1997)	Hepatitis A	Antibody titers are higher in females
Benjamin et al. (1992)	Rubella	Arthritis is 3.5 times more common in girls
Rebiere and Galy-Eyraud (1995)	Mumps	No sex difference in risk of developing vaccination meningitis

Pregnancy

Estradiol levels increase 100-fold and estriol levels increase 1,000-fold during human pregnancy. Within these ranges, estrogens upregulate immune functions, but clinically evident immunological changes during pregnancy are small. Pregnancy-specific proteins suppress lymphocyte function. Changes differ at different stages of pregnancy, with no apparent general pattern. Cutaneous and humoral immune responses to specific microbial antigens are selectively depressed, as are leukocyte chemotaxis and adhesion. Overall, during pregnancy the immune system deviates markedly from that during the nonpregnant state; the long-term effects, if any, of this deviation on women's biology or health are unknown. Specific infections, such as those caused by the measles virus, appear to be particularly virulent in pregnant women.

The striking sex difference in many autoimmune disorders is incompletely understood. A new aspect under study is the role of fetal cells transferred to the maternal blood (microchimerism) (Bianchi, 2000) and their persistence postpartum, in some instances for decades, in the pathogenesis of scleroderma (also called systemic sclerosis, a connective tissue disorder that leads to fibrosis of skin and internal organs). In women with scleroderma who had given birth to at least one son before disease onset, male DNA was detected more often and in larger amounts in their blood than in their normal sisters who had given birth to one or more sons (Artlett et al., 1998; Nelson, 1998; Nelson et al., 1998). Persistent microchimerism of maternal lymphocytes in the circulation of offspring occurs as well, but its relationship, if any, to autoimmune disorders, is not yet known. The implications of the association between autoimmune disorders and fetal microchimerism are unknown. The findings, however, do indicate a profound biological difference between men and women that may be relevant to sex ratios of disease.

Abnormal Processes

Infectious Disease

General Principles   Males do not differ from females in terms of their responses to infections, regardless of whether the invading organism is a virus, bacterium, mycobacterium, or parasite. In experiments with animals in controlled settings, males are more susceptible to parasites, fungi, bacteria, and viruses (Klein, 2000), probably because of hormonal effects. Most sex differences in humans, however, are caused by differences in exposures (a societal level effect) instead of differences between males and females at the individual, organ, or cell level. The following are examples of sex differences caused by different exposures:

* *Exposure.* Sex differences in attack rates occur with kuru (a disease caused by a prion), in which, for cultural reasons, only females eat the infected tissue; tuberculosis, when it is contracted in prison or homeless shelters; and infection with human immunodeficiency virus (HIV) when it is transmitted by male homosexual intercourse or needle sharing.
* *Portal of entry.* Differences in genitourinary anatomies and local immune responses cause different clinical phenotypes of gonorrhea and herpes genitalis.
* *Organism load.* Sex differences in organism loads are especially relevant in HIV infection; in part, these differences are also a function of portal of entry.
* *Receptors.* In experimental coxsackievirus myocarditis, male mouse hearts contain more viral receptors and receive higher viral loads.

TABLE 5-7   Sex Differences in Viral Infections in Humans

Reference	Disease	Finding
Suligoi (1997)	HIV infection	Females are at higher risk of infection, but there is no difference in the rate of progression to AIDS
Swanson et al. (1995)	Herpes	Males have higher-risk behavior
Sullivan et al. (1999)	Rubella	Male/female incidence ratio = 2, likely because of lower immunization rates for boys
Benn et al. (1997)	Measles	Vitamin A affects the antibody concentration in males more than in females
Dollimore et al. (1997)	Measles	Same incidence in boys and girls, higher fatality rate in girls

- *Social response.* Clinical acknowledgment of illness, particularly in the face of stigma, may differ between males and females, as may compliance with therapy. Tuberculosis and leprosy in developing countries are examples.
- *Response to therapy.* Sex differences in response to therapy are discussed below in terms of drug metabolism.

Virus   In humans, sex differences in viral illnesses are primarily due to differences in behavior, such as vaccination rates or exposure (Table 5-7). The apparent higher rate of fatality from measles in girls is not explained, and the different effects of vitamin A on antibody titers in males and females are controversial. In animals, sex differences of virus effects occur in both directions.

Bacteria   Bacterial diseases affect males and females approximately equally. Even in the conversion of acute to chronic Lyme disease (an illness that closely resembles autoimmune disease), the incidence and severity in males and females are similar (Pena and Strickland, 1999).

Mycobacteria, Fungi, and Parasites   Males animals are slightly more susceptible to infection with mycobacteria, fungi, and parasites (Klein, 2000). In humans, sex-specific rates of infection with mycobacteria, fungi, and parasites are approximately equal; most differences can be explained by differences in exposures (Table 5-8).

Leprosy and Chagas' disease induce lupus autoantibodies and tuberculosis induces rheumatoid factor, but these diseases do not induce clinical autoimmune disease in humans. Data are scant, but infected males

TABLE 5-8 Sex Differences in Mycobacterial, Fungal, and Parasitic Diseases

Reference	Disease	Finding
Holmes et al. (1998)	Tuberculosis	Disease rates are higher in males; young women progress from infection to disease more frequently
Hudelson (1996)	Tuberculosis	Females have more exposure risk, are less compliant with therapy
Freire et al. (1998)	Leprosy	Ninety-four percent of antineutrophil cytoplasmic antibody-positive patients are male
Rao et al. (1996)	Leprosy	Longer delay in identifying skin changes in women
Corredor Arjona et al. (1999)	Trypanosomiasis, Chagas' disease	No sex differences in positivity by enzyme-linked immunosorbent assay
Albarracin-Veizaga et al. (1999)	Chagas' disease	Females are more frequently seropositive
Michael et al. (1996)	Filariasis	More prevalent in males
Rogier et al. (1999)	Malaria	Incidences are the same in boys and girls

and females do not differ in their autoimmune responses to these diseases.

Autoimmune Disease

Definition, Classification, and Female/Male Ratios In autoimmunity the immune response is directed against host antigens instead of foreign invaders. The host antigens are either localized, as in thyroid and skin diseases, or ubiquitous, as in lupus. Autoimmunity characterizes the prototypical diseases whose occurrences differ by sex. Autoimmune diseases pose the central question for the study of such sex differences: what mechanisms explain discrepancies in disease occurrences by sex? Explaining sexual dimorphisms in autoimmune diseases will likely bring to light heretofore unknown important biological differences between females and males.

Autoimmunity is defined to occur when an antibody binds to or reacts with an autoantigen (an extract of a normal tissue). Cell-mediated mechanisms may participate in autoimmunity (Draca, 1995; Marchetti et al., 1998; Olff, 1999; Wilder, 1995). Other causes of autoimmunity include immunization and passive transfer of antibodies in animal models or participation of the major histocompatibility complex (MHC). There is no consensus definition, however. The different definitions and classifications partly explain why different diseases are named autoimmune diseases in standard medical texts. Most authorities agree that thyroid and

TABLE 5-9   Female/Male Ratios Associated with
Common Autoimmune Diseases

Disease	Female/Male Ratio
Hashimoto thyroiditis	10
Primary biliary cirrhosis	9
Chronic active hepatitis	8
Graves' hyperthyroidism	7
Systemic lupus erythematosus[a]	6
Scleroderma	3
Rheumatoid arthritis	2.5
Idiopathic thrombocytopenic purpura[a]	2
Multiple sclerosis	2
Autoimmune hemolytic anemia	2
Pemphigus	1
Type I diabetes[a]	1
Pernicious anemia	1
Ankylosing spondylitis	0.3
Goodpasture nephritis/pneumonitis	0.2

NOTE: Not all diseases are predominant in females.
  [a]Age specific.

rheumatic diseases are autoimmune diseases; they differ about inflammatory bowel disease, multiple sclerosis, some skin diseases, and juvenile-
onset diabetes.

Some autoimmune diseases are strikingly predominant in females,
others are not predominant in either sex, and still others are predominant
in males. Table 5-9 lists several such diseases. The female/male ratios
vary 50-fold. Predominance in females applies to some, but not all, of
these diseases.

The label "predominant in females" is commonly used for human
illness and refers to sex differences in incidence. By contrast, in parallel
diseases in experimental animals, the term often refers to differences in
disease severity. In human autoimmune diseases, severity is similar in
females and males.

Environmental Causes of Autoimmunity   The likelihood that environmental factors (toxins and infections) induce autoimmune disease is supported by the diseases and circumstances listed in Table 5-10. In several
exogenously induced mimics of autoimmune disease, sex differences in
disease occurrence are caused by exposure differences. These diseases are
described here.

Drug-induced lupus (Yung et al., 1997) and toxin-induced scleroderma-like disease (Abaitua Borda et al., 1998; Shulman, 1990) loosely
resemble but are not identical to idiopathic autoimmune diseases, sug-

TABLE 5-10 Autoimmune Diseases in Which Environmental Triggers Are Prominent

Agent	Disease	Sex
Toxin	Scleroderma-like disease	M, F[a]
	Drug-induced lupus	M
Infection	Cryoglobulinemia	F
	Chronic Lyme disease	–
	Fogo selvagem	–
	B27 spondyloarthropathy	M
	Subacute bacterial endocarditis	–
	Acute rheumatic fever	–

NOTE: M, males; F, females; –, no sex predominance.

[a]Industrial causes (polyvinyl chloride, mining) are predominant in males; toxic product causes (cooking oil, tryptophan) are predominant in females.

gesting that exogenous agents cause idiopathic autoimmune disease. More males than females take drugs that induce lupus (male predominant), and more males are exposed to silica inducers of scleroderma-like disease (male predominant). In Spain it was found that more females were exposed to the contaminated cooking oil that causes a scleroderma-like illness (female predominant). More females than males took contaminated L-tryptophan, a putatively natural antidepressant; the resulting epidemic of eosinophilia-myalgia syndrome was predominant in females. Chronic Lyme disease is a self-perpetuating autoimmune illness that is initiated by but that does not require the persistence of live *Borrelia burgdorferi* organisms (Carlson et al., 2000). Its incidence has no sex difference, yet it closely resembles rheumatoid arthritis, whose incidence does have a sex difference. Fogo selvagem, or Brazilian endemic pemphigus foliaceus, is transmitted by a black fly bite and is presumed to be caused by an infectious agent passed at the time of the bite. Fogo selvagem shows no sex preference (Hans-Filho et al., 1999), but spontaneous pemphigus foliaceus, which occurs elsewhere in the world, is predominant in females. Contact dermatitis may be predominant in females, but differential exposure to allergens is the likely cause (Kwangsukstith and Maibach, 1995).

The possibility that infection induces rheumatic autoimmune disease is widely (Miller et al., 2000; Montgomery et al., 1999) but not universally (Ringrose, 1999) accepted. It is unknown how infections induce different diseases by sex (other than by different exposure rates). Potential male-female differences in the processing of infecting organisms, differences in vulnerable periods, or differences in threshold immune responses still apply.

Hormonal Causes of Autoimmunity, Including Life Events   Case reports of clinical exacerbation or remission of autoimmune diseases after castration or hormone treatment suggest that gonadal hormone modulation plays an important role in disease severity in individuals but constitutes weak evidence for sexual dimorphisms in disease incidences in populations (Lahita, 1999). Studies of the effects of postmenopausal estrogen or oral contraceptive therapy on autoimmune disease incidence most often show that such therapy has little effect (Petri and Robinson, 1997). Synoviocyte estrogen receptors may be target organs in rheumatoid arthritis (Castagnetta et al., 1999), a possible explanation for the predominance of this illness in females. However, chronic Lyme disease causes a similar joint inflammation but is not predominant in females, and ankylosing spondylitis also causes a similar joint inflammation, but it is predominant in males. Androgens have no apparent role in ankylosing spondylitis (Giltay et al., 1999). Although experimental feminization worsens autoimmune diseases in animal models and experimental masculinization ameliorates autoimmune diseases in animal models, variations in both severity and incidence are found.

Rheumatoid arthritis goes into remission during pregnancy, contradicting the theory of estrogen-enhanced immunological activity. The remission of rheumatoid arthritis is likely due to a human leukocyte antigen (HLA) mismatch between mother and fetus rather than to pregnancy-associated hormones (Nelson et al., 1993; Ostensen, 1999). Multiple sclerosis also goes into remission during pregnancy (Confavreux et al., 1998). Although it is often cited that pregnancy induces the flare-up of lupus, lupus in fact does not worsen or worsens only slightly during pregnancy (Lockshin, 1993). Estrogen replacement therapy, oral contraceptives, and ovulation induction do not worsen lupus (Guballa et al., 2000).

Insight can be gained through the study of rheumatoid arthritis and multiple sclerosis through the study of pregnancy and events during gestation as well as during the postpartum period. In these two diseases, clinical symptoms frequently lessen substantially and can even abate during the third trimester of pregnancy, but the diseases flare soon after delivery.

At the cell level gonadal hormones modulate the immune response. Why and how (if it influences disease incidence at all) this effect influences disease incidence is unclear. Estrogen could play a permissive role, allowing survival of forbidden autoimmune clones. A threshold mechanism, that is, a specific level of estrogen at a vulnerable time, could explain the increase in incidence, but no such threshold has been postulated, tested, or demonstrated in humans. Hormones may also influence the frequency of autoimmune disease in males and females in ways that are independent of the immune system. It is possible that sex differences in the endothelium are critical for disease initiation. A still undiscovered sex difference related to, for example, ovulation- or menstruation-related cytokines, apoptosis of nonimmunological cells, or the presence of vaginal flora or the immune response to vaginal flora may be responsible for the different disease experiences of the two sexes.

Genetic Causes of Autoimmunity Evidence supporting the concept of genetic control of autoimmunity consists of studies with families and twins, the HLA types associated with specific illnesses, the identification of genes that enhance disease susceptibility, and transgenic experiments in which illness is induced in experimental animals (Seldin et al., 1990). Evidence of this type is particularly strong for spondyloarthropathy (Taurog et al., 1999), rheumatoid arthritis, and lupus.

HLA types by themselves do not explain the sexual dimorphism of the genetic causes of autoimmunity (Chen et al., 1999; Greenbaum et al., 2000), although sex differences in HLA-associated disease expression may occur (Lambert et al., 2000). For each haplotype associated with a sexually dimorphic autoimmune disease, there is another haplotype associated with an autoimmune disease that is not sexually dimorphic. For instance, HLA B27 is associated with both spondyloarthropathy (female/male ratio, 0.3) and uveitis (female/male ratio, 1.0), whereas DR3 is associated with Graves' disease (female/male ratio, 7.0), systemic lupus erythematosus (female/male ratio, 6.0), and myasthenia gravis (females/male ratio, 1.0).

With the exception of the CD40 ligand, few putative autoimmune markers identified to date are on the X or Y chromosome. No conclusive evidence for imprinting or X-chromosome inactivation differences exists for autoimmune diseases. The X chromosome has no role in human ankylosing spondylitis (Hoyle et al., 2000). Non-MHC genes may be relevant. In a mouse model of diabetes, mutation of a tissue or a developmental stage-specific proteasome product shows sex differences (Hayashi and Faustman, 1999). The sexual dimorphism of T-cell trafficking may be due to sex-determined cell surface markers or might be secondary to genomic or nongenomic effects.

Life Stage Causes of Autoimmunity Most diseases that are predominant in females cluster in the young-adult years, whereas autoimmune diseases that affect younger or older patients are more evenly divided between the sexes (Table 5-11).

Characteristics of young adulthood that may explain the predominance of a disease in females include the chronobiological effects of menstrual cycles, gonadal hormones, threshold effects, vascular responses, immune responses, vaginal flora, and other as yet unknown variables. Very little experimental work has considered these topics.

TABLE 5-11   Peak Ages of Various Autoimmune Diseases

Disease	Female/Male Ratio	Age (year)
Hashimoto thyroiditis	10	**30-50**
Primary biliary cirrhosis	9	30-75
Chronic active hepatitis	8	**30-50**
Graves' hyperthyroidism	7	**30-50**
Takayasu's arteritis	6	**10-30**
Systemic lupus	6	**15-45**
Idiopathic thrombocytopenic purpura[a]	3	**20-30**
Myasthenia gravis[a]	3	**20-30**
Scleroderma	3	**30-50**
Rheumatoid arthritis[b]	2.5	**20-40**
Dermatomyositis[a]	2.3	1-15
Poststreptococcal glomerulonephritis	2	5-15
Multiple sclerosis	2	**20-35**
Idiopathic thrombocytopenic purpura[a]	1	2-5
Henoch-Schönlein purpura[a]	1	2-5
Insulin-dependent diabetes mellitus	1	2-15
Ulcerative colitis	1	**15-40**
Henoch-Schönlein purpura[a]	1	30-65
Dermatomyositis[a]	1	40-60
Pernicious anemia	1	40-80
Rapidly progressive glomerulonephritis	1	50-70
Myasthenia gravis[a]	1	50-80
Bullous pemphigoid	1	60-75
Giant cell arteritis	0.5	50-90
Immunoglobulin A nephropathy	0.4	10-30
B27 spondyloarthropathy	0.3	**20-50**
Amyotrophic lateral sclerosis	0.3	40-70
Goodpasture nephritis/pneumonitis	0.2	**15-35**

NOTE: Ages that signify "young adulthood" are indicated in boldface. Higher female/male ratios cluster in young adulthood, as do very low female/male ratios.

[a]Two age peaks are listed.

[b]Some studies list an older age range.

SOURCE: Beeson (1994).

Animal Models of Autoimmunity   Animal models of autoimmune disease give mixed messages about the causes of sex differences in autoimmunity. Table 5-12 displays some relevant data for three animal models of human autoimmune diseases, two of which are predominant in females and one of which is dominant in males. Some information is dated and can be challenged by new technology.

Animal models of autoimmune disease use immunization, inbreeding, and transgenic and gene knockout methods. In the model of thyroiditis, different strains of mice and rats are variably susceptible, implying strong genetic control of this disease. Only young adult mice and rats were studied, however. In one rat strain, susceptibility was predominant in females. On the basis of backcross experiments, the X chromosome determines susceptibility. In mice, estrogen enhanced the antithyroid antibody titer (a marker of disease) but not thyroiditis itself. The severity of induced thyroiditis was also found to vary with diet. Thus, genetic, X-chromosome, hormonal, and extrinsic factors may influence the occurrence of thyroiditis.

In mouse models of spontaneous lupus, the incidence and severity of lupus are predominant in NZB × NZW (F1) strain females, whereas they are sex neutral in MRL *lpr/lpr* mice and are predominant in males of the BXSB strain. In animal models, spontaneous autoimmune lupus develops in young adulthood, implying that maturation or cumulative damage is required for disease expression. At maturation, susceptible mouse strains have more numerous and more avid estrogen receptors on lymphoid and uterine tissues than nonsusceptible strains, an explanation of strain susceptibility differences by strain but not of susceptibility differences by sex. Castration and replacement experiments demonstrate estrogen enhancement and testosterone suppression of spontaneous disease. When animals are raised in a germfree environment, however, neither the phenotype nor the disease incidence changes, except that females tend to have higher autoantibody levels than males. Raising animals in a germfree, antigenfree environment ameliorates disease. Males and females in germfree environments are affected equally. Gene knockout experiments give conflicting results. Of the two studies listed, one shows a markedly worse occurrence of glomerulonephritis in females, whereas the other shows equal incidences of glomerulonephritis in both sexes. Thus, in experimental lupus, genetic, hormonal, life stage, and environmental factors all appear to be relevant and sex differences remain unexplained.

The human HLA B27 gene transgenically expressed in rats induces a phenotype with features of psoriasis and ankylosing spondylitis. In a germfree environment, the spondylitis does not occur but the psoriasis does. Introduction of specific gastrointestinal pathogens to the germfree animal induces the spondylitis. The predominance of psoriasis and spondylitis in males is true of this model, as it is of the disease in humans. Genitourinary anatomy, sex hormones, immune response, and unknown factors are possible explanations.

In summary, animal models suggest that autoimmune diseases have specific genetic, hormonal, life stage, and environmental causes. The human sex differences are not reproduced in many of the animal models, but no attempt has been made to understand why.

TABLE 5-12   Animal Models of Human Autoimmune Diseases

Model	Method	Animal	Female/Male Ratio
Thyroiditis	Immunization with thyroglobulin	Mouse	F = M
	Immunization with thyroglobulin	Rat	F > M
Lupus	Spontaneous disease	Mouse	F > M
	Spontaneous disease	Mouse	F = M

Gene	Hormone	Life Stage	Environment
Inbred strains (MHC)	Estrogen enhances antibody level but not clinical disease in susceptible strains (Okayasu et al., 1981)	Young adults tested	Modified by diet (Bhatia et al., 1996)
Inbred strains, polygenic (not MHC), X chromosome (Lillehoj et al., 1981)	Castration; estrogen replacement increases severity and incidence in males	Young adults tested	
Inbred strains, MHC, comple-ment; other immune genes are relevant	Castration; estrogen replacement increases severity and incidence in males (Ahmed and Talal, 1999)	Disease develops in young adulthood (all strains); in the susceptible strain the estrogen receptor is more numerous and has a higher affinity at maturity (Dhaher et al., 2000)	Modified by diet
Inbred strains, MHC, comple-ment; other immune genes are relevant		Disease develops in young adulthood	Germfree; no difference in incidence or severity between males and females or conventionally raised controls (Unni et al., 1975); germfree, antigenfree males but not females have lower lymph node weights than conven-tional controls; the rate of glo merulonephritis is less in germ-free, antigenfree animals (Maldonado et al., 1999)

continued on next page

TABLE 5-12 Continued

Model	Method	Animal	Female/Male Ratio
	Gene knockout	Mouse	F > M
	Gene knockout	Mouse	F = M
Spondylopathy	Transgenic	Rat	F < M

NOTE: In human thyroiditis the female/male ratio is 9, in lupus the female/male ratio is 6, and in spondyloarthropathy the female/male ratio is 0.3. F, female; M, male.

Summary

Gonadal hormones can modulate the adaptive immune response, but hormone effects alone are unlikely to explain the excess incidence of autoimmune illness in females. If gonadal hormones play a role, they must do so through a threshold or permissive mechanism. Although susceptibility to autoimmune illness is regulated by genetic background, no genetic mechanism that would explain sexual dimorphism has yet been postulated. The epidemiological risk factors for the sex-discrepant autoimmune diseases—young age and female sex—are consistent with the differential exposures to causative agents between males and females, the existence of vulnerable periods in females, and threshold effects rather than cell- or organ-level differences in the biologies of females and males. A long period of latency between exposure and clinical disease is possible, complicating the search for etiologies that differ by sex.

A SPECTRUM OF SEX DIFFERENCES ACROSS A DISEASE: CORONARY HEART DISEASE

Coronary heart disease begins in utero, evolves through childhood, and emerges in middle and old age as a devastating and crippling problem. Plaques of cholesterol and other cellular materials are deposited in

Gene	Hormone	Life Stage	Environment
p21, antibody slightly worse in females; severe glomerulonephritis in females (Balomenos et al., 2000)		Disease develops in young adulthood	
DNase I, antibody slightly worse in females (Napirei et al., 2000)		Disease develops in young adulthood	
MHC		Disease develops in young adulthood	Germfree; intestinal bacteria are required for phenotype; more frequent in males (Taurog et al., 1999)

the inner lining of the coronary arteries and over time compromise the flow of blood, causing cell and organ death—myocardial infarction.

Coronary heart disease is a major cause of death in the United States (National Center for Health Statistics, 1999). In general, women manifest symptoms 10 to 20 years later than men (National Center for Health Statistics, 1999) and have a higher prevalence of primary risk factors (Becker et al., 1994; Greenland et al., 1991; Steingart et al., 1991). Men, however, die at an earlier age.

Advances in knowledge about heart disease have led to steady declines in the rates of mortality from heart disease. Yet, many questions remain, and none is more compelling than the differences between the sexes.

Sex Differences in Development of Coronary Heart Disease

The etiologies of coronary heart disease encompass the environment, genetics, age, and lifestyle.

Environment

The most important environmental agents influencing coronary heart disease are diet, drugs, airborne toxins, and, possibly, infectious agents;

and the effects of these agents may be synergistic. For example, overeating or obesity and a sedentary lifestyle promote high blood pressure, high cholesterol, and diabetes, which are major risk factors for coronary heart disease in both males and females. Yet, susceptibilities and responses vary by sex.

Genetics

Dyslipidemias are among the strongest genetic contributors to coronary heart disease (Goldstein et al., 1973a,b; Hazzard et al., 1973). Familial hypercholesterolemia (FH) is a low-density lipoprotein (LDL) cholesterol disorder caused by a genetic defect of the LDL receptor on cells. It is autosomal dominant and is more severe in homozygotes because of a gene dosage effect (Goldstein et al., 1995).

Homozygotic defects occur in about 1 in 1 million individuals, and such individuals present with cholesterol levels that range from 650 to 1,000 milligrams per deciliter (mg/dl); heterozygotic defects occur in about 1 in 500 individuals, and such individuals present with cholesterol levels that range from 350 to 550 mg/dl (Goldstein et al., 1995). Homozygotes develop atherosclerosis, which leads to coronary heart disease and death usually before age 20. Sex differences are undocumented in homozygotes but do occur among heterozygotes; heterozygous males die about 10 years earlier than heterozygous females (Table 5-13). In the FH heterozygote population, the age differences in incidence between the sexes are comparable to those for the general population.

Age

Sex differences in heart disease mortality occur over the life span

TABLE 5-13 Estimated Risk of Symptoms of Coronary Heart Disease and Death from Myocardial Infarction in Heterozygotes at Different Ages

	Percent			
	Male Heterozygotes		Female Heterozygotes	
Age (years)	Symptoms	Deaths	Symptoms	Deaths
40	20	—	3	0
50	45	25	20	2
60	75	50	45	15
70	—	80	75	30

SOURCE: Goldstein et al. (1995, p. 1986).

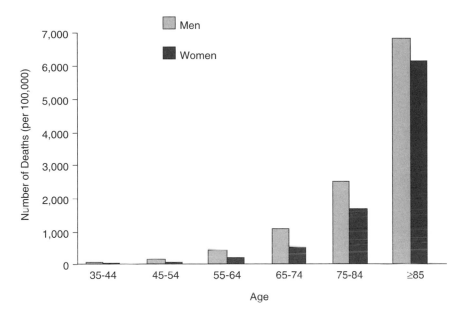

FIGURE 5-3 Death rates for diseases of the heart by age and sex, 1995–1997. Source: National Center for Health Statistics (1999).

between women and men (Figure 5-3). The Barker hypothesis postulates that the genesis of coronary heart disease may begin in utero, perhaps in response to malnutrition and stress (Barker, 2000; see also Chapter 3). The fetus may adapt to the lack of critical nutrients or an excess of maternal stress hormones by permanently altering metabolic, endocrine, and cardiovascular systems in such a manner as to promote atherosclerosis later in life (Barker, 1999).

Several longitudinal studies have demonstrated sex differences in coronary heart disease. The Framingham Heart Study, initiated in 1948 (Dawber et al., 1951), demonstrated that cardiovascular differences exist between the sexes. For example, it established the classical risk factor concept for coronary heart disease. This landmark study showed that a raised serum total cholesterol level, high blood pressure (systolic and diastolic), and smoking increase the risk of developing coronary heart disease in men and women in a graded fashion. Women develop coronary heart disease about 10 years later than men and women's risk is smaller.

The Bogalusa Heart Study followed African-American and Caucasian children over time, beginning in the 1960s, demonstrating that sex differences in risks for coronary heart disease begin at an early age.

The longitudinal Tromso Heart Study (Norway) (Stensland-Bugge et al., 2000) reexamined 3,000 middle-aged women and men in Norway 15 years after an initial examination. Hypertension, total cholesterol levels, high-density lipoprotein (HDL) cholesterol levels, and body mass index independently predicted increased carotid intimal thickness in both women and men. However, triglyceride levels were an independent risk factor in women but not men, whereas physical activity and smoking were independent risk factors in men but not women.

The National Health and Nutrition Examination Survey is a federal epidemiological follow-up study that has collected national data on U.S. residents since the 1960s and that provides evidence of the incidence and prevalence of a variety of health indicators by age, race, and sex (National Center for Health Statistics, 2000b). These data again show differences in cardiovascular disease incidence between the sexes and among racial and ethnic groups. For example, the age-adjusted risk for incident coronary heart disease is higher in African-American women ages 20 to 54 years than in Caucasian women of the same age and lower in African-American men than in Caucasian men of the same age (Gillum et al., 1997).

In terms of risk factors, men have higher prevalences of hypertension, cigarette smoking (until age 65), and excess weight, whereas women have higher prevalences of elevated serum cholesterol levels and obesity (National Center for Health Statistics, 2000a). Regarding the age-specific prevalences of hypertension and serum cholesterol levels greater than 240 mg/dl, men have a higher prevalence than women until about their late 40s and early 50s. After that, the prevalence is higher in women.

These studies underscore the fact that coronary heart disease begins early in life, that it continues across the life span, and that sex differences exist. What they do not demonstrate is why such differences exist.

Cigarette Smoking

Many airborne toxins that are absorbed through the respiratory system predispose an individual to the development of coronary heart disease. One of the most pervasive and lethal of these agents is cigarette smoke.

Cigarette smoking is more frequent among men than women, especially in African Americans (National Center for Health Statistics, 1999) (Table 5-14).

Data from the Centers for Disease Control and Prevention indicate that both men and women who smoke have three times the risk of dying from heart disease as individuals who do not smoke. In women, smoking (Baron et al., 1988; Michnovicz et al., 1986) promotes susceptibility to early menopause and to a number of diseases, including coronary heart disease.

TABLE 5-14 Smoking Prevalence by Race and Sex, 1998

	Percent	
	African American	Caucasian
Males	29	26
Females	21	23

SOURCE: National Center for Health Statistics (1999).

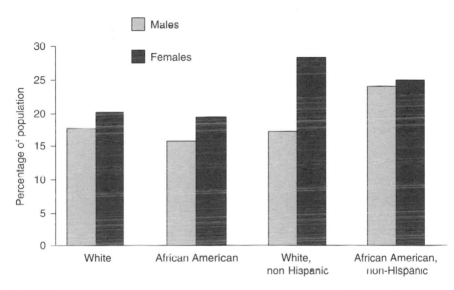

FIGURE 5-4 Age-adjusted high serum cholesterol levels (> 240 mg/dl) among individuals ages 20 to 74 years, by sex and race, 1988–1994 Source: National Center for Health Statistics (1999).

Cholesterol

Sex differences exist in the levels of lipoprotein subfractions of cholesterol: LDL cholesterol, HDL cholesterol, and very-low-density lipoprotein (VLDL) cholesterol (Figure 5-4 and 5-5).

Before menopause, women have higher HDL cholesterol ("good cholesterol") levels and lower LDL cholesterol ("bad cholesterol") levels. During the peri- and postmenopausal periods, however, LDL cholesterol levels rise and HDL cholesterol levels drop. Rates of death from heart disease rise with age in both men and women, but the rate of ascent rises more sharply in women as menopause ensues.

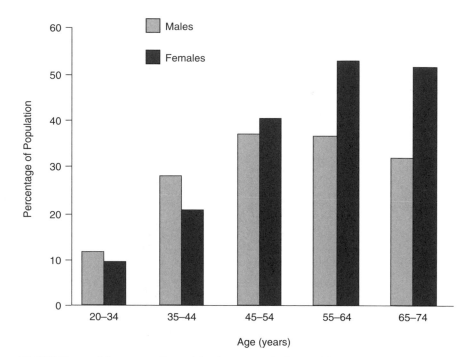

FIGURE 5-5 Non-age-adjusted high serum cholesterol levels (>240 mg/dl) by sex and age. Source: National Center for Health Statistics (1999).

Estrogen affords women a protective advantage against coronary heart disease before menopause. 17-β-Estradiol increases HDL cholesterol levels and decreases LDL cholesterol levels, stimulates nitric oxide, and inhibits vasoconstricting factors (Collins, 2000). These factors may operate independently or synergistically (Collins, 2000). Estrogen also prevents calcium influx through ion channels in the membranes of vascular smooth muscle cells, preventing vessel contraction.

During perimenopause estrogen levels begin to decline and continue to do so through menopause, and HDL cholesterol levels fall as LDL cholesterol levels rise. Hepatic LDL cholesterol receptor activity may explain these changes (Semenkovich and Ostlund, 1987). Another explanation for the increased incidence of cardiovascular disease after menopause is that the LDL cholesterol particles may become denser and therefore less protective (Campos et al., 1988; Haffner et al., 1993).

High triglyceride levels present a greater risk to women than to men. HDL cholesterol levels may be a better predictor than LDL cholesterol levels of coronary heart disease risk in women (Gordon et al., 1989; Jacobs et al., 1990).

As noted above, endogenous estrogen present in premenopausal women appears to have a cardioprotective effect. Observational studies of postmenopausal women taking hormone replacement therapy, and experimental studies with animals, demonstrate that unopposed estrogen has a strong effect in preventing atherosclerosis and its clinical sequelae (Barrett-Connor, 1998a; Barrett-Connor and Grady, 1998). These studies however have not been supported in two large clinical trials of estrogen combined with progestin in women with established coronary disease (Hulley et al., 1998; Herrington et al., 2000). Other clinical trials including women both with and without established coronary disease are currently in progress. As a result, the issue of whether hormone replacement therapy has cardioprotective effects must be considered unresolved.

Hypertension

The causes of hypertension are unknown (Williams, 1991), yet studies suggest multiple factors, polygenetic and environmental. Essential hypertension is the most common form, and it affects a substantial portion of the U.S. population. Risk factors for hypertension include age, sex, smoking, diet, elevated blood cholesterol levels, obesity, diabetes, sedentary lifestyle, and family history.

Hypertension is both a risk factor for coronary heart disease and a disease itself. As a result of hypertension, the heart wall thickens and its function declines. There are differences in the association of hypertension and coronary heart disease by sex (Fiebach et al., 1989; Kannel et al., 1976; Sigurdsson et al., 1984) and race (Johnson et al., 1986).

Men have higher blood pressure levels than women (National Center for Health Statistics, 2000a, p. 245). Height differences as well as differences in mass contribute to differences in blood pressure between men and women. The genesis of hypertension in adulthood often occurs in childhood, and weight is a greater predictor for hypertension in girls than in boys (Cook et al., 1997).

Blood pressure is higher during the follicular phase than during the luteal phase of the menstrual cycle in both normotensive and hypertensive women (Dunne et al., 1991). African-American women respond to stress with a higher diastolic pressure and higher plasma epinephrine levels during the follicular phase than during the luteal phase, but Caucasian women (and men of all ethnicities) do not exhibit any significant change in blood pressure over the course of a month (Ahwal et al., 1997; Mills et al., 1996). These results have been disputed by investigators (Litschauer et al., 1998), who believe that the differences may be caused by an interaction of sex and task characteristics (cause of stress).

The angiotensin-converting enzyme deletion-insertion polymorphism appears to be associated with systemic hypertension in Caucasian men

(O'Donnell et al., 1998). In Japanese men but not Japanese women there is a similar association between angiotensin-converting enzyme gene polymorphism and hypertension (Higaki et al., 2000).

Two hypertension-associated conditions are sex specific: preeclampsia and hypertension of pregnancy. Both conditions are characterized by increasing levels of hypertension as pregnancy progresses and are most common in the last trimester. Both are serious and can be fatal. Whether either of these conditions progresses to coronary heart disease is not understood, although two studies have shown that such a relationship exists (Croft and Hannaford, 1989; Rosenberg et al., 1983).

Diabetes Mellitus

Diabetes mellitus is a risk factor for coronary heart disease and is an example of the sex differences in the risk for coronary heart disease. Premenopausal women, who are not typically at risk for coronary heart disease, are at risk if they have type I (juvenile) or type II (adult-onset, non-insulin-dependent) diabetes mellitus (Figure 5-6).

Rates of mortality from coronary heart disease are two to four times greater in diabetic men than nondiabetic men and three to seven times greater in diabetic women than nondiabetic women (Barrett-Connor and Wingard, 1983; Kannel and Abbott, 1987; Manson et al., 1991; Pan et al., 1986). Diabetes may negate estrogen receptor binding and thereby mitigate the positive estrogenic effect (Ruderman and Haudenschild, 1984).

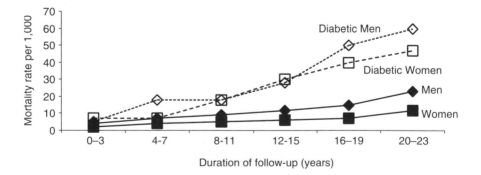

FIGURE 5-6 Mortality from coronary heart disease and diabetes in men and women ages 25 to 64. Source: Krolewski et al. (1991). Reprinted, with permission, from A. S. Krolewski, J. H. Warram, P. Valsania, B. C. Martin, L. M. Laffel, and A. R. Christlieb. 1991. Evolving natural history of coronary artery disease in diabetes mellitus. *American Journal of Medicine* 90:56S–61S. Copyright 1991 by Elsevier Science Ltd.

Diabetes of pregnancy may represent a risk for the development of non-insulin-dependent diabetes mellitus after pregnancy. Current evidence suggests that gestational diabetes is a risk factor for coronary heart disease (Mestman, 1988; O'Sullivan, 1984; Stowers, 1984).

Differences in Presentation of Coronary Heart Disease

The manifestations of coronary heart disease vary in presentation and intensity between women and men (Table 5-15).

Coronary heart disease presents in women 10 to 15 years later than it does in men.

Women often have comorbidities, such as congestive heart failure, hypertension, diabetes, and others. Diabetic women are particularly vulnerable to complications after a myocardial infarction (Greenland et al., 1991).

More men present with myocardial infarction as the initial manifestation of the disease, but the event is more often fatal in women (Greenland et al., 1991; Kannel and Abbott, 1987; Lerner and Kannel, 1986; Murabito et al., 1993; Wenger, 1985). Women admitted with acute myocardial infarction are more likely, on average, to be older than men being admitted and therefore have more severe coronary artery disease. However, in the Framingham study, nearly 66 percent of sudden deaths due to coronary heart disease in women occurred in those with no previous symptoms of disease (Mosca et al., 1999).

TABLE 5-15 Complications of Acute Myocardial Infarctions, by Sex

Complication	Percent		
	Females (N = 1,524)	Males (N = 4,315)	P value
Mechanical complications			
Angina in hospital	8.2	8.8	NS[a]
Congestive heart failure on admission	26.8	24.4	0.02
Cardiogenic shock	11.1	7.4	<0.002
Arrhythmic complications			
Sinus tachycardia	3.2	3.1	NS
Supraventricular arrhythmia	12.1	13.0	NS
Atrioventricular block	12.6	10.0	NS
Ventricular tachycardia	12.9	19.0	<0.005
Ventricular fibrillation	5.8	7.4	0.11
Cardiac arrest	9.8	6.6	<0.0005

[a]NS, not significant.
SOURCE: Greenland et al. (1991).

Among individuals with myocardial infarction, men more often present with ventricular tachycardia and women more often present with cardiogenic shock and cardiac arrest (Greenland et al., 1991; Milner et al., 1999).

Although many women present with "classical" signs and symptoms, some do not. Women are less likely to present with severe chest pain than men and at the time of diagnosis are more likely to be experiencing congestive heart failure (events that may be age rather than sex related).

Sex Differences in Treatment of Coronary Heart Disease (Myocardial Infarction)

Women do not fare as well as men after a myocardial infarction for the following reasons:

- Women with myocardial infarctions are older.
- Women have more "silent" myocardial infarctions.
- Men have larger collateral circulations.

After a myocardial infarction, women younger than 65 years of age are more than twice as likely to die as men of the same age (Vaccarino et al., 1999). Possible explanations include the following:

–Diabetes, heart failure, and stroke are more prevalent in younger women.

–Plaque erosions are more common in premenopausal women who die.

–Arterial narrowing is less and reactive platelets levels are higher in younger women.

–Women are less likely to be given effective interventions, such as aspirin, beta-blockers, and thrombolytic agents.

Differences also extend to the use of different diagnostic and therapeutic procedures, in that women have fewer diagnostic procedures (O'Farrel et al., 2000; Shaw et al., 1994; Steingart et al., 1991; Vaccarino et al., 2001; Wong et al., 2001). A great deal has been posited about whether women are discriminated against or whether mitigating factors account for the differences in assessment of women for coronary heart disease. Certainly, tests for coronary heart disease are more frequently conducted for men.

- Women have less obstructive disease at earlier ages than men, and thus, the noninvasive tests have less predictive value for women (Wenger, 1994).

• Subclinical disease, which occurs in younger women, is two to three times more likely to be myocardial infarction or stroke (Kuller et al., 1995).

• Women have a smaller coronary artery size (lumen). This reduces the possibility of angiography or angioplasty and bypass surgery and thus of diagnosis and a better outcome (Sheifer et al., 2000). However, the technology is gradually changing to accommodate this need.

A 1991 study examined such differences in Massachusetts and Maryland (Ayanian and Epstein, 1991). The findings confirm that women are less likely than men to undergo diagnostic and therapeutic procedures (Table 5-16). Men were between 15 and 45 percent more likely to undergo selected procedures. The investigators (Ayanian and Epstein, 1991) suggest several reasons for such discrepancies:

• physician perception of the severity of the disease in men versus women;
• physician perception of the risks and efficacies of diagnostic and therapeutic procedures between men and women (women have higher rates of mortality after the use of procedures);
• higher rates of admission for women with an absence of true coronary heart disease versus the rates for women with ischemic symptoms;
• patient's perceptions and preferences (women may be more willing to adhere to a lifestyle of medications and limitations than to face surgery); and
• bias in health care delivery.

TABLE 5-16 Male:Female Odds Ratios for Use of Diagnostic Procedures for Coronary Heart Disease

| Disease | Mean (Range) Odds Ratio | | | |
| | Massachusetts | | Maryland | |
	Angiography	Revascularization	Angiography	Revascularization
Any coronary heart disease	1.28 (1.22–1.35)	1.45 (1.35–1.55)	1.15 (1.08–1.22)	1.27 (1.16–1.40)
Myocardial infarction	1.39 (1.23–1.58)	1.31 (1.10–1.51)	1.29 (1.10–1.51)	1.40 (1.02–1.91)

NOTE: Odds ratios were calculated by multiple logistic regression, with adjustment for principal diagnosis, age, secondary diagnosis of congestive heart failure or diabetes mellitus, race, and insurance status.
SOURCE: Ayanian and Epstein (1991).

Racial and ethnic differences exist between the sexes. A surveillance of hospital admissions for myocardial infarction and of in-hospital and out-of-hospital deaths due to coronary heart disease between 1987 and 1994, showed that Caucasian men had the greatest average annual decrease in rates of mortality from coronary heart disease and myocardial infarction, followed by Caucasian women, African-American women, and African-American men. No differences in rates of hospitalization for a first myocardial infarction were evident between men and women over the time studied. Furthermore, over the time period studied, the rate of reinfarction decreased and the rate of survival increased (Rosamond et al., 1998).

Summary

Sex differences in the development, recognition, and treatment of coronary heart disease exist across the life span. There is mounting evidence that these differences are not solely related to hormones. Scientists and clinicians have just begun to appreciate and address these differences by studying the earliest stages of development and the subsequent effects of the internal and external environments. Research to date, however, has posed as many questions as it has answered.

FINDINGS AND RECOMMENDATIONS

Findings

Many diseases affect both sexes, and the diseases often have different frequencies or presentations in males and females; therefore, different preventive, diagnostic, and treatment approaches may be required for males and females. Exposures, susceptibilities, responses to initiating agents, energy metabolism, genetic predisposition, and responses to therapeutic agents are important factors in understanding how each sex responds to insult, injury, disease progression, and treatment (Figure 5-7)

Compounds that may be differentially internalized by males and females include

- foods for energy and nutrients, including vitamins and minerals;
- drugs for diagnostic, prophylactic, therapeutic, or recreational purposes;
- environmental compounds to which exposure is either purposeful (preservatives in foods) or inadvertent (pollutants or secondhand cigarette smoke); and
- microorganisms that act as pathogens or commensals.

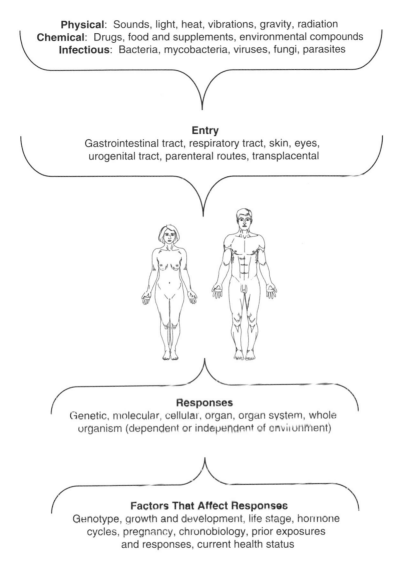

Physical: Sounds, light, heat, vibrations, gravity, radiation
Chemical: Drugs, food and supplements, environmental compounds
Infectious: Bacteria, mycobacteria, viruses, fungi, parasites

Entry
Gastrointestinal tract, respiratory tract, skin, eyes,
urogenital tract, parenteral routes, transplacental

Responses
Genetic, molecular, cellular, organ, organ system, whole
organism (dependent or independent of environment)

Factors That Affect Responses
Genotype, growth and development, life stage, hormone
cycles, pregnancy, chronobiology, prior exposures
and responses, current health status

FIGURE 5-7 External agents.

These compounds can enter the body via the placenta, gastrointestinal tract, respiratory tract, eyes, urogenital tract, the transdermal route, or the parenteral route. Portals of entry can differ between the sexes, affecting types and incidences of disease.

In addition, individuals are exposed to environmental factors such as sensory stimuli (sounds, light, heat), forces (vibration, gravity), and radiation.

Exposures and responses to exogenous agents may be influenced by growth and development; other aging processes; reproductive events; body size and composition; cumulative exposures, prior responses, and current health status; and genotype.

Some exogenous factors (e.g., vitamins) are essential, whereas others are of no apparent consequence and some (e.g., cigarette smoke) are detrimental. Some factors are beneficial at low doses but harmful at high doses (e.g., ultraviolet radiation). It is essential to understand whether males and females respond differently to these various substances, whether they do so at various stages in their life spans, and if so, how and with what implications.

A continuing challenge is the identification of sex differences in health and illness that are methodologically robust, hereafter referred to (provocatively) as "true" sex differences. Different biological, lifestyle, and social structural contexts for males and females can lead to spurious inferences about sex. Even the most methodologically valid comparisons are potentially susceptible to biased interpretations, intentional or not.

Exposure, susceptibility, responses to initiating agents, energy metabolism, and responses to therapeutic agents matter and must be considered in any consideration of sex differences in health and disease. However, in many instances these differences in disease manifestations and health outcomes cannot be explained by the obvious anatomical or sex hormone differences between males and females. In some instances, societal practices and beliefs, independent of biological sex, account for the differences, but in other instances, the differences remain unexplained. The following recommendation is presented as a result of these considerations.

Recommendation

RECOMMENDATION 6: Monitor sex differences and similarities for all human diseases that affect both sexes.

Investigators should

- **consider sex as a biological variable in all biomedical and health-related research; and**
- **design studies that will**
  −control for exposure, susceptibility, metabolism, physiology (cycles), and immune response variables;
  −consider how ethical concerns (e.g., risk of fetal injury) constrain study designs and affect outcomes; and
  −detect sex differences across the life span.

Also see Recommendation 3 (in Chapter 3) for a discussion of the need to mine cross-species information.

6

The Future of Research on Biological Sex Differences: Challenges and Opportunities

ABSTRACT

Being male or female is an important fundamental variable that should be considered when designing and analyzing basic and clinical research. Historically, the terms sex and gender have been loosely—and sometimes inappropriately—used in the reporting of research results, a situation that should be remedied through further clarification. Conducting studies that account for sex differences might require innovative designs, methods, and model systems, all of which might require additional resources. Studies that rely on biological materials would benefit from a determination and disclosure of the sex of origin of the material, and clinical researchers should attempt to identify the endocrine status of research subjects. Longitudinal studies should be designed to allow analysis of data by sex. Once studies are conducted, data regarding sex differences, or the lack thereof, should be readily available in the scientific literature. Interdisciplinary efforts are needed to conduct research on sex differences.

A common, recurring message emerged as the committee addressed the current state of knowledge about sex differences in health and illness and scientific evidence related to sex differences in health and illness and as it met with scientific experts from diverse disciplines. This message is that sex—that is, being male or female—is an important basic human variable that should be considered when designing and analyzing the results of studies in all areas and at all levels of biomedical and health-related research. Differences in health and illness between individuals are influenced not only by individuals' genetic and physiological constitutions but also by environmental and experiential factors, all of which interact. As discussed in Chapter 2, the cells of males and females have many basic biochemical differences, and many of these stem from genetic rather than hormonal differences. As reviewed in Chapters 3 and 4, sex differences are evident and evolve across the life span; however, these differences cannot be attributed solely to sex hormones.

In addition, naturally occurring variations in sexual differentiation and development can provide unique opportunities to obtain a better understanding of the basic differences and the similarities between and within the sexes. As described in Chapter 5, the incidence and severity of disease vary between the sexes and may be related to differences in exposures, portals of entry and processing, and cellular responses. One of the most compelling reasons for looking at what is known about the biology of sex differences is that there are striking differences in human disease that are not explained at this time.

In addition to assessing the available scientific data on sex differences in health and illness, the sponsors asked the committee to consider current and potential barriers to progress, including ethical, financial, sociological, and scientific factors. Committee members raised a wide variety of concerns during the committee discussions. It is the committee's opinion that meeting the challenges described in the following sections will, in particular, help to advance scientific knowledge about sex differences in health and illness.

TERMINOLOGY

One of the first barriers that the committee faced was the inconsistent and often confusing use of the terms *sex* and *gender* in the scientific literature and the popular press.

Use of *sex* and *gender* varies widely among disciplines and authors (National Institutes of Health, Office of Research on Women's Health, 1999a; Kim and Nafziger, 2000). Anthropologists Walker and Cook (1998) consider the distinction between *sex* and *gender* in their field of anthropology to be very important, as it is possible to determine sex by analyzing skeletal remains and to obtain information on gender roles through the study of artifacts. A 1998 study by Walker and Cook demonstrates that although the rate of use of the term *sex* in the biomedical literature has not changed significantly since the late 1960s, the rate of use of the term *gender* has increased markedly, especially since the early 1980s (Walker and Cook, 1998). Upon further examination, they found that most articles published in the late 1960s and early 1970s made a distinction between *sex* and *gender*. However, among the more recent articles that Walker and Cook surveyed in their examination of articles indexed in MedLine under both *sex* and *gender*, more than half did not distinguish between the terms. Haig (2000) obtained similar results on examination of the use of *sex* and *gender* in a sampling of the Science Citation Index.

The term *gender* first appeared in the medical and biological literature in the 1960s in publications of research on the individual psychology of "gender identity" and "gender role" (Hampson and Hampson, 1961; Money and Ehrhardt, 1996). Later, in part as a result of the feminist movement, *gender* came to refer to a set of power relationships in society (Lorber, 1994, pp. 30–31). The resulting use of gender as both an individual characteristic and a social institution, however, leads to significant confusion.

Synonymous use of *sex* and *gender* is common in health-related government guidelines and regulations. The final U.S. Food and Drug Administration rule entitled Investigational New Drug Applications and New Drug Applications establishes in law the requirement that applications for approval of new drugs contain "effectiveness and safety data for important demographic subgroups, specifically *gender*, age, and racial subgroups" (21 CFR Parts 312 and 314, U.S. Department of Health and Human Services, 1998, p. 6854 [emphasis added]). In contrast, a May 2000 U.S. General Accounting Office (GAO) report, *Women's Health: NIH Has Increased Its Efforts to Include Women in Research*, uses *sex* when referring to an analysis of the results of different clinical studies conducted with women and men and notes that *gender* is used to discuss culturally shaped variations (U.S. General Accounting Office, 2000).

The use of *sex* and *gender* as synonyms in science is apparent throughout the literature. According to the current scientific literature, rats, mice, guinea pigs, other research animals, and even plants have gender. Animals may have social behaviors and roles often associated with one or the other sex; however, most published reports are using gender as a synonym for sex, and investigators have not developed animals models that mimic the uniquely human trait of gender.

Medical textbooks perpetuate the confusion. *Harrison's Principles of Internal Medicine*, the quintessential internal medicine text, uses sex and gender interchangeably. In a discussion of demographic factors and disease, *Harrison's* states that "by definition, many disorders of the reproductive tract occur exclusively in one *gender*," but later in the same paragraph it states, "other conditions occur regularly in both *sexes*, but predominate or tend to be more severe in one or the other" (Ernster and Colford, 1998, p. 14 [emphasis added])

The interchangeable use of *sex* and *gender* tends to cause confusion not only in the scientific community but also among policy makers and the general public. Consistent usage across disciplines would aid in the accurate measurement and reporting of differences between men and women and help to communicate clearly how the differences apply to biomedical research, patient care, and policy.

RECOMMENDATION 7: Clarify use of the terms *sex* and *gender*.

Researchers should specify in publications their use of the terms *sex* and *gender*. To clarify usage and bring some consistency to the literature, the committee recommends the following:

   • **In the study of human subjects, the term *sex* should be used as a classification, generally as male or female, according to the reproductive organs and functions that derive from the chromosomal complement.**

   • **In the study of human subjects, the term *gender* should be used to refer to a person's self-representation as male or female, or how that person is responded to by social institutions on the basis of the individual's gender presentation.**

   • **In most studies of nonhuman animals the term *sex* should be used.**

RESEARCH TOOLS AND RESOURCES

More Complex Studies and Additional Resources for Research

Differences between the sexes may be modest, yet the differences may still result in different outcomes or may point to significant and larger underlying mechanisms of sex differences. Detection of modest differences may require studies with more complex experimental designs, the use of more complex model systems, and the use of more subjects to achieve statistical power; and, thus, in some cases detection of modest differences may require additional financial resources.

A recent example is a large population-based study (O'Donnell et al., 1998) that demonstrates an association and genetic linkage of the angiotensin-converting enzyme (ACE) locus with hypertension and with diastolic blood pressure in men but not women. Existing data on the association of the ACE locus and blood pressure or hypertension have been conflicting. O'Donnell and colleagues have suggested that "many prior studies may have had inadequate power to detect the modest contribution that might be expected from an individual genetic factor to complex traits such as blood pressure" (O'Donnell et al., 1998, p. 1766). They also note that differences in the genetic makeup or environmental exposures of the different study populations may also play a role in the different results observed.

Another example relates to sex differences in sensitivity to noxious stimuli, which overall are relatively small but whose underlying mechanisms are wide-ranging and significant for many aspects of treatment (see Chapter 4 and Berkley [1997a,b]).

RECOMMENDATION 8: Support and conduct additional research on sex differences.

Because differences between the sexes are pervasive across all subdisciplines of biology, all research sponsors should encourage research initiatives on sex differences. Research sponsors and peer-review committees should recognize that research on sex differences may require additional resources.

Information from the Published Literature

Information on sex differences can be difficult to glean from the published literature. In 1999, the U.S. Congress asked GAO to assess the National Institutes of Health's (NIH's) progress in conducting research on women's health in the decade since publication of the 1990 GAO report on the inclusion of women in clinical trials. Over the course of its audit, GAO experienced difficulties in determining whether analysis of data by sex is occurring. Even when scientists do analyze data by sex, the results are not always published. Often, when an analysis reveals no difference in outcome by sex, journal editors omit this information and generally discourage researchers from including such information in the results (U.S. General Accounting Office, 2000). GAO noted that the deficiency in reporting the outcomes of studies by sex appeared to be due in part to a lack of documentation of negative findings. In addition, when sex differences are reported, they may not be appropriately indexed by abstracting and indexing services, making it difficult to identify articles of interest (Montgomery and Sherif, 2000).

In fact, very few journals have any information or guidelines regarding analysis of data by subpopulations, such as sex, in their instructions for authors. Many journals refer to the "Uniform Requirements for Manuscripts Submitted to Biomedical Journals" by the International Committee of Medical Journal Editors, which states that when writing about methods, researchers should describe their "selection of the observational or experimental subjects (patients or laboratory animals, including controls) clearly. Identify the age, sex, and other important characteristics of the subjects" (International Committee of Medical Journal Editors, 1997, p. 311). However, the uniform requirements do not say anything about "age, sex, or other important characteristics of subjects" in the requirements for the statistics, results, or discussion sections of articles.

The *Journal of the National Cancer Institute* (*JNCI*) has taken the lead in encouraging authors to include information on and analyses of subjects by sex. In October 2000, *JNCI* amended its Information for Authors to say, "Where appropriate, clinical and epidemiological studies should be analyzed to see if there is an effect of sex or any of the major ethnic groups. If there is no effect, that should be stated so in Results" (Arnold, 2000; *Journal of the National Cancer Institute*, 2000). On the basis of the recent GAO report and other related reports, encouraging the inclusion of "negative data" (the absence of a finding of a sexual dimorphism may be an indication of a similarity between the sexes) would be an important step. The phrase "where appropriate" regarding the need for analysis by sex, however, may be interpreted and applied quite differently by different researchers.

RECOMMENDATION 9: Make sex-specific data more readily available.

Journal editors should encourage researchers to include in their reports descriptions of the sex ratios of the research population and to specify the extent to which analyses of the data by sex were included in the study. If there is no effect (absence of a sex difference), that should be stated in the results and researchers should give an informative statistic (e.g., means and standard deviations, t-test value for comparison, exact P value) rather than simply indicating that the comparison was not statistically significant. Reporting of exact statistics allows the findings to be taken into account far more effectively in later meta-analyses. When designing or updating databases of scientific journal articles and other information, informatics developers should devise ways of reliably accessing sex-specific data.

Information on Sex of Origin of Cell and Tissue Culture Material

All somatic cells have a full complement of chromosomes, including the sex chromosomes. Despite this, useful information on the sex of origin of cell lines or tissue cultures is often lacking in the literature. Data suggest that many cells throughout the body display sex specificity. For example, human primary osteoblasts (a type of bone cell) isolated from pre- and postmenopausal women show age-dependent changes in their expression of biochemical markers and responsiveness to hormones that are not observed in the same bone cells from younger or older men (Katzburg et al., 1999). Receptors for sex hormones are present on a wide variety of cells. Arterial wall macrophages derived from circulating blood monocytes are known to take up lipoproteins and to form large foam cells. Such foam cell formation is an early event in atherosclerosis, and recent research suggests that the earlier onset and higher incidence of atherosclerosis in men may be related to the presence of androgen receptors on the immune cells and androgen-mediated lipid loading (McCrohon et al., 2000).

A great deal of research on human cell lines involves newborn foreskin cells, which are obligatorily male. There is no equivalent source of female newborn tissue. Reviewers often ask whether the genital location of foreskin fibroblasts or keratinocytes modifies their behavior and makes them invalid models for the behaviors of cells derived from a nongenital location, but reviewers do not ask if male versus female sex is similarly relevant. The fetal fibroblast-like cell lines commonly used in aging research (e.g., WI-38 and IMR-90 cells) are nowhere characterized as male versus female, nor has anyone questioned the relevance of cellular sex in studies with these lines. (The large number of malignant immortal cell lines available from the American Type Culture Collection and similar sources are rarely identified by sex, but even if they were it would be extremely difficult to interpret differences among donor lines, as the expression of many genes is presumably abnormal by virtue of the malignant transformation process.)

Few to no data are available for determination of whether cell sex matters when studying such functions as cell life span and the response to stresses. Information about the sex of origin of cells and tissues, however, could be very useful and even critical for interpretation of results and for comparison of results across disciplines. Because the sex of the source of eukaryotic cells used in research can readily be determined by DNA sequencing, it need not remain an unknown. Many published studies, however, do not report such information even when it is known.

RECOMMENDATION 10: Determine and disclose the sex of origin of biological research materials.

The origins and sex chromosome constitutions of cells or tissue cultures used for cell biological, molecular biological, or biochemical experiments should be stated when they are known. Attempts should be made to discern the sex of origin when it is unknown. Journal editors should encourage inclusion of such information in Materials and Methods sections as standard practice.

(The committee acknowledges that inclusion of people, animals, or cells and tissues of or from both sexes in all studies is not always feasible or appropriate. Rather, the committee is urging researchers to regard sex, that is, being male or female, as an important basic human variable that should be considered when designing, analyzing, and reporting findings from studies in all areas and at all levels of biomedical research. Determining and disclosing the sex of origin of biological research materials are important steps in that direction.)

Lack of Data on Sex Differences Across the Life Span from Longitudinal Studies

The health status of males and females can vary considerably, both within and between the sexes, across the life span—from intrauterine development to old age. Several longitudinal studies, some spanning more than 40 years, have provided vitally important data that demonstrate sex differences, ranging from genetic differences to differences in diagnostic and therapeutic interventions, as individuals age (such as the Framingham Study and the Bogalusa Heart Study [Berenson et al., 1992; Dawber et al., 1951; Kannel et al., 1976; O'Donnell et al., 1998]). These studies have provided such information not only about the original participants but about their offspring as well. Those studies, however, were designed with specific disease end points, such as the risk factors for and the development of coronary artery disease, thereby precluding consideration of many other relevant developmental issues and other diseases, disorders, and conditions. Unfortunately, few such longitudinal studies exist. As a result, the lack of longitudinal studies has limited understanding in particular of sex differences throughout the life span.

RECOMMENDATION 11: Longitudinal studies should be conducted and should be constructed so that their results can be analyzed by sex.

Lack of Consideration of Hormonal Variability

Data on cycles (menstrual, circadian, etc.) are often lacking. Most studies with women do not define which part of the cycle the participants were in at the time of study, note the participants only by age and not whether they are pre- or postmenopausal, or are based on only one cycle.

Furthermore, characterization of the phases of estrous and menstrual cycles across studies is inconsistent and can lead to considerable confusion. For example, in studies with humans some investigators assess a phenomenon or condition during the luteal phase and take their measures near the end of that phase, when progesterone levels are dropping or are at low levels, whereas others take their measures near the midpoint of the luteal phase, when progesterone levels are rising or are at their peak.

Problems with timing the menstrual cycle for research are not insurmountable, and several studies (including studies determining timing of the menstrual cycle for surgery for breast cancer prognosis) are under way (Hagen and Hrushesky, 1998; Jatoi, 1998; Macleod et al., 2000).

RECOMMENDATION 12: Identify the endocrine status of research subjects (an important variable that should be considered, when possible, in analyses).

INTERDISCIPLINARY AND COLLABORATIVE RESEARCH

Uniformity in Application of Federal Regulations

Interpretation and application of federal regulations regarding protection of human subjects are at the discretion of university and industry institutional review boards (IRBs) and can be highly variable. For example, current federal guidance describes policies for inclusion of women in research protocols that may be applied more restrictively at the discretion of local IRBs. Similarly, the policies for the use of research animals set by institutional animal care and use committees (IACUCs) vary by institution. Thus, the ability to study sex differences is not uniform across institutions, and there is a question of fairness, as some oversight bodies allow procedures that others do not. This lack of uniformity can inhibit collaborative work between institutions with different IRB and IACUC regulations.

Uncertainties about how best to protect women in their childbearing years contribute significantly to the inconsistencies in the application of guidelines. A 1999 statement by the Committee on Ethics of the American College of Obstetricians and Gynecologists (ACOG) notes the valid concerns for the well-being of the fetus but states that "the resulting sense of restraint has limited the growth of knowledge in some areas of normal physiology, pathophysiology, and therapeutic approaches during pregnancy" (Chervenak and McCullough, 1999, p. 206). The ACOG committee affirmed the need for research with pregnant women and offered guidelines for selecting, informing, and caring for pregnant women in clinical research studies.

IRBs are a topic of great interest to the members of the Institute of Medicine (IOM) Clinical Research Roundtable (www.iom.edu/crr). In addition, the Office of Human Research Protection of the U.S. Department of Health and Human Services has commissioned IOM to do a two-part study on the future of IRBs. The first report will be a 6-month fast-track study that addresses accreditation standards for IRBs (expected release date, summer 2001). The second part will be a full-length study of the overall structure and functioning of activities used to protect human subjects and the criteria used to evaluate the performance of activities used to protect human subject (expected release date, fall 2002).

The committee is encouraged by the attention that the problems of IRBs will receive from these two IOM activities and looks forward to their published proceedings and recommendations.

Opportunities for Interdisciplinary Collaboration

The need for greater use of interdisciplinary collaboration in not unique to the study of sex differences. The committee refers the reader to the recent IOM report *Bridging Disciplines in the Brain, Behavioral, and Clinical Sciences* (Institute of Medicine, 2000). Although the report is primarily concerned with brain research, the discussion of the issues and barriers related to interdisciplinary research and training and to translational research is relevant to the study of sex differences as well. The committee that prepared that report concluded that researchers sometimes perceive interdisciplinary research as impure or "second rate," with each discipline having a sense of superiority and believing others to be less rigorous. Moreover, students fear that interdisciplinary training will not properly prepare them for a career.

The National Research Council's Committee on National Needs for Biomedical and Behavioral Sciences noted in its recent report (National Research Council, 2000) that the number of researchers in the basic biomedical workforce is sufficient to meet the nation's needs. It also encouraged NIH to gradually shift the focus of its predoctoral programs from single-discipline to interdisciplinary training and increase opportunities for postdoctoral training through interdisciplinary training grants.

In the study of sex differences, synergy is needed between and among basic scientists, epidemiologists, social scientists, and clinical researchers. There is a need for better translational—or bench-to-bedside—research. Data on interlevel integration (cellular, to animal, to human) are often limited. At the human level, collaboration across medical specialties is also needed.

As noted in a 1994 IOM report, *Women and Health Research*, such collaborations can be difficult as researchers from different disciplines look at different points along a causal pathway, use different tools, and obtain different results (Institute of Medicine, 1994). Strategies for more effective communication and cooperation are needed.

As an example of mutual benefits that can come from interdisciplinary research, consider epidemiology and basic biological research. Epidemiological studies can be used to identify areas in which basic research is needed. Information about environmental exposures that affect disease risk and pathogenesis could point to genes and biological mechanisms that modify risk. In the opposite and equally beneficial scenario, understanding the biological basis of differences or similarities could help identify unrecognized environmental risk factors (Hoover, 2000). Collection of better data on exposures, including multiple exposures, could enhance analysis.

RECOMMENDATION 13: Encourage and support interdisciplinary research on sex differences.

Interdisciplinary research is generally accepted as valuable and important. Opportunities for interdisciplinary collaboration to enhance the understanding of sex differences, however, have not been fully realized. The committee recommends the continued development of interdisciplinary research programs and strategies for more effective communication and cooperation to achieve the following goals:

- synergy between and among basic scientists, epidemiologists, social scientists, and clinical researchers;
- enhanced collaboration across medical specialties; and
- better translational—or bench-to-bedside—research and interlevel integration of data (cellular, to animal, to human).

NON-HEALTH-RELATED IMPLICATIONS OF RESEARCH ON SEX DIFFERENCES IN HEALTH

Lack of Awareness That the Consequences of Genetics and Physiology May Be Amenable to Change

A problem with discussing sex differences is that such differences, when shown to have a genetic or physiological influence, are thought to be immutable. Such sex differences are interpreted as being a direct result of chromosomes. Since an individual's sex chromosomes, either XX or XY, cannot be changed, people tend to think that differences between the sexes are also unchangeable (Valian, 1998). Valian (1998) notes that "it is odd that we should interpret sex differences as immutable, when we do not accept biology as destiny in other aspects of human existence" (p. 67) and cites aging as an example. The human life span is set by biology, but people do not accept the average life span as their fate. Biology incorporates mutually interacting factors, from genetic to psychosocial, across the life span. Great amounts of time and many resources are put into research on understanding mechanisms of disease and developing cures. People eat certain foods, take vitamins, exercise, and take preventive treatments such as vaccines, all in attempts to prolong life.

Discriminatory Practices Based on Sex Differences

Historically, studies on race, ethnicity, age, nationality, religion, and sex have led to discriminatory practices. Participants in the Research Designs and Gender working group at the NIH Scientific Meeting and Public Hearing on Influences of Sex and Gender on Health in 1996 noted that in the past it has been difficult to publish findings on sex differences. "The paucity of studies on neuroendocrine aspects of female functions may be attributable to a belief that it was not politically correct to acknowledge different functioning at different times of the month for fear of discrimination based on the differences" (National Institutes of Health, Office of Research on Women's Health, 1999d, p. 97).

Scientific research is not separate from other practices of society. Bias in interpretation or reporting by observers is well documented in the social sciences but is less obvious in the basic and clinical sciences. Yet, scientific theories, questions, and data are also subject to biased interpretation (Institute of Medicine, 1994). Such biases and the tendency to perceive one sex (classically, males), race, age group, or other subpopulation to be the norm can portray differences displayed by others as "deviant" (Institute of Medicine, 1994). To acknowledge and explore nonreproductive aspects of sex differences in health and illness requires a view of males and females as different but equally "legitimate" biological entities without respect to whether there is (or should be) equivalence or equality in all other domains.

RECOMMENDATION 14: Reduce the potential for discrimination based on identified sex differences.

The committee noted that, historically, studies on race, ethnicity, age, nationality, religion, and sex have sometimes led to discriminatory practices. The committee believes, therefore, that these historical practices should be taken into consideration so that they will not be repeated. The past should not limit the future of research but should serve as a guide to its use. Ethical research on the biology of sex differences is essential to the advancement of human health and should not be constrained.

References

Abad-Santos, F., A. Carcas, P. Guerra, C. Govantes, C. Montuenga, E. Gomez, A. Fernandez, and J. Frias. 1996. Evaluation of sex differences in the pharmacokinetics of ranitidine in humans. *Journal of Clinical Pharmacology* 36:748–751.

Abaitua Borda, I., R. M. Philen, M. Posada de la Paz, A. Gomez de la Camara, M. Diez Ruiz-Navarro, O. Gimenez Ribota, J. Alvargonzalez Soldevilla, B. Terracini, S. Severiano Pena, C. Fuentes Leal, and E. M. Kilbourne. 1998. Toxic oil syndrome mortality: the first 13 years. *International Journal of Epidemiology* 27:1057–1063.

Abdel Malek, V. 1998. Regulation of human pigmentation by ultraviolet light and by endocrine, paracrine, and autocrine hormones. In: *The Pigmentary System: Physiology and Pathophysiology.* J. J. Nordland, R. E. Boissy, V. J. Hearing, R. A. King, and J.-P. Ortonne, eds. New York: Oxford University Press.

Achermann, J. C., M. Ito, P. C. Hindmarsh, and J. L. Jameson. 1999. A mutation in the gene encoding steroidogenic factor-1 causes XY sex reversal and adrenal failure in humans. *Nature Genetics* 22:125–126.

Affleck, G., H. Tennen, F. J. Keefe, J. C. Lefebvre, S. Kashikar-Zuck, K. Right, K. Starr, and D. S. Caldwell. 1999. Everyday life with osteoarthritis or rheumatoid arthritis: independent effects of disease and gender on daily pain, mood, and coping. *Pain* 83:601–609.

Ahmed, S. A., and N. Talal. 1999. Effects of sex hormones on immune responses and autoimmune diseases: an update, pp. 333–338. In: *The Decade of Autoimmunity.* Y. Shoenfeld, ed. Amsterdam: Elsevier.

Ahwal, W. N., P. J. Mills, D. A. Kalshan, and R. A. Nelesen. 1997. Effects of race and sex on blood pressure and hemodynamic stress response as a function of menstrual cycle. *Blood Pressure Monitoring* 2:161–167.

Albarracin-Veizaga, H., M. E. Carvalho, and E. M. Nascimenta. 1999. Chagas disease in an area of recent occupation in Cochabamba, Bolivia. *Revista de Saude Publica* 33:230–236.

Alkayed, N. J., I. Harukuni, A. S. Kimes, E. D. London, R. J. Traystman, and P. D. Hurn. 1998. Gender-linked brain injury in experimental stroke. *Stroke* 29:159–165.

Alkayed, N. J., S. J. Murphy, R. J. Traystman, P. D. Hurn, and V.M. Miller. 2000. Neuroprotective effects of female gonadal steroids in reproductively senescent female rats. *Stroke* 31:161–168.

Aloisi, A. A. 2000. Sensory effects of gonadal hormones, pp. 7–24. *In: Sex, Gender, and Pain.* R. B. Fillingim, ed. Seattle: IASP Press.

American Journal of Medicine. 1993. Consensus Development Conference: diagnosis, prophylaxis, and treatment of osteoporosis. *American Journal of Medicine* 94:646–650.

Amir, R. E., I. B. Van den Veyver, M. Wan, C. Q. Tran, U. Francke, and H. Y. Zoghbi. 1999. Rett syndrome is caused by mutations in X-linked MECP2, encoding methyl-CpG-binding protein 2. *Nature Genetics* 23:185–188.

Ammon, E., C. Schafer, U. Hofmann, and U. Klotz. 1996. Disposition and first-pass metabolism of ethanol in humans: is it gastric or hepatic and does it depend on gender? *Clinical Pharmacology and Therapeutics* 59:503–513.

Andersen, S. L., and M. H. Teicher. 2000. Sex differences in dopamine receptors and their relevance to ADHD. *Neuroscience and Biobehavioral Reviews* 24:137–141.

Andersson, A. M., A. Juul, J. H. Petersen, J. Müller, N. P. Groome, and N. E. Skakkebaek. 1997. Serum inhibin B in healthy pubertal and adolescent boys: relation to age, stage of puberty, and follicle-stimulating hormone, luteinizing hormone, testosterone and estradiol levels. *Journal of Clinical Endocrinology and Metabolism* 82:3976–3981.

Anton, A. H. 1960. The relationship between the binding of sulfonamides to albumin and their antibacterial efficacy. *Journal of Pharmacology and Experimental Therapy* 129:282–290.

Arato, M., E. Frecska, D. J. Maccrimmon, R. Guscott, B. Saxena, K. Tekes, and L. Tothfalusi. 1991. Serotonergic interhemispheric asymmetry: neurochemical and pharmaco-EEG evidence. *Progress in Neuropsychopharmacology and Biological Psychiatry* 15:759–764.

Arnold, A. P., and S. M. Breedlove. 1985. Organizational and activational effects of sex hormones on vertebrate brain and behavior: a re-analysis. *Hormones and Behavior* 19:469–498.

Arnold, K. 2000. Journal to encourage analysis by sex/ethnicity. *Journal of the National Cancer Institute* 92:1561.

Artlett, C. M., J. B. Smith, and S. A. Jimenez. 1998. Identification of fetal DNA and cells in skin lesions from women with systemic sclerosis. *New England Journal of Medicine* 338:1186–1191.

Atabani, S., G. Landucci, M. W. Steward, H. Whittle, J.G. Tilles, and D.N. Forthal. 2000. Sex-associated differences in the antibody-dependent cellular cytotoxicity antibody response to measles vaccine. *Clinical and Diagnostic Laboratory Immunology* 7:111–113.

Ayanian, J. Z., and A. M. Epstein. 1991. Differences in the use of procedures between women and men hospitalized for coronary heart disease. *New England Journal of Medicine* 325:221–225.

Bachevalier, J., and C. Hagger. 1991. Sex differences in the development of learning abilities in primates. *Psychoneuroendocrinology* 16:177–188.

Balomenos, D., J. Martin-Caballero, M. I. Garcia, I. Prieto, J. M. Flores, M. Serrano, and A. C. Martinez. 2000. The cell cycle inhibitor p21 controls T-cell proliferation and sex-linked lupus development. *Nature Medicine* 6:171–176.

Bardhan, K. D., G. Bodemar, H. Geldof, E. Schutz, A. Heath, J. G. Mills, and L. A. Jacques. 2000. A double-blind, randomized, placebo-controlled dose-ranging study to evaluate the efficacy of alosetron in the treatment of irritable bowel syndrome. *Alimentary Pharmacology and Therapeutics* 14:23–34.

Barker, D. J. 1995. The Wellcome Foundation Lecture, 1994. The fetal origins of adult disease. *Proceedings of the Royal Society of London. Series B: Biological Sciences* 262:37–43.

Barker, D. J. 1997. Fetal nutrition and cardiovascular disease in later life. *British Medical Bulletin* 53:96–108.

Barker, D. J. 1999. Fetal origins of cardiovascular disease. *Annals of Medicine* 31(Suppl. 1): 3–6.

Barker, D. J., A. W. Shiell, M. E. Barker, and C. M. Law. 2000. Growth in utero and blood pressure levels in the next generation. *Journal of Hypertension* 18:843–846.

Barker, D. J. 2000. In utero programming of cardiovascular disease. *Theriogenology* 53: 555–574.

Baroiller, J.-F., Y. Guiguen, and A. Fostier. 1999. Endocrine and environmental aspects of sex differentiation in fish. *Cellular and Molecular Life Sciences* 55:910–931.

Baron, J. A., P. Adams, and M. Ward. 1988. Cigarette smoking and other correlates of cytologic estrogen effect in postmenopausal women. *Fertility and Sterility* 50:766–771.

Barrett-Connor, E. 1998a. Hormone replacement therapy. *British Medical Journal* 317: 457–461.

Barrett-Connor, E. 1998b. Rethinking estrogen and the brain. *Journal of the American Geriatric Society* 46:918–920.

Barrett-Connor, E., and D. Grady. 1998. Hormone replacement therapy, heart disease, and other considerations. *Annual Review of Public Health* 19:55–72.

Barrett-Connor, E., and D. Kritz-Silverstein. 1993. Estrogen replacement therapy and cognitive function in older women. *Journal of the American Medical Association* 269:2637–2641.

Barrett-Connor, E., and D. L. Wingard. 1983. Sex differential in ischemic heart disease mortality in diabetics: a prospective population-based study. *American Journal of Epidemiology* 118:489–496.

Barton, N. H., and B. Charlesworth. 1998. Why sex and recombination? *Science* 281: 1986–1990.

Becker, J. B. 1999. Gender differences in dopaminergic function in striatum and nucleus accumbens. *Pharmacology, Biochemistry, and Behavior* 64:803–812.

Becker, R. C., M. Terrin, R. Ross, G. L. Knatterud, P. Desvigne-Nickens, J. M. Gore, and E. Braunwald. 1994. Comparison of clinical outcomes for women and men after myocardial infarction. The Thrombolysis in Myocardial Infarction Investigators. *Annals of Internal Medicine* 120:638–645.

Beeson, P. B. 1994. Age and sex associations of 40 autoimmune diseases. *American Journal of Medicine* 96:457–462.

Beierle, I., B. Meibohm, and H. Derendorf. 1999. Gender differences in pharmacokinetics and pharmacodynamics. *International Journal of Clinical Pharmacology and Therapeutics* 37:529–547.

Belayev, L., O. F. Alonso, R. Busto, W. Zhao, and M. D. Ginsburg. 1996. Middle cerebral artery occlusion in the rat by intraluminal suture. Neurological and pathological evaluation of an improved model. *Stroke* 27:1616–1622.

Belmont, J. W. 1996. Genetic control of X inactivation and processes leading to X-inactivation skewing. *American Journal of Human Genetics* 58:1101–1108.

Belpaire, F. M., P. Wynant, P. Van Trapppen, M. Dhont, A. Verstraete, and M. G. Bogaert. 1995. Protein binding of propranolol and verapamil enantiomers in maternal and foetal serum. *British Journal of Clinical Pharmacology* 39:190–193.

Benbow, C. P. 1988. Sex differences in mathematical reasoning ability in intellectually talented preadolescents: their nature, effects, and possible causes. *Behavioral and Brain Sciences* 11:169–232.

Benderly, B. L. 1997. *In Her Own Right: The Institute of Medicine's Guide to Women's Health Issues*. Washington, DC:National Academy Press.

Benjamin, C. M., G. C. Chew, and A. J. Silman. 1992. Joint and limb symptoms in children after immunisation with measles, mumps, and rubella vaccine. *British Medical Journal* 304:1075–1078.

Benn, C. S., P. Aaby, C. Bale, J. Olsen, K. F. Michaelsen, E. George, and H. Whittle. 1997. Randomised trial of effect of vitamin A supplementation on antibody response to measles vaccine in Guinea-Bissau, West Africa. *Lancet* 350:101–105.

Bennink, R., M. Peeters, V. Van den Maegdenbergh, B. Geypens, P. Rutgeerts, M. De Roo, and L. Mortelmans. 1998. Comparison of total and compartmental gastric emptying and antral motility between healthy men and women. *European Journal of Nuclear Medicine* 25:1293–1299.

Bennink, R., M. Peeters, V. Van den Maegdenbergh, B. Geypens, P. Rutgeerts, M. De Roo, and L. Mortelmans. 1999. Evaluation of small-bowel transit for solid and liquid test meal in healthy men and women. *European Journal of Nuclear Medicine* 26:1560–1566.

Bentham, G., and A. Aase. 1996. Incidence of malignant melanoma of the skin in Norway, 1955–1989: associations with solar ultraviolet radiation, income and holidays abroad. *International Journal of Epidemiology* 25:1132–1138.

Benton, R. E., M. Sale, D. A. Flockhardt, and R. L. Woosley. 2000. Greater quinidine-induced QTc interval prolongation in women. *Clinical Pharmacology and Therapeutics* 67:413–418.

Berenbaum, S. A. 1998. How hormones affect behavioral and neural development: introduction to the special issue on gonadal hormones and sex differences in behavior. *Developmental Neuropsychology* 14:175–196.

Berenbaum, S. A. 2000. Psychological outcome in congenital adrenal hyperplasia, pp. 186–199. *In: Therapeutic Outcome of Endocrine Disorders: Efficacy, Innovation, and Quality of Life*. B. Stabler and B. B. Bercy, eds. New York: Springer.

Berenbaum, S. A., and S. M. Resnick. 1997. Early androgen effects on aggression in children and adults with congenital adrenal hyperplasia. *Psychoneuroendocrinology* 22:505–515.

Berenbaum, S. A., and E. Snyder. 1995. Early hormonal influences on childhood sex-typed activity and playmate preference: implications for the development of sexual orientation. *Developmental Psychology* 31:31–42.

Berenson, G. S., W. A. Wattigney, R. E. Tracey, W. P. Newman III, S. R. Srinivasan, L. S. Webber, E. R. Dalferes, Jr., and J. P. Strong. 1992. Atherosclerosis of the aorta and coronary arteries and cardiovascular risk factors in persons aged 6 to 30 years and studied at necropsy (The Bogalusa Heart Study). *American Journal of Cardiology* 70:851–858.

Berkley, K. J. 1997a. Female vulnerability to pain and the strength to deal with it. *Behavioral and Brain Sciences* 20:473–479.

Berkley, K. J. 1997b. Sex differences in pain. *Behavioral and Brain Sciences* 20:371–380.

Berkley, K. J. 2000. Female pain versus male pain, pp. 373–381. *In: Sex, Gender, and Pain*, R. B. Fillingim, ed. Seattle: IASP Press.

Berkley, K. J., and A. Holdcroft. 1999. Sex and gender differences in pain, pp. 951–965. *In: Textbook of Pain*, 4th ed., P. D. Wall and R. Melzack, eds. Edinburgh: Churchill Livingstone.

Bernardi, R. R., L. C. Dermentzoglou, T. L. Russell, S. P. Schmaltz, J. L. Barnett, K. M. Jarvenpaa, and J. B. Dressman. 1990. Upper gastrointestinal (GI) pH in young, healthy men and women. *Pharmacology Research* 7:756–761.

Berry, K., H. M. Wisniewski, L. Svarz-Bein, and S. Baez. 1975. On the relationship of brain vasculature to production of neurological deficit and morphological changes following acute unilateral common carotid artery ligation in gerbils. *Journal of Neurological Science* 25:75–92.

Bhatia, S. K., N. R. Rose, B. Schofield, A. Lafond-Walker, and R. C. Kuppers. 1996. Influence of diet on the induction of experimental autoimmune thyroid disease. *Proceedings of the Society for Experimental Biology and Medicine* 213:294–300.

Bianchi, D. W. 2000. Fetomaternal cell trafficking: a new cause of disease? *American Journal of Medical Genetics* 91:22–28.

Bilezikian, J. P., A. Morishima, J. Bell, and M. M. Grumbach. 1998. Increased bone mass as a result of estrogen therapy in a man with aromatase deficiency. *New England Journal of Medicine* 339:599–603.

Biro, F. M., A. W. Lucky, G. A. Huster, and J. A. Morisson. 1995. Pubertal staging in boys. *Journal of Pediatrics* 127:100–102. (Erratum, 127:674.)

Björntorp, P. A. 1996. The regulation of adipose tissue distribution in humans. *International Journal of Obesity and Related Metabolic Disorders* 20:291–302.

Björntorp, P. A. 1989. Sex differences in the regulation of energy balance with exercise. *American Journal of Clinical Nutrition* 49(Suppl. 5):958–961.

Black, A. J., J. Topping, B. Durham, R. G. Farquharson, and W. D. Fraser. 2000. A detailed assessment of alterations in bone turnover, calcium homeostasis, and bone density in normal pregnancy. *Journal of Bone Mineral Research* 15:557–563.

Blackless, M., A. Charuvastra, A. Derryck, A. Fausto-Sterling, K. Lauzanne, and E. Lee. 2000. How sexually dimorphic are we? Review and synthesis. *American Journal of Human Biology* 12:151–166.

Blum, W. F., P. Englaro, S. Hanitsch, A. Juul, N. T. Hertel, J. Muller, N. E. Skakkebaek, M. L. Heiman, M. Birkett, A. M. Attanasio, W. Kiess, and W. Rascher. 1997. Plasma leptin levels in healthy children and adolescents: dependence on body mass index, body fat mass, gender, pubertal stage, and testosterone. *Journal of Clinical Endocrinology and Metabolism* 82:2904–2910.

Boklage, C. E. 1985. Interactions between same-sex dizygotic fetuses and the assumptions of Weinberg difference method epidemiology. *American Journal of Human Genetics* 37:591–605.

Booth, A., G. Shelley, A. Mazur, G. Tharp, and R. Kittok. 1989. Testosterone, and winning and losing in human competition. *Hormones and Behavior* 23:556–571.

Bouchard, C. 1992. Genetic aspects of human obesity, pp. 343–351. In: *Obesity*. P. Björntorp and B. N. Brodoff, eds. Philadelphia: J. B. Lippincott Company.

Boulos, B. M., L. E. Davis, C. H. Almond, and C. R. Sirtori. 1971. Comparison among sulfanilamide concentrations in the fetal, umbilical, maternal blood and amniotic fluid. *Archives of International Pharmacodynamic Therapy* 191:142–146.

Bradley, L. A., and G. S. Alarcón. 2000. Sex-related influences in fibromyalgia, pp. 281–307. In: *Sex, Gender, and Pain*, R. B. Fillingim, ed. Seattle: IASP Press.

Bradley, S. J., G. D. Oliver, A. B. Chernick, and K. J. Zucker. 1998. Experiment of nurture: ablatio penis at 2 months, sex reassignment at 7 months, and a psychosexual follow-up in young adulthood. *Pediatrics* 102:e9.

Bradshaw, H. B., and K. J. Berkley. 2000. Estrous changes in responses of rat gracile nucleus neurons to stimulation of skin and pelvic viscera. *Journal of Neuroscience* 20:7722–7727.

Braidman, I., C. Baris, L. Wood, P. Selby, J. Adams, A. Freemont, and J. Hoyland. 2000. Preliminary evidence for impaired estrogen receptor-alpha protein expression in osteoblasts and osteocytes from men with idiopathic osteoporosis. *Bone* 26:423–427.

Breedlove, S. M. 1994. Sexual differentiation of the human nervous system. *Annual Review of Psychology* 45:389–418.

Broman, K. W., J. C. Murray, V. C. Sheffield, R. L.White, and J. L. Weber. 1998. Comprehensive human genetic maps: individual and sex-specific variation in recombination. *American Journal of Human Genetics* 63:861–869.

Brooks-Gunn, J., J. A. Graber, and R. L. Paikoff. 1994. Studying links between hormones and negative affect: models and measures. *Journal of Research on Adolescence* 4:469–486.

Brown, A. S., and E. S. Susser. 1997. Sex differences in prevalence of congenital neural defects after periconceptional famine exposure. *Epidemiology* 8:55–58.

Brown, E. A., M. L. Shelley, and J. W. Fisher. 1998. A pharmacokinetic study of occupational and environmental benzene exposure with regard to gender. *Risk Analysis* 18:205–213.

Brown, L., and R. Langer. 1988. Transdermal delivery of drugs. *Annual Review of Medicine* 39:221–229.

Buchanan, C. M., J. S. Eccles, and J. B. Becker. 1992. Are adolescents the victims of raging hormones: evidence for activational effects of hormones on moods and behavior at adolescence. *Psychological Bulletin* 111:62–107.

Bulletti, C., K. DeZiegler, E. Giacomucci, V. Polli, S. Rossi, S. S. Alfieri, and C. Flamigni. 1997. Vaginal drug delivery: the first uterine pass effect. *Annals of the New York Academy of Sciences* 828:285–290.

Bussey, K., and A. Bandura. 1999. Social cognitive theory of gender development and differentiation. *Psychological Review* 106:676–713.

Buyse, G., K. Waldek, C. Verpoorten, H. Björk, P. Casaer, and K.E. Andersson. 1998. Intravesical oxybutinin for neurogenic bladder dysfunction: less systemic side effects due to reduced first pass metabolism. *Journal of Urology* 160:892–896.

Bynoe, M. S., C. M. Grimaldi, and B. Diamond. 2000. Estrogen up-regulates Bcl-2 and blocks tolerance induction of naïve B cells. *Proceedings of the National Academy of Sciences of the United States of America* 97:2703–2708.

Calvari, V., V. Bertini, A. De Grandi, G. Peverali, O. Zuffardi, M. Ferguson-Smith, J. Knudtzon, G. Camerino, G. Borsani, and S. Guioli. 2000. A new submicroscopic deletion that refines the 9p region for sex reversal. *Genomics* 65:203–212.

Camilleri, M., W. L. Hasler, H. P. Parkman, E. M. Quigley, and E. Soffer. 1998. Measurement of gastrointestinal motility in the GI laboratory. *Gastroenterology* 115:747–762.

Camilleri M., A. R. Northcutt, S. Kong, G. E. Dukes, D. McSorley, and A. W. Mangel. 2000. Efficacy and safety of alosetron in women with irritable bowel syndrome: a randomised, placebo-controlled trial. *Lancet* 355:1035–1040.

Campos, H., J. R. McNamara, P. W. Wilson, J. M. Ordovas, and E. J. Schaefer. 1988. Differences in low density lipoprotein subfractions and apolipoproteins in premenopausal and postmenopausal women. *Journal of Clinical Endocrinology and Metabolism* 67:30–35.

Cannon, J. G., and B. A. St. Pierre. 1997. Gender differences in host defense mechanisms. *Journal of Psychiatric Research* 31:99–113.

Capel, B. 2000. The battle of the sexes. *Mechanisms of Development* 92:89–103.

Caprio, M., E. Fabbrini, A. M. Isidori, A. Aversa, and A. Fabbri. 2001. Leptin in reproduction. *Trends in Endocrinology and Metabolism* 12:65–72.

Cardell, K., A. Fryden, and B. Normann. 1999. Intradermal hepatitis B vaccination in health care workers. Response rate and experiences from vaccination in clinical practise. *Scandinavian Journal of Infectious Diseases* 31:197–200.

Carlson, D., J. Hernandez, B. J. Bloom, J. Coburn, J. M. Aversa, and A. C. Steere. 2000. Lack of *Borrelia burgdorferi* DNA in synovial samples from patients with antibiotic treatment-resistant Lyme arthritis. *Arthritis and Rheumatism* 42:2705–2709.

Carpenter, W. H., T. Fonong, M. J. Toth, P. A. Ades, J. Calles-Escandon, J. D. Walston, and E. T. Poehlman. 1998. Total daily energy expenditure in free-living older African Americans and Caucasians. *American Journal of Physiology* 274:E96–E101.

Carrel, L., and H. F. Willard. 1999. Heterogeneous gene expression from the inactive X chromosome: an X-linked gene that escapes X inactivation in some human cell lines but is inactivated in others. *Proceedings of the National Academy of Sciences of the United States of America* 96:7364–7369.

Carrel, L., A. A. Cottle, K. C. Goglin, and H. F. Willard. 1999. A first-generation X-inactivation profile of the human X chromosome. *Proceedings of the National Academy of Sciences of the United States of America* 96:14440–14444.

Carter, C. S., A. C. DeVries, and L. L. Getz. 1995. Physiological substrates of mammalian monogamy: the prairie vole model. *Neuroscience and Biobehavioral Reviews* 19:303–314.

Caspi, A., and T. E. Moffitt. 1991. Individual differences are accentuated during periods of social change: the sample case of girls at puberty. *Journal of Personality and Social Psychology* 61:157–168.

Castagnetta, L., M. Cutolo, O. M. Granata, M. Di Falco, V. Bellavia, and G. Carruba. 1999. Endocrine end-points in rheumatoid arthritis. *Annals of the New York Academy of Sciences* 876:180–191.

Catalano, S. M., and C. J. Shatz. 1998. Activity-dependent cortical target selection by thalamic axons. *Science* 281:559–562.

Catts, H. W. 1986. Speech production/phonological deficits in reading-disordered children. *Journal of Learning Disabilities* 19:504–508.

Catts, H. W. 1989. Speech production deficits in developmental dyslexia. *Journal of Speech and Hearing Disorders* 54:422–428.

Charney, P., B. R. Meyer, W. H. Frishman, A. Ginsberg, and B. Eastwood. 1992. Gender, race, and genetic issues in cardiovascular pharmacotherapeutics. *In: Cardiovascular Pharmacotherapeutics.* W. H. Frishman and E. H. Sonnenblick, eds. New York: McGraw-Hill.

Cheek, A. O., P. Thomas, and C. V. Sullivan. 2000. Sex steroids relative to alternative mating behaviors in the simultaneous hermaphrodite *Serranus sublingarius* (Percifores: Serranidae). *Hormones and Behavior* 37:198–211.

Chen, X. Q., M. Bulbul, G. C. de Gast, A. M. van Loon, D. R. Nalin, and J. van Hattum. 1997. Immunogenicity of two versus three injections of inactivated hepatitis A vaccine in adults. *Hepatology* 26:260–264.

Chen, B. H., C. H. Chiang, S. R. Lin, M. G. Chao, and S. T. Tsai. 1999. The influence of age at onset and gender on the HLA-DQA1, DQB1 association in Chinese children with insulin-dependent diabetes mellitus. *Human Immunology* 60:1131–1137.

Chervenak, F. A., and L. B. McCullough. 1999. Ethical considerations in research involving pregnant women. *Women's Health Issues* 9:206–207.

Chiaramonte, M., S. Majori, T. Ngatchu, M. E. Moschen, V. Baldo, G. Renzulli, I. Simoncello, S. Rocco, T. Bertin, R. Naccarato, and R. Trivello. 1996. Two different dosages of yeast derived recombinant hepatitis B vaccines: a comparison of immunogenicity. *Vaccine* 14:135–137.

Cho, N. H., D. L. Silverman, T. A. Rizzo, and B. E. Metzger. 2000. Correlations between the intrauterine metabolic environment and blood pressure in adolescent offspring of diabetic mothers. *Journal of Pediatrics* 136:587–592.

Chowienczyk, P. J., G. F. Watts, J. R. Cockcroft, S. E. Brett, and J. M. Ritter. 1994. Sex differences in endothelial function in normal and hypercholesterolaemic subjects. *Lancet* 344:305–306.

Christy, N. P., and J. C. Shaver. 1974. Estrogens and the kidney. *Kidney International* 6:366–376.

Cicuttini, F., A. Forbes, K. Morris, S. Darling, M.M. Bailey, and S. Stuckey. 1999. Gender differences in knee cartilage volume as measured by magnetic resonance imaging. *Osteoarthritis and Cartilage* 7:265–271.

Clark, B. A., D. Elahi, and F. H. Epstein. 1990. The influence of gender, age, and the menstrual cycle on plasma atrial natriuretic peptide. *Journal of Clinical Endocrinology and Metabolism* 70:349–352.

Clark, M. M., and B. G. Galef, Jr. 1998. Effects of intrauterine position on the behavior and genital morphology of litter-bearing rodents. *Developmental Neuropsychology* 14:197–211.

Clayton, P. E., M. S. Gill, C. M. Hall, V. Tillmann, A. J. Whatmore, and D. A. Price. 1997. Serum leptin through childhood and adolescence. *Clinical Endocrinology* 46:727–733.

Clement, K., C. Vaisse, N. Lahlou, S. Cabrol, V. Pelloux, D. Cassuto, M. Gourmelen, C. Dina, J. Chambaz, J. M. Lacorte, A. Basdevant, P. Bougneres, Y. Lebouc, P. Froguel, and B. Guy-Grand. 1998. A mutation in the human leptin receptor gene causes obesity and pituitary dysfunction. *Nature* 392:398–401.

Colapinto, J. 2000. *As Nature Made Him: The Boy Who Was Raised as a Girl.* New York: Harper Collins.

Cole-Harding, S., A. L. Morstad, and J. R. Wilson. 1988. Spatial ability in members of opposite-sex twin pairs (abstract.) *Behavioral Genetics* 18:710.

Collaer, M. L., and M. Hines. 1995. Human behavioral sex differences: a role for gonadal hormones during early development? *Psychological Bulletin* 118:55–107.

Collen, M. J., J. D. Abdulian, and Y. K. Chen. 1994. Age does not affect basal gastric acid secretion in normal subjects or in patients with acid-peptic disease. *American Journal of Gastroenterology* 89:712–716.

Collins, L. C., M. F. Cornelius, R. L. Vogel, J. F. Walker, and B. A. Stamford. 1994. Effect of caffeine and/or cigarette smoking on resting energy expenditure. *International Journal of Obesity and Related Metabolic Disorders* 18:551–556.

Collins, P. 2000. The basic science of hormone replacement therapy. Presentation at the First International Congress on Heart Disease and Stroke in Women, May 2000, Victoria, British Columbia, Canada.

Confavreux, C., M. Hutchinson, M. M. Hours, P. Cortinovis-Tourniaire, T. Moreau, and the Pregnancy in Multiple Sclerosis Group. 1998. Rate of pregnancy-related relapse in multiple sclerosis. *New England Journal of Medicine* 339:285–291.

Conte, J. E., Jr., J. A. Golden, M. McQuitty, J. Kipps, E. T. Lin, and E. Zurlinden. 2000. Effects of AIDS and gender on steady-state plasma and intrapulmonary ethionamide concentrations. *Antimicrobial Agents and Chemotherapy* 44:1337–1341.

Cook, N. R., M. W. Gillman, B. A. Rosner, J. O. Taylor, and C. H. Hennekens. 1997. Prediction of young adult blood pressure from childhood blood pressure, height, and weight. *Journal of Clinical Epidemiology* 50:571–579.

Corredor Arjona, A., C. A. Alvarez Moreno, C. A. Agudelo, M. Bueno, M. C. Lopez, E. Caceres, P. Reyes, S. Duque Beltran, L.E. Gualdron, and M. M. Santacruz. 1999. Prevalence of Trypanosoma cruzi and Leishmania chagasi infection and risk factors in a Colombian indigenous population. *Revista do Instituto de Medicina Tropical de Sao Paulo* 41:229–234.

Cresswell, J. L., D. J. Barker, C. Osmond, P. Egger, D. I. Phillips, and R. B. Fraser. 1997. Fetal growth, length of gestation, and polycystic ovaries in adult life. *Lancet* 350:1131–1135.

Crews, D. 1993. The organizational concept and vertebrates without sex chromosomes. *Brain, Behavior, and Evolution* 42:202–214.

Crews, D. 2000. Sexuality: the environmental organization of phenotypic plasticity, pp. 473–499. *In: Reproduction in Context: Social and Environmental Influences on Reproductive Physiology and Behavior.* K. Wallen and J. E. Schneider, eds. Boston: MIT Press.

Crews, D., T. Wibbels, and W. H. N. Gutzke. 1989. Action of sex hormones on temperature-induced sex determination in the snapping turtle (*Chelydra serpentina*). *General and Comparative Endocrinology* 75:159–166.

Croft, P., and P. C. Hannaford. 1989. Risk factors for acute myocardial infarction in women: evidence from the Royal College of General Practitioners' oral contraception study. *British Medical Journal* 298:165–168.

Crouter, A. C., B. A. Manke, and S. M. McHale. 1995. The family context of gender intensification in early adolescence. *Child Development* 66:317–329.

Cullen, D. M., R. T. Smith, and M. P. Akhter. 2000. Time course for bone formation with long-term external mechanical loading. *Journal of Applied Physiology* 88:1943–1948.

Cutolo, A., A. Sulli, B. Seriolo, S. Accardo, and A. T. Masi. 1995. Estrogens, the immune response, and autoimmunity. *Clinical and Experimental Rheumatology* 13:217–226.

D'Agostino, P., S. Milano, C. Barbera, G. Di Bella, M. La Rosa, V. Ferlazzo, R. Farruggio, D.M. Miceli, M. Miele, L. Castagnetta, and E. Cillari. 1999. Sex hormones modulate inflammatory mediators produced by macrophages. *Annals of the New York Academy of Sciences* 876:426–429.

Daly, M., and M. Wilson. 1990. Is parent-offspring conflict sex-linked? Freudian and Darwinian models. *Journal of Personality* 58:163–189.

Damien, E., J. S. Price, and L. E. Lanyon. 2000. Mechanical strain stimulates osteoblast proliferation through the estrogen receptor in males as well as females. *Journal of Bone and Mineral Research* 15:2169–2177.

Daniels, R., S. Lowell, V. Bolton, and M. Monk. 1997. Transcription of tissue-specific genes in human preimplantation embryos. *Human Reproduction* 12:2251–2256.

Da Silva, J. A. 1999. Sex hormones and glucocorticoids: interactions with the immune system. *Annals of the New York Academy of Sciences* 876:102–117.

Datz, F. L., P. E. Christian, and J. Moore. 1987. Gender-related differences in gastric emptying. *Journal of Nuclear Medicine* 28:1204–1207.

Davis, K. D., C. L. Kwan, A. P. Crawley, and D. J. Mikulis. 1998. Functional MRI study of thalamic and cortical activations evoked by cutaneous heat, cold, and tactile stimuli. *Journal of Neurophysiology* 80:1533–1546.

Davison, J. M. 1987. Kidney function in pregnant women. *American Journal of Kidney Diseases* 9:248–252.

Dawber, T. R., G. F. Meadors, and F. E. J. Moore. 1951. Epidemiological approaches to heart disease: the Framingham Study. *American Journal of Public Health* 41:279–286.

Dawkins, K., and W. Z. Potter. 1991. Gender differences in pharmacokinetics and pharmacodynamics of psychotropics: focus on women. *Psychopharmacology Bulletin* 27:417–426.

Dean, B., K. Opeskin, G. Pavey, L. Naylor, C. Hill, N. Keks, and D. L. Copolov. 1995. [^{3}H]paroxetine binding is altered in the hippocampus but not the frontal cortex or caudate nucleus from subjects with schizophrenia. *Journal of Neurochemistry* 64:1197–1202.

DeFries, J. C., R. K. Olson, B. F. Pennington, and S. D. Smith. 1991. Colorado Reading Project: an update, pp. 53–70. In: *The Reading Brain: The Biological Basis of Dyslexia*. D. D. Duane and D. B. Gray, eds. Parkton, MD: York Press.

Denckla, M. B., and R. G. Rudel. 1976. Naming of object-drawings by dyslexic and other learning disabled children. *Brain and Language* 3:1–15.

Derbyshire, S. W. G. 1997. Sources of variation in assessing male and female responses to pain. *New Ideas in Psychology* 15:83–95.

de Wildt, S. N., G. L. Kearns, J. S. Leeder, and J. N. van den Anker. 1999. Cytochrome P450 3A: ontogeny and drug disposition. *Clinical Pharmacokinetics* 37:485–505

Dhaher, Y. Y., B. Greenstein, E. de Fougerolles Nunn, M. Khamashta, and G. R. Hughes. 2000. Strain differences in binding properties of estrogen receptors in immature and adult BALB/c and MRL/MP-lpr/lpr mice, a model of systemic lupus erythematosus. *International Journal of Immunopharmacology* 22:247–254.

Diamond, M., and H. K. Sigmundson. 1997. Sex reassignment at birth. Long-term review and clinical implications. *Archives of Pediatrics and Adolescent Medicine* 151:298–304.

Dias, V. C., B. Tendler, S. Oparil, P. A. Reilly, P. Snarr, and W. B. White. 1999. Clinical experience with transdermal clonidine in African-American and Hispanic-American patients with hypertension: evaluation from a 12-week prospective, open label clinical trial in community-based clinics. *American Journal of Therapeutics* 6:19–24.

Divoll, M., D. J. Greenblatt, J. S. Harmatz, and R. I. Shader. 1981. Effect of age and gender on disposition of temazepam. *Journal of Pharmaceutical Sciences* 70:1104–1107.

Dollimore, N., F. Cutts, F. N. Binka, D. A. Ross, S. S. Morris, and P. G. Smith. 1997. Measles incidence, case fatality, and delayed mortality in children with or without vitamin A supplementation in rural Ghana. *American Journal of Epidemiology* 146:646–654.

Donahoe, P. K., R. L. Cate, D. T. MacLaughlin, J. Epstein, A. F. Fuller, M. Takahashi, J. P. Coughlin, E. G. Ninfa, and L. A. Taylor. 1987. Müllerian inhibiting substance: gene structure and mechanism of action of a fetal regressor. *Recent Progress in Hormone Research* 43:431–467.

Dorland's Illustrated Medical Dictionary, 28th ed. 1994. Philadelphia: W. B. Saunders Co.

Draca, S. R. 1995. Endocrine-immunological homeostasis: the interrelationship between the immune system and and sex steroids involves the hypothalamo-pituitary-gonadal axis. Panminerva Medica 37:71–76.

Drake, W. M., D. Coyte, C. Comacho-Hubner, N. M. Jivanji, G. Kaltsas, D. F. Wood, P. J. Trainer, A. B. Grossman, G. M. Besser, and J. P. Monson. 1998. Optimizing growth hormone replacement therapy by dose titration in hypopituitary adults. Journal of Clinical Endocrinology and Metabolism 83:3913–3919.

Dressman, J. B., R. R. Berardi, L. C. Dermentzoglou, T. L. Russell, S. P. Schmaltz, J. L. Marnett, and K. M. Jarvenpaa. 1990. Upper gastrointestinal (GI) pH in young healthy men and women. Pharmaceutical Research 7:756–761.

Drici, M. D., T. R. Burklow, V. Haridasse, R. I. Glazer, and R. L. Woosley. 1996. Sex hormones prolong the QT interval and downregulate potassium channel expression in the rabbit heart. Circulation 94:1471–1474.

Drinkwater, B. L., K. Nilson, C. H. Chesnut, W. J. Bremner, S. Shainholtz, and M. B. Southworth. 1984. Bone mineral content of amenorrheic and eumenorrheic athletes. New England Journal of Medicine 311:277–281.

Dronamraju, K. 1964. R. Y-linkage in man. Nature 201:424–425.

Dubner, R., and M. A. Ruda. 1992. Activity-dependent neuronal plasticity following tissue injury and inflammation. Trends in Neurosciences 15:96–103.

Dunaif, A., K. R. Segal, D. R. Shelley, G. Green, A. Dobrjansky, and T. Licholai. 1992. Evidence for distinctive and intrinsic defects in insulin action in polycystic ovary syndrome. Diabetes 41:1257–1266.

Dunne, F. P., D. G. Barry, J. B. Ferriss, G. Grealy, and D. Murphy. 1991. Changes in blood pressure during the normal menstrual cycle. Clinical Science 81:515–518.

Ebert, S. N., X.K. Liu, and R. L. Woosley. 1998. Female gender as a risk factor for drug-induced cardiac arrhythmias: evaluation of clinical and experimental evidence. Journal of Women's Health 7:547–557.

Ehrhardt, A. A., and S. W. Baker. 1974. Fetal androgens, human central nervous system differentiation, and behavior sex differences, pp. 3351. In: Sex Differences in Behavior. R. C. Friedman, R. R. Richart, and R. L. Vande Weile, eds. New York: Wiley & Wilson.

Epting, L. K., and W. H. Overman. 1998. Sex-sensitive tasks in men and women: a search for performance fluctuations across the mentrual cycle. Behavioral Neuroscience 112:1304–1317.

Ernster, V. L., and J. M. Colford, Jr. 1998. Host and disease: influence of demographic and socioeconomic factors. In: Harrison's Principles of Internal Medicine, 14th ed. A. S. Fauci, E. Braunwald, K. J. Isselbacher, J. D. Wilson, J. B. Martin, D. L. Kasper, S. L. Hauser, and D. L. Longo, eds. New York: McGraw-Hill.

Evans, M. J., S. MacLaughlin, R. D. Marvin, and N. I. Abdou. 1997. Estrogen decreases in vitro apoptosis of peripheral blood mononuclear cells from women with normal menstrual cycles and decreases TNF-α production in SLE but not in normal cultures. Clinical Immunology and Immunopathology 82:258–262.

Eveleth, P. B., and J. M. Tanner. 1990. Worldwide Variation in Human Growth, pp. 212–221. Cambridge: Cambridge University Press.

Farlow, M. R., D. K. Lahiri, J. Poirier, J. Davignon, L. Schneider, and S. L. Hui. 1998. Treatment outcome of tacrine therapy depends on apolipoprotein genotype and gender of the subjects with Alzheimer's disease. Neurology 50:669–677.

Farooqi, I. S., S. A. Jebb, G. Langmack, E. Lawrence, C. H. Cheetham, A. M. Prentice, I. A. Hughes, M. A. McCamish, and S. O'Rahilly. 1999. Effects of recombinant leptin therapy in a child with congenital leptin deficiency. New England Journal of Medicine 341:879–884.

Fausto-Sterling, A. 2000. *Sexing the Body: Gender Politics and the Construction of Sexuality.* New York: Basic Books.

Ferguson-Smith, M. A., and P. N. Goodfellow. 1995. SRY and primary sex reversal syndromes. In: *The Metabolic and Molecular Basis of Inherited Disease,* 7th ed. C. R. Scriver, A. L. Beaudet, W. S. Sly, D. Valle, B. Childs, B. Vogelstein, and K. W. Kinzler, eds. New York: McGraw-Hill.

Fiebach, N. H., P. R. Hebert, M. J. Stampfer, G. A. Colditz, W. C. Willett, B. Rosner, F. E. Speizer, and C. H. Hennekens. 1989. A prospective study of high blood pressure and cardiovascular disease in women. *American Journal of Epidemiology* 130:646–654.

Fillingim, R. B., ed. 2000. *Sex, Gender, and Pain.* Seattle: IASP Press.

Fillingim, R. B., and W. Maixner. 2000. Sex-related factors in temporomandibular disorders, pp. 309–325. In: *Sex, Gender, and Pain.* R. B. Fillingim, ed. Seattle: IASP Press.

Fillingim, R. B., and T. J. Ness. 2000. The influence of menstrual cycle and sex hormones on pain responses in humans, pp. 191–207. In: *Sex, Gender, and Pain.* R. B. Fillingim, ed. Seattle: IASP Press.

Finkelstein, J. W., E. J. Susman, V. M. Chinchilli, S. J. Kunselman, M. R. D'Arcangelo, J. Schwab, L. M. Demers, L. S. Liben, G. Lookingbill, and H. E. Kulin. 1997. Estrogen or testosterone increases self-reported aggressive behaviors in hypogonadal adolescents. *Journal of Clinical Endocrinology and Metabolism* 82:2433–2438.

Fischette, C. T., A. Biegon, and B. S. McEwen. 1984. Sex steroid modulation of the serotonin behavioral syndrome. *Life Sciences* 35:1197–1206.

Fisher, E. M., P. Beer-Romero, L. G. Brown, A. Ridley, J. A. McNeil, J. B. Lawrence, H. F. Willard, F. R. Bieber, and D. C. Page. 1990. Homologous ribosomal protein genes on the human X and Y chromosomes: escape from X inactivation and possible implications for Turner syndrome. *Cell* 63:1205–1218.

Fitch, R. H., and V. H. Denenberg. 1998. A role for ovarian hormones in sexual differentiation of the brain. *Behavioral and Brain Sciences* 21:311–327.

Flechtner-Mors, M., H. H. Ditschuneit, I. Yip, and G. Adler. 1999. Sympathetic modulation of lipolysis in subcutaneous adipose tissue: effects of gender and energy restriction. *Journal of Laboratory and Clinical Medicine* 134:33–41.

Flegal, K. M., M. D. Carroll, R. J. Kuczmarski, and C. L. Johnson. 1998. Overweight and obesity in the United States: prevalence and trends, 1960–1994. *International Journal of Obesity and Related Metabolic Disorders* 22:39–47.

Fodor, J. A. 1983. *The Modularity of Mind.* Cambridge, MA: MIT Press.

Forger, N. G. 1998. Sex differentiation, psychological, pp. 421–430. In: *Encyclopedia of Reproduction.* E. Knobil and J. D. Neill, eds. San Diego: Academic Press.

Forthal, D. N., G. Landucci, A. Habis, M. Laxer, M. Javato-Laxer, J. G. Tilles, E. N. Janoff. 1995. Age, sex, and household exposure are associated with the acute measles-specific antibody-dependent cellular cytotoxicity response. *Journal of Infectious Diseases* 172:1587–1591.

Francis, R. C. 1992. Sexual liability in teleosts: developmental factors. *Quarterly Review of Biology* 67:1–18.

Francis, J. S., and V. P. Sybert. 1997. Incontinentia pigmenti. *Seminars in Cutaneous Medicine and Surgery* 16:54–60.

Francois, I., and F. de Zegher. 1997. Adrenarche and fetal growth. *Pediatric Research* 41: 440–442.

Freedman, R. R., and R. Girgis. 2000. Effects of menstrual cycle and race on peripheral vascular alpha-adrenergic responsiveness. *Hypertension* 35:795–799.

Freire, B. F., A. A. Ferraz, E. Nakayama, S. Ura, and T. T. Queluz. 1998. Anti-neutrophil cytoplasmic antibodies (ANCA) in the clinical forms of leprosy. *International Journal of Leprosy and Other Mycobacterial Diseases* 66:475–482.

Gaillard, R. C., and E. Spinedi. 1998. Sex- and stress-steroids interactions and the immune system: evidence for a neuroendocrine-immunological sexual dimorphism. *Domestic Animal Endocrinology* 15:345–352.

Gallagher, A. M., R. De Lisi, P. C. Holst, A. V. McGillicuddy-DeLisi, M. Morely, and C. Cahalan. 2000. Gender differences in advanced mathematical problem solving. *Journal of Experimental Child Psychology* 75:165–190.

Gandhi, S. K., J. Gainer, D. King, and N. Brown. 1998. Gender affects renal vasoconstrictor response to Ang I and Ang II. *Hypertension* 31:90–96.

Garcia-Duran, M., T. de Frutos, J. Diaz-Recasens, G. Garcia-Galvez, A. Jimenez, M. Monton, J. Farre, L. Sanchez de Miguel, F. Gonzalez-Fernandez, M. D. Arriero, L. Rico, R. Garcia, S. Casado, and A. Lopez-Farre. 1999. Estrogen stimulates neuronal nitric oxide synthase protein expression in human neutrophils. *Circulation Research* 85:1020–1026.

Garland, M. 1998. Pharmacology of drug transfer across the placenta. *Obstetrics and Gynecology Clinics of North America* 25:21–42.

Garnero, P., E. Hausherr, M. C. Chapuy, C. Marcelli, H. Grandjean, C. Muller, C. Cormier, G. Breart, P. J. Meunier, and P. D. Delmas. 1996. Markers of bone resorption predict hip fracture in elderly women: the EPIDOS Prospective Study. *Journal of Bone and Mineral Research* 11:1531–1538.

Gaudry, S. E., D. S. Sitar, D. D. Smyth, J. K. McKenzie, and F. Y. Aoki. 1993. Gender and age as factors in the inhibition of renal clearance of amantadine by quinine and quinidine. *Clinical Pharmacology and Therapeutics* 54:23–27.

Gear, R. W., C. Miaskowski, N. C. Gordon, S. M. Paul, P. H. Heller, and J. D. Levine. 1996. Kappa-opioids produce significantly greater analgesia in women than in men. *Nature Medicine* 2:1248–1250.

Gear, R. W., C. Miaskowski, N. C. Gordon, S. M. Paul, P. H. Heller, and J. D. Levine. 1999. The kappa opioid nalbuphine produces gender- and dose-dependent analgesia and antianalgesia in patients with postoperative pain. *Pain* 83:339–345.

Gelnar, P. A., B. R. Krauss, P. R. Sheehe, N. M. Szeverenyi, and A. V. Apkarian. 1999. A comparative fMRI study of cortical representations for thermal painful, vibrotactile, and motor performance tasks. *NeuroImage* 10:460–482.

Giamberardino, M. A. 2000. Sex-related and hormonal modulation of visceral pain, pp. 135–163. *In: Sex, Gender, and Pain*. R. Fillingim, ed. Seattle: IASP Press.

Giamberardino, M. A., K. J. Berkley, S. Iezzi, P. de Bigontina, and L. Vecchiet. 1997. Pain threshold variations in somatic wall tissues as a function of menstrual cycle, segmental site and tissue depth in non-dysmenorrheic women, dysmenorrheic women and men. *Pain* 71:187–197.

Giamberardino, M. A., G. Affaitati, R. Lerza, L. Vecchiet, and K. J. Berkley. 1999. The impact of painful gynecological conditions on pain of urological origin. *Society of Neuroscience Abstracts* 25:143.

Giedd, J. N., F. X. Castellanos, J. C. Rajapakse, A. C. Vaituzis, and J. L. Rapoport. 1987. Sexual dimorphism of the developing human brain. *Progress in Neuro-psychopharmacology and Biological Psychiatry* 21:1185–1201.

Gilchrest, B. A., M. S. Eller, A. C. Geller, and M. Yaar. 1999. The pathogenesis of melanoma induced by ultraviolet radiation. *New England Journal of Medicine* 340:1341–1348.

Gill, R. C., K. L. Bowes, and Y. J. Kingma. 1985. Effect of progesterone on canine colonic smooth muscle. *Gastroenterology* 88:1941–1947.

Gill, R. C., P. D. Murphy, H. R. Hooper, K. L. Bowes, and Y. J. Kingma. 1987. Effect of menstrual cycle on gastric emptying. *Digestion* 36:168–174.

Gillette, J. R. 1973. Overview of drug-protein binding. *Annals of the New York Academy of Sciences* 226:6–17.

Gillum, R. F., M. E. Mussolino, and J. H. Madans. 1997. Coronary heart disease incidence and survival in African-American women and men. The NHANES I Epidemiological Follow-up Study. *Annals of Internal Medicine* 127:111–118.

Gilmore, D. A., J. Gal, J. G. Gerber, and A. S. Nies. 1992. Age and gender influence the stereoselective pharmacokinetics of propranolol. *Journal of Pharmacology and Experimental Therapeutics* 261:1181–1186.

Giltay, E. J., D. van Schaardenburg, L. J. Gooren, C. Popp-Sijders, and B. A. Dijkmans. 1999. Androgens and ankylosing spondylitis: a role in the pathogenesis? *Annals of the New York Academy of Sciences* 876:340–364.

Gintzler, A. R., and N.-J. Liu. 2000. Ovarian sex steroids activate antinociceptive systems and reveal gender-specific mechanisms, pp. 89–108. *In: Sex, Gender, and Pain*. R. B. Fillingim, ed. Seattle: IASP Press.

Godwin, J., D. Crews, and R. R. Warner. 1996. Behavioural sex change in the absence of gonads in a coral reef fish. *Proceedings of the Royal Society of London* 263:1683–1688.

Goldberg, R., D. Goff, L. Cooper, R. Luepker, J. Zapka, V. Bittner, S. Osganian, D. Lessard, C. Cornell, A. Meshack, C. Mann, J. Gilliland, and H. Feldman. 2000. Age and sex differences in presentation of symptoms among patients with acute coronary disease: the REACT Trial. Rapid Early Action for Coronary Treatment. *Coronary Artery Disease* 11:399–407.

Goldsmith, L. A., and E. H. Epstein, Jr. 1999. Genetics in Relation to the Skin. *In: Fitzpatick's Dermatology in General Medicine*. 5th edition. I. M. Freedberg, A. Z. Eisen, and K. Wolff, eds. New York: McGraw Hill.

Goldstein, A., L. Aronow, and S. M. Kalman. 1969. *Principles of Drug Action*, p. 189. New York: Paul B. Hoebner, Inc.

Goldstein, J. L., W. R. Hazzard, H. G. Schrott, E. L. Bierman, and A. G. Motulsky. 1973a. Hyperlipidemia in coronary heart disease. I. Lipid levels in 500 survivors of myocardial infarction. *Journal of Clinical Investigation* 52:1533–1543.

Goldstein, J. L., H. G. Schrott, W. R. Hazzard, E. L. Bierman, and A. G. Motulsky. 1973b. Hyperlipidemia in coronary heart disease. II. Genetic analysis of lipid levels in 176 families and delineation of a new inherited disorder, combined hyperlipidemia. *Journal of Clinical Investigation* 52:1544–1568.

Goldstein, J. L., H. H. Hobbs, and M. S. Brown. 1995. *Familial Hypercholesterolemia in the Metabolic and Molecular Bases of Inherited Disease*. Vol. II. C. R. Scrivner, A. S. Beaudet, W. S. Sly, and D. Valle, eds. New York: McGraw-Hill.

Gonda, I. 2000. The ascent of pulmonary drug delivery. *Journal of Pharmaceutical Sciences* 89:940–945.

Goran, M. I. 2000. Energy metabolism and obesity. *Medical Clinics of North America* 84:347–362.

Gordon, D. J., J. L. Probstfield, R. J. Garrison, J. D. Neaton, W. P. Castelli, J. D. Knoke, D. R. Jacobs Jr., S. Bangdiwali, and H. A. Tyroler. 1989. High density lipoprotein cholesterol and cardiovascular disease. Four prospective American studies. *Circulation* 79:8–15.

Gordon, H. W., and P. A. Lee. 1993. No difference in cognitive performance between phases of the menstrual cycle. *Psychoneuroendocrinology* 18:521–531.

Gorski, R. A., J. H. Gordon, J. E. Shryne, and A. M. Southam. 1978. Evidence for a morphological sex difference within the medial preoptic area of the rat brain. *Brain Research* 148:333–439.

Gottlieb, G. 1997. *Synthesizing Nature-Nurture: Prenatal Roots of Instinctive Behavior*. Mahwah, NJ: Lawrence Erlbaum Associates.

Govaert, T. M., G. J. Dinant, K. Aretz, N. Masurel, M. J. Sprenger, and J. A. Knottnerus. 1993. Adverse reactions to influenza vaccine in elderly people: randomised double blind placebo controlled trial. *British Medical Journal* 307:988–990.

Goy, R. W., and B. S. McEwen. 1980. *Sexual Differentiation of the Brain.* London: Oxford University Press.

Goy, R. W., F. B. Bercovitch, and M. C. McBrair. 1988. Behavioral masculinization is independent of genital masculinization in prenatally androgenized female rhesus macaques. *Hormones and Behavior* 22:552–571.

Graber, J. A., P. M. Lewinsohn, J. R. Seeley, and J. Brooks-Gunn. 1997. Is psychopathology associated with the timing of pubertal development? *Journal of the American Academy of Child and Adolescent Psychiatry* 36:1768–1776.

Greenbaum C. J., D. A. Schatz, D. Cuthberson, A. Zeidler, G. S. Eisenbarth, and J. P. Krischer. 2000. Islet cell antibody-positive relatives with human leukocyte antigen DQA*0102, DQB*0602: identification by the Diabetes Prevention Trial-type 1. *Journal of Clinical Endocrinology and Metabolism* 85:1255–1260.

Greenblatt, D. J., M. Divoll, J. S. Harmatz, and R. I. Shader. 1980. Oxazepam kinetics: effects of age and sex. *Journal of Pharmacology and Experimental Therapeutics* 215:86–91.

Greenblatt, D. J., D. R. Abernethy, R. Matlis, J. S. Harmatz, and R. I. Shader. 1984. Absorption and disposition of ibuprofen in the elderly. *Arthritis and Rheumatism* 27:1066–1069.

Greenland, P., H. Reicher-Reiss, U. Goldbourt, and S. Behar. 1991. In-hospital and 1-year mortality in 1,524 women after myocardial infarction—comparison with 4,315 men. *Circulation* 83:484–491.

Greiff, J. M., and D. Rowbotham. 1994. Pharmacokinetic drug interactions with gastrointestinal motility modifying agents. *Clinical Pharmacokinetics* 27:447–461.

Griffin, J. E., M.J. McPhaul, D. Russell, and J. D. Wilson. 1995. The androgen resistance syndromes: 5α-reductase deficiency, testicular feminization, and related disorders, pp. 1919–1944. *In: The Metabolic and Molecular Basis of Inherited Disease*, 7th ed. C. R. Scriver, A. L. Beaudet, W.A. Sly, and D. Valle, eds. New York: McGraw-Hill.

Grimshaw, G. M., G. Sitarenios, and J. A. Finegan. 1995. Mental rotation at 7 years: relations with prenatal testosterone levels and spatial play experience. *Brain and Cognition* 29: 85–100.

Grodstein, F., J. E. Manson, G. A. Colditz, W. C. Willett, F. E. Speizer, and M. J. Stampfer. 2000. A prospective, observational study of postmenopausal hormone therapy and primary prevention of cardiovascular disease. *Annals of Internal Medicine* 133:933–941.

Gron, G., A. P. Wunderlich, M. Spitzer, R. Tomczak, and M. W. Riepe. 2000. Brain activation during human navigation: gender-different neural networks as substrate of performance. *Nature Neuroscience* 3:404–408.

Gross, A. S., B. Heuer, and M. Eichelbaum. 1988. Stereoselective protein binding of verapamil enantiomers. *Biochemical Pharmacology* 37:4623–4627.

Groswasser, Z., M. Cohen, and O. Keren. 1998. Female TBI patients recover better than males. *Brain Injury* 12:805–808.

Grumbach, M. M. 2000. Estrogen, bone, growth and sex: a sea change in conventional wisdom. *Journal of Pediatric Endocrinology and Metabolism* 13(Suppl. 6):1439–1455.

Grumbach, M. M., and R. J. Auchus. 1999. Estrogen: consequences and implications of human mutations in synthesis and action. *Journal of Clinical Endocrinology and Metabolism* 84:4677–4694.

Grumbach, M. M., and F. A. Conte. 1998. Disorders of sex differentiation, pp. 1303–1425. *In: Williams Textbook of Endocrinology*, 9th ed. J. D. Wilson, D. W. Foster, H. M. Kronenberg, and P. R. Larsen, eds. Philadelphia: W. B. Saunders Co.

Grumbach, M. M., and P. D. Gluckman. 1994. The human fetal hypothalamus and pituitary gland: the maturation of neuroendocrine mechanisms controlling the secretion of fetal pituitary growth hormone, prolactin, gonadotropin, adrenocorticotropin-related peptides, and thyrotropin, pp. 193–261. *In: Maternal-Fetal Endocrinology*, 2nd ed. D. Tulchinsky and A. B. Little, eds. Philadelphia: W. B. Saunders Co.

Grumbach, M. M., and S. L. Kaplan. 1990. The neuroendocrinology of human puberty: an ontogenetic perspective, pp. 1–62. In: Control of the Onset of Puberty. M. M. Grumbach, P. C. Sizonenko, and M.L. Aubert, eds. Baltimore: Williams & Wilkins.

Grumbach, M. M., and D. M. Styne. 1998. Puberty: ontogeny, neuroendocrinology, physiology, and disorders, pp. 1509–1625. In: Williams Textbook of Endocrinology, 9th ed. J. D. Wilson, D. W. Foster, H. M. Kronenberg, and P. R. Larsen, eds. Philadelphia: W. B. Saunders Co.

Gryback, P., E. Naslund, P. M. Hellstrom, H. Jacobsson, and L. Backman. 1996. Gastric emptying of solids in humans: improved evaluation by Kaplan-Meier plots, with special reference to obesity and gender. European Journal of Nuclear Medicine 23:1562–1567.

Guballa, N., L. Sammaritano, S. Schwartzman, J. Buyon, and M. D. Lockshin. 2000. Ovulation induction and in vitro fertilization in systemic lupus erythematosus and antiphospholipid syndrome. Arthritis and Rheumatism 43:550–556.

Guinee, D. G. Jr., W. D. Travis, G. E. Trivers, V. M. De Benedetti, H. Cawley, J. A. Welsh, W. P. Bennett, J. Jett, T. V. Colby, H. Tazelaar, S. L. Abbondanzo, P. Pairolero, V. Trastek, N. E. Caporaso, L. A. Litto, and C. C. Harris. 1995. Gender comparisons in human lung cancer: anaylsis of p53 mutations, anti-p53 serum antibodies and C-erbB-2 expression. Carcinogenesis 16:993–1002.

Gupta, S. K., L. Atkinson, T. Tu, and J. A. Longstreth. 1995. Age and gender related changes in stereoselective pharmacokinetics and pharmacodynamics of verapamil and norverapamil. British Journal of Clinical Pharmacology 40:325–331.

Gutierrez-Adan, A., M. Oter, B. Martinez-Madrid, B. Pintado, and J. De La Fuente. 2000. Differential expression of two genes located on the X chromosome between male and female in vitro-produced bovine embryos at the blastocyst stage. Molecular Reproduction and Development 55:146–151.

Haarbo, J., D. F. Hansen, and C. Christiansen. 1991. Hormone replacement therapy prevents coronary artery disease in ovariectomized cholesterol-fed rabbits. Acta Pathologica, Microbiologica, et Immunologica Scandinavica 99:721–727.

Haffner, S. M., L. Mykkanen, R. A. Valdez, M. Paidi, M. P. Stern, and B. V. Howard. 1993. LDL size and subclass pattern in a biethnic population. Arteriosclerosis and Thrombosis 13:1623–1630.

Hagen, A. A., and W. J. Hrushesky. 1998. Menstrual timing of breast cancer surgery. American Journal of Surgery 175:245–261.

Haig, D. 2000. Of sex and gender. Nature Genetics 25:373.

Haldane, J. B. S. 1935. The rate of spontaneous mutation of a human gene. Journal of Genetics 31:317–326.

Hall, E. D., K. E. Pazara, and K. L. Linseman. 1991. Sex differences in postischemic neuronal necrosis in gerbils. Journal of Cerebral Blood Flow and Metabolism 11:292–298.

Hall, J. A., and J. D. Carter. 1999. Gender-stereotype accuracy as an individual difference. Journal of Personality & Social Psychology 77:350–359.

Halpern, D. F. 2000. Sex Differences in Cognitive Abilities, 3rd ed. Mahwah, NJ: Lawrence Erlbaum Associates.

Hampson, E. In press. Sex differences in human brain and cognition: the influence of sex steroids in early and adult life. In: Behavioral Endocrinology, 2nd ed. J. B. Becker, S. M. Breedlove, D. Crews, and M. McCarthy, eds. Cambridge, MA: MIT Press/Bradford Books.

Hampson, E. 1990a Variations in sex-related cognitive abilities across the menstrual cycle. Brain and Cognition 14:26–43.

Hampson, E. 1990b. Estrogen-related variations in human spatial and articulatory-motor skills. Psychoneuroendocrinology 15:97–111.

Hampson, E., and D. Kimura. 1988. Reciprocal effects of hormonal fluctuations on human motor and perceptual-spatial skills. Behavioral Neuroscience 102:456–459.

Hampson, E., and D. Kimura. 1992. Sex differences and hormonal influences on cognitive function in humans, pp. 357–398. *In: Behavioral Endocrinology.* J. B. Becker, S. M. Breedlove, and D. Crews, eds. Cambridge, MA: MIT Press.

Hampson, E., J. F. Rovet, and D. Altmann. 1998. Spatial reasoning in children with congenital adrenal hyperplasia due to 21-hydroxylase deficiency. *Developmental Neuropsychology* 14:299–320.

Hampson, J. L., and J. G. Hampson. 1961. The ontogenesis of sexual behavior in man. *In: Sex and Internal Secretions.* W. C. Young and G. W. Corner, eds. Baltimore: Williams & Wilkins.

Hanley, N. A., S. G. Ball, M. Clement-Jones, D. M. Hagan, T. Strachan, S. Lindsay, S. Robson, H. Ostrer, K. L. Parker, and D. I. Wilson. 1999. Expression of steroidogenic factor 1 and Wilms' tumor 1 during early human gonadal development and sex determination. *Mechanisms of Development* 87:175–180.

Hanley, N. A., D. M. Hagan, M. Clement-Jones, S. G. Ball, T. Strachan, L. Salas-Cortes, K. McElreavey, S. Lindsay, S. Robson, P. Bullen, H. Ostrer, and D. I. Wison. 2000. SRY, SOX9, and DAX1 expression patterns during human sex determination and gonadal development. *Mechanisms of Development* 91:403–407.

Hans-Filho, G., V. Aoki, E. Rivitti, D. P. Eaton, M. S. Lin, and L. A. Diaz. 1999. Endemic pemphigus foliaceus (fogo selvagem)—1998: the Cooperative Group on Fogo Selvagem Research. *Clinics in Dermatology* 17:225–235.

Harris, R. Z., L. Z. Benet, and J. B. Schwartz. 1995. Gender effects in pharmacokinetics and pharmacodynamics. *Drugs* 50:222–239.

Haseltine, F. O., and B. G. Jacobson, eds. 1997. *Women's Health Research: A Medical and Policy Primer.* Washington, DC: Health Press International.

Haskell, S. G., E. D. Richardson, and R. I. Horwitz. 1997. The effect of estrogen replacement therapy on cognitive function in women: a critical review of the literature. *Journal of Clinical Epidemiology* 50:1249–1264.

Hassink, S. G., D. V. Sheslow, E. de Lancey, I. Opentanova, R. V. Considine, and J. F. Caro. 1996. Serum leptin in children with obesity: relationship to gender and development. *Pediatrics* 98(2 Pt 1):201–203.

Hassold, T., S. Sherman, and P. Hunt. 2000. Counting cross-overs: characterizing meiotic recombination in mammals. *Human Molecular Genetics* 9:2409–2419.

Havlichek, D., Jr., K. Rosenman, M. Simms, and P. Guss. 1997. Age-related hepatitis B seroconversion rates in health care workers. *American Journal of Infection Control* 25: 418–420.

Hayashi, T., and D. Faustman. 1999. NOD mice are defective in proteasome production and activation of NF-kappaB. *Molecular and Cellular Biology* 19:8646–8659.

Hazzard, W. R., J. L. Goldstein, M. G. Schrott, A. G. Motulsky, and E. L. Bierman. 1973. Hyperlipidemia in coronary heart disease. III. Evaluation of lipoprotein phenotypes of 156 genetically defined survivors of myocardial infarction. *Journal of Clinical Investigation* 52:1569–1577.

Heard, E., P. Clerc, and P. Avner. 1997. X-chromosome inactivation in mammals. *Annual Review of Genetics* 31:571–610.

Hebbard, G. S., W. M. Sun, F. Bochner, and M. Horowitz. 1995. Pharmacokinetic considerations in gastrointestinal motor disorders. *Clinical Pharmacokinetics* 28:41–66.

Heegaard, A., H. L. Jorgensen, A. W. Vestergaard, C. Hassager, and S. H. Ralston. 2000. Lack of influence of collagen type Ialpha1 Sp1 binding site polymorphism on the rate of bone loss in a cohort of postmenopausal Danish women followed for 18 years. *Calcified Tissue International* 66:409–413.

Henney, J. E. 2000. From the food and drug administration. *Journal of the American Medical Association* 283:2779.

Herman-Giddens, M. E., E. J. Slora, R. C. Wasserman, C. J. Bourdony, M. V. Bhapkar, G. G. Koch, and C. M. Hasemeier. 1997. Secondary sexual characteristics and menses in young girls seen in office practice: a study from the Pediatric Research in Office Settings network. *Pediatrics* 99:505–512.

Hermansson, G., and R. Silvertsson,. 1996. Gender-related differences in gastric emptying rate of solid meals. *Digestive Diseases and Sciences* 41:1994–1998.

Herrington D. M., D. M. Reboussin, K. B. Brosnihan, P. C. Sharp, S. A. Shumaker, T. E. Snyder, C. D. Furberg, G. J. Kowalchuk, T. D. Stuckey, W. J. Rogers, D. H. Givens, and D. Waters. 2000. Effects of estrogen replacement on the progression of coronary-artery atherosclerosis. *New England Journal of Medicine* 343:522–529.

Heymsfield, S. B., Z. Wang, R. N. Baumgartner, and R. Ross. 1997. Human body composition: advances in models and methods. *Annual Review of Nutrition* 17:527–558.

Hier, D. B., and W. F. Crowley, Jr. 1982. Spatial ability in androgen-deficient men. *New England Journal of Medicine* 306:1202–1205.

Higaki, J., S. Baba, T. Katsuya, N. Sato, K. Ishikawa, T. Mannami, J. Ogata, and T. Ogihara. 2000. Deletion allele of angiotensin-converting enzyme gene increases risk of essential hypertension in Japanese men: the Suita Study. *Circulation* 101:2060–2065.

Hill, J. O., and J. C. Peters. 1998. Environmental contributors to the obesity epidemic. *Science* 280:1371–1374.

Hill, J. P., and M. E. Lynch. 1983. The intensification of gender-related role expectations during early adolescence, pp. 201–228. In: *Girls at Puberty: Biological and Psychosocial Perspectives*. J. Brooks-Gunn and A. C. Petersen, eds. New York: Plenum Press.

Hines, M. 1990. Gonadal hormones and human cognitive development, pp. 51–63. In: *Hormones, Brain and Behavior in Vertebrates. 1. Sexual Differentiation, Neuroanatomical Aspects, Neurotransmitters and Neuropeptides*, Vol. 1. J. Balthazart, ed. Basel: Karger.

Hiort, O., and P. M. Holterhus. 2000. The molecular basis of male sexual differentiation. *European Journal of Endocrinology* 142:101–110.

Hobart, J. A., and D. R. Smucker. 2000. The female athlete triad. *American Family Physician* 61:3357–3364.

Holbrook, T. L. 1985. *The Frequency of Occurrence, Impact and Cost of Muscoskeletal Conditions in the United States*. Chicago: American Academy of Orthopedic Surgeons.

Holm, P., H. T. Andersen, G. Arroe, and S. Stender. 1998. Gender gap in aortic cholesterol accumulation in cholesterol-clamped rabbits: role of the endothelium and mononuclear-endothelial cell interaction. *Circulation* 98:2731–2737.

Holmes, C. B., H. Hausler, and P. Nunn. 1998. A review of sex differences in the epidemiology of tuberculosis. *International Journal of Tuberculosis and Lung Disease* 2:96–104.

Holroyd, K. A., and G. L. Lipchik. 2000. Differences in recurrent headache disorders: over view and significance, pp. 251–279. In: *Sex, Gender, and Pain*. R. B. Fillingim, ed. Seattle: IASP Press.

Hoover, R. N. 2000. Cancer—nature, nurture, or both (editorial). *New England Journal of Medicine* 343:135–136.

Horlick, M. B., M. Rosenbaum, M. Nicolson, L. S. Levine, B. Fedun, J. Wang, R. N. Pierson, Jr., and R. L. Leibel. 2000. Effect of puberty on the relationship between circulating leptin and body composition. *Journal of Clinical Endocrinology and Metabolism* 85: 2509–2518.

Horowitz, M., G. J. Maddern, B. E. Chatterton, P. J. Collins, P. E. Harding, and D. J. Shearman. 1984. Changes in gastric emptying rates with age. *Clinical Science* 67:213–218.

Horowitz, M., G. J. Maddern, B. E. Chatterton, P. J. Collins, O. M. Pertucco, R. Seamark, and D. J. Shearman. 1985. The normal menstrual cycle has no effect on gastric emptying. *British Journal of Obstetrics and Gynaecology* 92:743–746.

Horst, R. L., J. P. Goff, and T. A. Reinhardt. 1997. Calcium and vitamin D metabolism during lactation. *Journal of Mammary Gland Biology and Neoplasia* 2:253-263.

Hoyenga, K. B., and K. T. Hoyenga. 1982. Gender and energy balance: sex differences in adaptations for feast and famine. *Physiology and Behavior* 28:545–563.

Hoyle, E., S. H. Laval, A. Calin, B. P. Wordsworth, and M. A. Brown. 2000. The X-chromosome and susceptibility to ankylosing spondylitis. *Arthritis and Rheumatism* 43: 1353–1355.

Hudelson, P. 1996. Gender differences in tuberculosis: the role of socio-economic and cultural factors. *Tubercle and Lung Disease* 77:391–400.

Hulley, S., D. Grady, T. Bush, C. Furburg, D. Herrington, B. Riggs, and E. Vittinghoff. 1998. Randomized trial of estrogen plus progestin for secondary prevention of coronary heart disease in postmenopausal women. Heart and Estrogen/Progestin Replacement Study (HERS) Research Group. *Journal of the American Medical Association* 280:605–613.

Hulst, L. K., J. C. Fleishaker, G. R. Peters, J. D. Harry, D. M. Wright, and P. Ward. 1994. Influence of sex, menstrual cycle and oral contraception on the disposition of nitrazepam. *British Journal of Clinical Pharmacology* 13:319–324.

Hunt, P. A., and R. LeMaire. 1992. Sex-chromosome pairing: evidence that the behavior of the pseudoautosomal region differs during male and female meiosis. *American Journal of Human Genetics* 50:1162–1170.

Huopio, J., H. Kroger, R. Honkanen, S. Saarikoski, and E. Alhava. 2000. Risk factors for perimenopausal fractures: a prospective study. *Osteoporosis International* 11:219–227.

Hurst, L. D., and H. Ellegren. 1998. Sex biases in the mutation rate. *Trends in Genetics* 14: 446–452.

Hutson, W. R., R. L. Roehrkasse, and A. Wald. 1989. Influence of gender and menopause on gastric emptying and motility. *Gastroenterology* 96:11–17.

Hyde, J. S., and M. C. Linn. 1988. Gender differences in verbal ability: a meta-analysis. *Psychological Bulletin* 104:53–69.

Hyde, R. J., and R. P. Feller. 1981. Age and sex effects on taste of sucrose, NaCl, citric acid and caffeine. *Neurobiology of Aging* 2:315–318.

Ibáñez, L., N. Potau, M. Zampolli, N. Pratt, R. Virdis, E. Vicens-Calvet, and A. Carrascosa. 1996. Hyperinsulinemia in postpubertal girls with a history of premature pubarche and functional ovarian hyperandrogenism. *Journal of Clinical Endocrinology and Metabolism* 81:1237–1243.

Ibáñez, L., N. Potau, I. Francois, and F. de Zegher. 1998. Precocious pubarche, hyperinsulinism, and ovarian hyperandrogenism in girls: relation to reduced fetal growth. *Journal of Clinical Endocrinology and Metabolism* 83:3558–3562.

Ibáñez, L., N. Potau, M. V. Marcos, and F. de Zegher. 1999a. Exaggerated adrenarche and hyperinsulinism in adolescent girls born small for gestational age. *Journal of Clinical Endocrinology and Metabolism* 84:4739–4741.

Ibáñez, L., N. Potau, and F. de Zegher. 1999b. Precocious pubarche, dyslipidemia, and low IGF binding protein-1 in girls: relation to reduced prenatal growth. *Pediatric Research* 46:320–322.

Ibáñez, L., N. Potau, and F. de Zegher. 2000. Ovarian hyporesponsiveness to follicle stimulating hormone in adolescent girls born small for gestational age. *Journal of Clinical Endocrinology and Metabolism* 85:2624–2626.

Ingvar, M., and J.-C. Hsieh. 1999. The image of pain, pp. 215–233. *In: Textbook of Pain*, 4th ed. P. D. Wall and R. Melzack, eds. Edinburgh: Churchill Livingstone.

Institute of Medicine. 1992. *Body Composition and Physical Performance, Applications for the Military Services*. B. M. Marriott and J. Grumstrup-Scott, eds. Washington, DC: National Academy Press.

Institute of Medicine. 1993. *Veterans at Risk: The Health Effects of Mustard Gas and Lewisite*. C. M. Pechura and D. P. Rall, eds. Washington, DC: National Academy Press.

Institute of Medicine. 1994. *Women and Health Research*, Vol. 1. *Ethical and Legal Issues of Including Women in Clinical Studies*. A. C. Mastroianni, R. Faden, and D. Federman, eds. Washington, DC: National Academy Press.

Institute of Medicine. 1996. *In Her Lifetime: Female Morbidity and Mortality in Sub-Saharan Africa*. C. P. Howson, P. F. Harrison, D. Hotra, and M. Law, eds. Washington, DC: National Academy Press.

Institute of Medicine. 1998. *Assessing Readiness in Military Women. The Relationship of Body Composition, Nutrition and Health*. Washington, DC: National Academy Press.

Institute of Medicine. 2000. *Bridging Disciplines in the Brain, Behavioral, and Clinical Sciences*. T. C. Pellmar and L. Eisenberg, eds. Washington, DC: National Academy Press.

International Committee of Medical Journal Editors. 1997. Uniform requirements for manuscripts submitted to biomedical journals. *New England Journal of Medicine* 336:309–315.

International Human Genome Sequencing Consortium. 2001. Initial sequencing and analysis of the human genome. *Nature* 409:860–921.

International SNP Map Working Group. 2001. A map of human genome sequence variation containing 1.42 million single nucleotide polymorphisms. *Nature* 409:928–933.

Irwin, M. 1999. Immune correlates of depression. *Advances in Experimental Medicine and Biology* 461:1–24.

Ishida, N., M. Kaneko, and R. Allada. 1999. Biological clocks. *Proceedings of the National Academy of Sciences of the United States of America* 96:8819–8820.

Ito, I., T. Hayashi, K. Yamada, M. Kuzuya, M. Naito, and A. Iguchi. 1995. Physiological concentration of estradiol inhibits polymorphonuclear leukocyte chemotaxis via a receptor mediated system. *Life Sciences* 56:2247–2253.

Iverson, C. (chair). 1998. *American Medical Association Manual of Style: A Guide for Authors and Editors*, 9th ed. Baltimore: Williams & Wilkins.

Jacobs, D., M. X. Tang, Y. Stern, M. Sano, K. Marder, K. L. Bell, P. Schofield, G. Dooneief, B. Gurland, and R. Mayeux. 1998. Cognitive function in nondemented older women who took estrogen after menopause. *Neurology* 50:368–373.

Jacobs, D. R., Jr., I. L. Mebane, S. I. Bangdiwala, M. H. Criqui, and H. A. Tyroler. 1990. High density lipoprotein cholesterol as a predictor of cardiovascular disease mortality in men and women: the follow-up study of the Lipid Research Clinics Prevalence Study. *American Journal of Epidemiology* 131:32–47.

James, W. P. 1995. A public health approach to the problem of obesity. *International Journal of Obesity and Related Metabolic Disorders* 19:S37–S45.

James, G. D., J. E. Sealey, M. Alderman, S. Ljungman, F. B. Mueller, M. S. Pecker, and J. H. Laragh. 1988. A longitudinal study of urinary creatinine and creatinine clearance in normal subjects. Race, sex, and age differences. *American Journal of Hypertension* 1:124–131.

Jann, M. W., T. L. ZumBrunnen, S. N. Tenjarla, E. S. Ward, Jr., and D. J. Weidler. 1998. Relative bioavailability of ondansetron 8-mg oral tablets versus two extemporaneous 16-mg suppositiories: formulation and gender differences. *Pharmacotherapy* 18:288–294.

Jaquet, D., J. Leger, D. Chevenne, P. Czernichow, and C. Levy-Marchal. 1999. Intrauterine growth retardation predisposes to insulin resistance but not to hyperandrogenism in young women. *Journal of Clinical Endocrinology and Metabolism* 84:3945–3949.

Jatoi, I. 1998. Timing of surgery for primary breast cancer with regard to the menstrual phase and prognosis. *Breast Cancer Research and Treatment* 52:217–225.

Jegalian, K., and D. C. Page. 1998. A proposed path by which genes common to mammalian X and Y chromosomes evolve to become X inactivated. *Nature* 394:776–780.

Jochemsen, R., M. van der Graaff, J. K. Boeijinga, and D. D. Breimer. 1982. Influence of sex, menstrual cycle and oral contraception on the disposition of nitrazepam. *British Journal of Clinical Pharmacology* 13:319–324.

Johnson, J. L., E. F. Heineman, G. Heiss, C. G. Hames, H. A. Tyroler. 1986. Cardiovascular disease risk factors and mortality among black women and white women aged 40-64 years in Evans County, Georgia. *American Journal of Epidemiology* 123:209–220.

Jones, L. V. 1984. White-black achievement differences: the narrowing gap. *American Psychologist* 39:1207–1213.

Jordan, A. S., P. G. Catcheside, R. S. Orr, F. J. O'Donoghue, N. A. Saunders, and R. D. McEvoy. 2000. Ventilatory decline after hypoxia and hypercapnia is not different between healthy young men and women. *Journal of Applied Physiology* 88:3–9.

Josefsson, E., A. Tarkowski, and H. Carlsten. 1992. Anti-inflammatory properties of estrogen. I. In vivo suppression of leukocyte production in bone marrow and redistribution of peripheral blood neutrophils. *Cellular Immunology* 142:67–78.

Josso, N., R. L. Cate, J.Y. Picard, B. Vigier, N. di Clemente, C. Wilson, S. Imbeaud, R. B. Pepinsky, D. Guerrier, and L. Boussin. 1993. Anti-Müllerian hormone: the Jost factor. *Recent Progress in Hormone Research* 48:1–59.

Journal of the National Cancer Institute. 2000. Information for authors. *Journal of the National Cancer Institute* 92:1621.

Kailasam, M. T., J. A. Martinez, J. H. Cervenka, S. S. C. Yen, D. T. O'Connor, and R. J. Parmer. 1998. Racial differences in renal kallikrein excretion: effect of the ovulatory cycle. *Kidney International* 54:1652–1658.

Kamel, H. K., H. M. Perry III, and J. E. Morley. 2001. Hormone replacement therapy and fractures in older adults. *Journal of the American Geriatrics Society* 49:179–187.

Kamm, M. A., M. J. Farthing, and J. E. Lennard-Jones.1989. Bowel function and transit during the menstrual cycle. *Gut* 30:605–608.

Kammer, G. M., and G. C. Tsokos. 1998. Emerging concepts of the molecular basis for estrogen effects on T lymphocytes in systemic lupus erythematosus. *Clinical Immunology and Immunopathology* 89:192–195.

Kanda, N., T. Tsuchida, and K. Tamaki. 1999. Estrogen enhancement of anti-double-stranded DNA antibody and immunoglobulin G production in peripheral blood mononuclear cells from patients with systemic lupus erythematosus. *Arthritis and Rheumatism* 42:328–337.

Kanikkannan, N., K. Kandimalla, S. S. Lamba, and M. Singh. 2000. Structure-activity relationship of chemical penetration enhancers in transdermal drug delivery. *Current Medicinal Chemistry* 7:593–608.

Kannel, W. B., and R. D. Abbott. 1987. Incidence and prognosis of myocardial infarction in women: the Framingham study. *In: Coronary Heart Disease in Women: Proceedings from the NHLBI Workshop.* E. D. Eaker, B. Packard, M. K. Wenger, and K. Nanette, eds. New York: Haymarket Doyma.

Kannel, W. B., D. McGee, and T. Gordon. 1976. A general cardiovascular risk profile: the Framingham Study. *American Journal of Cardiology* 38:46–51.

Kaplan, R. M., and P. Erickson. 2000. Gender differences in quality-adjusted survival using a Health-Utilities Index. *American Journal of Preventive Medicine* 18:77–82.

Kaplan, S. L., and M. M. Grumbach. 1978. Pituitary and placental gonadotropins and sex steroids in the human and sub-human fetus. *Clinics in Endocrinology and Metabolism* 7:487–511.

Kashuba, A. D., and A. N. Nafziger. 1998. Physiological changes during the menstrual cycle and their effects on the pharmacokinetics and pharmacodynamics of drugs. *Clinical Pharmacokinetics* 34:203–218.

Kato, I., P. Toniolo, A. Zeleniuch-Jacquotte, R. E. Shore, K. L. Koenig, A. Akhmedkhanov, and E. Riboli. 2000. Diet, smoking and anthropometric indices and postmenopausal bone fractures: a prospective study. *International Journal of Epidemiology* 29:85–92.

Katz, L. C., and C. J. Shatz. 1996. Synaptic activity and the construction of cortical circuits. *Science* 274:1133–1138.

Katzburg, S., M. Lieberherr, A. Ornoy, B. Y. Klein, D. Hendel, and D. Somjen. 1999. Isolation and hormonal responsiveness of primary cultures of human bone-derived cells: gender and age differences. *Bone* 25:667–673.

Kennedy, A., T. W. Gettys, P. Watson, P. Wallace, E. Ganaway, Q. Pan, and W. T. Garvey. 1997. The metabolic significance of leptin in humans: gender-based differences in relationship to adiposity, insulin sensitivity, and energy expenditure. *Journal of Clinical Endocrinology and Metabolism* 82:1293–1300.

Kent-First, M., A. Muallem, J. Shultz, J. Pryor, K. Roberts, W. Nolten, L. Meisner, A. Chandley, G. Gouchy, L. Jorgensen, T. Havighurst, and J. Grosch. 1999. Defining regions of the Y-chromosome responsible for male infertility and identification of a fourth AZF region (AZFd) by Y-chromosome microdeletion detection. *Molecular Reproduction and Development* 53:27–41.

Kerns, K. A., and S. A. Berenbaum. 1991. Sex differences in spatial ability in children. *Behavior Genetics* 21:383–396.

Kessler, S. 1998. *Lessons from the Intersexed.* New Brunswick, NJ: Rutgers University Press.

Khetawat, G., N. Faraday, M. L. Nealen, K. V. Vijayan, E. Bolton, S. J. Noga, and P. F. Bray. 2000. Human megakaryocytes and platelets contain the estrogen receptor beta and androgen receptor (AR): testosterone regulates AR expression. *Blood* 95:2289–2296.

Khosla, S., L. J. Melton III, and B. L. Riggs. 1999. Osteoporosis: gender differences and similarities. *Lupus* 8:393–396.

Khosla, S., L. J. Melton III, E. J. Atkinson, W. M. O'Fallon, G. G. Klee, and B. L. Riggs. 1998. Relationship of serum sex steroid levels and bone turnover markers with bone mineral density in men and women: a key role for bioavailable estrogen. *Journal of Clinical Endocrinology and Metabolism* 83:2266–2274.

Kim, J. S., and A. N. Nafziger. 2000. Is it sex or is it gender? (commentary). *Clinical Pharmacology and Therapeutics* 68:1–3.

Kim, S., and R. R. Voskuhl. 1999. Decreased IL-12 production underlies the decreased ability of male lymph node cells to induce experimental autoimmune encephalomyelitis. *Journal of Immunology* 162:5561–5568.

Kimura, D. 1995. Estrogen replacement therapy may protect against intellectual decline in postmenopausal women. *Hormones and Behavior* 29:312–321.

Kirschstein, R. L. 2000. Testimony before the Subcommittee on Public Health of the Senate Committee on Health, Education, Labor, and Pensions, July 26, Washington, DC. Provided by Office of the Director, National Institutes of Health, Rockville, MD.

Kjeldsen, S. E., R. E. Kolloch, G. Leonetti, J. M. Mallion, A. Zanchetti, D. Elmfeldt, I. Warnold, and L. Hansson. 2000. Influence of gender and age on preventing cardiovascular disease by antihypertensive treatment and acetylsalicylic acid. The HOT study. Hypertension Optimal Treatment. *Journal of Hypertension* 18:629–642.

Klein, K. O., J. Baron, M. J. Colli, D. P. McDonnell, and G. B. Cutler, Jr. 1994. Estrogen levels in childhood determined by an ultrasensitive recombinant cell bioassay. *Journal of Clinical Investigation* 94:2475–2480.

Klein, S. L. 2000. The effects of hormones on sex differences in infection: from genes to behavior. *Neuroscience and Biobehavioral Reviews* 24:627–638.

Knight, L. C., H. P. Parkman, K. L. Brown, M. A. Miller, D. M. Trate, A. H. Maurer, and R. S. Fisher. 1997. Delayed gastric emptying and decreased antral contractility in normal premenopausal women compared with men. *American Journal of Gastroenterology* 92:968–975.

Koh, H. K., D. R. Miller, A. Geller, R. W. Clapp, M. B. Mercer, and R. A. Lew. 1992. Who discovers melanoma? Patterns from a population-based survey. *Journal of the American Academy of Dermatology* 26:914–919.

Koh, H. K., A. C. Geller, D. R. Miller, B. B. Davis, and R. A. Lew. 1995. Skin cancer: prevention and control. *In: Cancer Prevention and Control.* P. Greenwald, B. S. Kramer, and D. L. Weed, eds. New York: Marcel Dekker.

Kohen, F., L. Abel, A. Sharp, Y. Amir-Zaltsman, D. Somjen, S. Luria, G. Mor, A. Knyszynski, H. Thole, and A. Globerson. 1998. Estrogen-receptor expression and function in thymocytes in relation to gender and age. *Developmental Immunology* 5:277–285.

Koopman, P. 1999. Sry and Sox 9: mammalian testis-determining genes. *Cellular and Molecular Life Sciences* 55:839–856.

Koopman, P., J. Gubbay, N. Vivian, P. Goodfellow, and R. Lovell-Badge. 1991. Male development of chromosomally female mice transgenic for Sry. *Nature* 351:117–121.

Kosary, C. L., L. A. G. Ries, B. A. Miller, B. F. Hankey, A. Harras, and B. K. Edwards, eds. 1996. *SEER Cancer Statistics Review, 1973–1992: tables and graphs.* NIH Publication No. 96-2789. Bethesda, MD: National Cancer Institute.

Kramer, M. S. 2000. Invited commentary: association between restricted fetal growth and adult chronic disease: Is it causal? Is it important? *American Journal of Epidemiology* 52:605–608.

Kristjansson, F., and S. B. Thorsteinsson. 1991. Disposition of alprazolam in human volunteers. Differences between genders. *Acta Pharmaceutica Nordica* 3:249–250.

Krolewski, A. S., J. H. Warram, P. Valsania, B. C. Martin, L. M. Laffel, and A. R. Christlieb. 1991. Evolving natural history of coronary artery disease in diabetes mellitus. *American Journal of Medicine* 90:56S–61S.

Kubota, K., N. Kubota, G. L. Pearce, and W. H. Inman. 1996. ACE inhibitor-induced cough, an adverse drug reaction unrecognised for several years in prescription-event monitoring. *European Journal of Clinical Pharmacology* 49:431–437.

Kubota, T., C. F. McTiernan, C. S. Frye, S. E. Slawson, B. H. Lemster, A. P. Koretsky, A. J. Demetris, and A. M. Feldman. 1997. Dilated cardiomyopathy in transgenic mice with cardiac-specific overexpression of tumor necrosis factor-alpha. *Circulation Research* 81:627–635.

Kuhlkamp, V., J. Mermi, C. Mewis, and L. Seipel. 1997. Efficacy and proarrhythmia with the use of *d,l*-sotalol for sustained ventricular tachyarrhythmias. *Journal of Cardiovascular Pharmacology* 29:373–381.

Kuller, L. H., L. Shemanski, B. M. Psaty, N. O. Borhani, J. Gardin, M. N. Haan, D. H. O'Leary, and P. J. Savage. 1995. Subclinical disease as an independent risk factor for cardiovascular disease. *Circulation* 92:720-726.

Kumanyika, S. K. 1998. Obesity in African Americans: biobehavioral consequences of culture. *Ethnicity and Disease* 8:93–96.

Kuslys, T., B. S. Vishwanath, F. J. Frey, and B. M. Frey. 1996. Differences in phospholipase A2 activity between males and females and Asian Indians and Caucasians. *European Journal of Clinical Investigation* 26:310–315.

Kwangsukstith, C., and H. I. Maibach. 1995. Effect of age and sex on the induction and elicitation of allergic contact dermatitis. *Contact Dermatitis* 33:289–298.

Lahita, R. G. 1999. The role of sex hormones in systemic lupus erythematosus. *Current Opinions in Rheumatology* 11:352–356.

Lahn, B. T., and D. C. Page. 1997. Functional coherence of the human Y chromosome. *Science* 278:675–680.

Lahn, B. T., and D. C. Page. 1999. Four evolutionary strata on the human X chromosome. *Science* 286:964–967.

Lambert, N. C., O. Distler, U. Muller-Ladner, T. S. Tylee, D. E. Furst, and J. L. Nelson. 2000. HLA-DQA1 *0501 is associated with diffuse systemic sclerosis in Caucasian men. *Arthritis and Rheumatism* 43:2005–2010.

Lancet. 2001. An overstretched hypothesis? (editorial) *The Lancet* 357:405.

Lamon-Fava, S. 2000. Complete and selective estrogenic effects on lipids and cardiovascular disease. *Current Atherosclerosis Reports* 2:72–75.

Lander, E. S. 1996. The new genomics: global views of biology. *Science* 274:536–539.

Lange, N., J. N. Giedd, F. X. Castellanos, A. C. Vaituzis, and J. L. Rapoport. 1997. Variability of human brain structure size: ages 4–20 years. *Psychiatry Research* 74:1–12.

Latham, K. E., B. Patel, F. D. Bautista, and S. M. Hawes. 2000. Effects of X chromosome number and parental origin on X-linked gene expression in preimplantation mouse embryos. *Biology of Reproduction* 63:64–73.

Laubach, M., J. Wessberg, and M. A. Nicolelis. 2000. Cortical ensemble activity increasingly predicts behaviour outcomes during learning of a motor task. *Nature* 405:567–571.

Lauderdale, D. S., and P. J. Rathouz. 2000. Body mass index in a US national sample of Asian Americans: effects of nativity, years since immigration and socioeconomic status. *International Journal of Obesity and Related Metabolic Disorders* 24:1188–1194.

Laws, A., H. M. Hoen, J. V. Selby, M. F. Saad, S. M. Haffner, and B. V. Howard. 1997. Differences in insulin suppression of free fatty acid levels by gender and glucose tolerance status. Relation to plasma triglyceride and apolipoprotein B concentrations. Insulin Resistance Atherosclerosis Study (IRAS) Investigators. *Arteriosclerosis, Thrombosis, and Vascular Biology* 17:64–71.

Lefly, D. L., and B. F. Pennington. 1991. Spelling errors and reading fluency in compensated adult dyslexics. *Annals of Dyslexia* 41:143–162.

Legato, M. J. 1997. Gender-specific aspects of obesity. *International Journal of Fertility and Women's Medicine* 42:184–197.

Lehmann, M. H., S. Hardy, D. Archibald, B. Quart, and D. J. MacNeil. 1996. Sex difference in risk of torsades de pointes with d,1-sotalol. *Circulation* 15:2535–2541.

LeResche, L. 1999. Gender considerations in the epidemiology of chronic pain, pp. 43-52. In: *Epidemiology of Pain.* I. K. Crombie, P. R. Croft, S. J. Linton, L. LeResche., and M. Von Korff, eds. Seattle: IASP Press.

Lerner, D. J., and W. B. Kannel. 1986. Patterns of coronary heart disease morbidity and mortality in the sexes: a 26-year follow-up of the Framingham population. *American Heart Journal* 111:383–390.

Leveille, S. G., B. W. Penninx, D. Melzer, G. Ismirlian, and J. M. Guralnik. 2000. Sex differences in the prevalence of mobility disability in old age: the dynamics of incidence, recovery and mortality. *Journals of Gerontology Series B, Psychological Sciences and Social Sciences* 55:S41–S50.

Leveroni, C. L., and S. A. Berenbaum. 1998. Early androgen effects of interest in infants: evidence from children with congenital adrenal hyperplasia. *Developmental Neuropsychology* 14:321–340.

Levy, G. 1998. Predicting effective drug concentrations for individual patients. Determinants of pharmacodynamic variability. *Clinical Pharmacokinetics* 34:323–333.

Lew, K. H., E. A. Ludwig, M. A. Mildad, K. Donovan, E. Middleton, Jr., J. J. Ferry, and W. J. Jusko. 1993. Gender-based effects on methylprednisolone pharmacokinetics and pharmacodynamics. *Clinical Pharmacology and Therapeutics* 54:402–414.

Liberman, A. M., and I. G. Mattingly. 1989. A specialization for speech perception. *Science* 243:489–494.

Liberman, A. M. 1989. Reading is hard just because listening is easy. In: *Wenner-Gren International Symposium Series: Brain and Reading.* C. von Euler, I. Lundberg, and G. Lennerstrand, eds. New York: Stockton Press.

Likitmaskul, S., C. T. Cowell, K. Donaghue, D. J. Kreutzmann, N. J. Howard, B. Blades, and M. Silink. 1995. "Exaggerated adrenarche" in children presenting with premature adrenarche. *Clinical Endocrinology* 42:265–272.

Lillehoj, H. S., K. Beisel, and N. R. Rose. 1981. Genetic factors controlling the susceptibility to experimental autoimmune thyroiditis in inbred rat strains. *Journal of Immunology* 127:654–659.

Linn, M. C., and A. C. Petersen. 1985. Emergence and characterization of sex differences in spatial ability: a meta-analysis. *Child Development* 56:1479–1498.

Lisse, I. M., P. Aaby, H. Whittle, H. Jensen, M. Engelmann, and L. B. Christensen. 1997. T-lymphocyte subsets in West African children: impact of age, sex, and season. *Journal of Pediatrics* 130:77–85.

Litschauer, B., S. Zauchner, K. H. Huemer, and A. Kafka-Lutzow. 1998. Cardiovascular, endocrine, and receptor measures as related to sex and menstrual cycle phase. *Psychosomatic Medicine* 60:219–226.

Liu, D., J. Diorio, J. C. Day, D. D. Francis, and M. J. Meaney. 2000. Maternal care, hippocampal synaptogenesis and cognitive development in rats. *Nature Neuroscience* 3:799–806.

Lockhart, D. J., and E. A. Winzeler. 2000. Genomics, gene expression and DNA arrays. *Nature* 405:827–836.

Lockshin, M. D. 1993. Does lupus flare during pregnancy? *Lupus* 2:1–2.

Lockshin, R. A. 1999. Gender differences: the perspective from biology. *Lupus* 8:361–364.

Loebstein, R., A. Lalkin, and G. Koren. 1997. Pharmacokinetic changes during pregnancy and their clinical relevance. *Clinical Pharmacokinetics* 33:328–343.

Lonnqvist, F., A. Thorne, V. Large, and P. Arner. 1997. Sex differences in visceral fat lipolysis and metabolic complications of obesity. *Arteriosclerosis, Thrombosis, and Vascular Biology* 17:1472–1480.

Lorber, J. 1994. *Paradoxes of Gender*. New Haven: Yale University Press.

Lumey, L. H. 2001. Glucose tolerance in adults after prenatal exposure to famine (letter to the editor). *Lancet* 357:472–473.

Lyon, M. F. 1999. Imprinting and X-chromosome inactivation. *Results and Problems in Cell Differentiation* 25:73–90.

Lytton, H., and D. M. Romney. 1991. Parents' differential socialization of boys and girls: a meta-analysis. *Psychological Bulletin* 109:267–296.

Maccoby, E. E. 1998. *The Two Sexes: Growing up Apart, Coming Together*. Cambridge, MA: Harvard University Press.

Maccoby, E. E., and C. N. Jacklin. 1974. *The Psychology of Sex Differences*. Sanford, CA: Stanford University Press.

Macdonald, J. L., R. J. Herman, and R. K. Verbeek. 1990. Sex-difference and the effects of smoking and oral contraceptive steroids on the kinetics of diflunisal. *European Journal of Clinical Pharmacology* 38:175–179.

MacKichan, J. J. 1992. Influence of protein binding and use of unbound (free) drug concentrations, pp. 1–48. In: *Applied Pharmacokinetics, Principles of Therapeutic Drug Monitoring*, revised 3rd ed. W. E. Evans, J. J. Schentag, and W. Jusko, eds. Vancouver, British Columbia, Canada: Applied Therapeutics, Inc.

Macleod, J., R. Fraser, and N. Horeczko. 2000. Menses and breast cancer: does timing of mammographically directed core biopsy affect outcome? *Journal of Surgical Oncology* 74:232–236.

Madsen, J. L. 1992. Effects of gender, age and body mass index on gastrointestinal transit times. *Digestive Diseases and Sciences* 37:1548–1553.

Makkar, R. R., B. S. Fromm, R. T. Steinman, M. D. Meissner, and M. H. Lehmann. 1993. Female gender as a risk factor for torsades de pointes associated with cardiovascular drugs. *Journal of the American Medical Association* 270:2590–2597.

Malagelada, R., R. Azpiroz, and F. Mearin. 1993. Gastroduodenal motor function in health and disease. In: *Gastrointestinal Disease: Pathophysiology/Diagnosis/Management*, M. H. Sleisenger and J. S. Fordtran, eds. Philadelphia: W. B. Saunders Co.

Maldonado, M. A., V. Kakkanaiah, G. C. MacDonald, F. Chen, E. A. Reap, E. Balish, W. R. Farkas, J. C. Jennette, M. P. Madaio, B. I. Kotzin, P. I. Cohen, and R. A. Eisenberg. 1999. The role of environmental antigens in the spontaneous development of autoimmunity in MRLlpr mice. *Journal of Immunology* 162:6322–6330.

Manolagas, S. C. 2000. Birth and death of bone cells: basic regulatory mechanisms and implications for the pathogenesis and treatment of osteoporosis. *Endocrinology Review* 21:115–137.

Manson, J. E., G. A. Colditz, M. J. Stampfer, W. C. Wilett, A. S. Krolewski, B. Rosner, R. A. Arky, F. E. Speizer, and C. H. Hennekens. 1991. A prospective study of maturity-onset diabetes mellitus and risk of coronary heart disease and stroke in women. *Archives of Internal Medicine* 151:1141–1147.

Manton, K. G. 2000. Gender differences in cross-sectional and cohort age dependence of cause-specific mortality: the United States, 1962–1995. *Journal of Gender-Specific Medicine* 3:47–54.

Marazziti, D., A. Rossi, L. Palego, A. Barsanti, M. Carrai, G. Giannaccini, P. Serra, A. Lucacchini, and G. B. Cassano. 1998a. Effect of aging and sex on the [3H]-paroxetine binding to human platelets. *Journal of Affectional Disorders* 50:11–15.

Marazziti, D., L. Palego, A. Rossi, and G. B. Cassano. 1998b. Gender-related seasonality of human platelet phenolsulfotransferease activity. *Neuropsychobiology* 38:1–5.

Marchetti, B., F. Gallo, Z. Farinella, C. Tirolo, N. Testa, C. Romeo, and M.C. Morale. 1998. Luteinizing hormone-releasing hormone is a primary signaling molecule in the neuroimmune network. *Annals of the New York Academy of Sciences* 840:205–248.

Marie, P. J., and E. Zerath. 2000. Role of growth factors in osteoblast alterations induced by skeletal unloading in rat. *Growth Factors* 18:1–10.

Marti-Henneberg, C., F. Capdevila, V. Arija, S. Perez, G. Cuco, B. Vizmanos, and J. Fernandez-Ballart. 1999. Energy density of the diet, food volume and energy intake by age and sex in a healthy population. *European Journal of Clinical Nutrition* 53:421–428.

Mashiah, A., V. Berman, H. H. Thole, S. S. Rose, S. Pasik, H. Schwarz, and J. Ben-Hur. 1999. Estrogen and progesterone receptors in normal and varicose saphenous veins. *Cardiovascular Surgery* 7:327–331.

Mathias, J. R., and M. H. Clench. 1998. Relationship of reproductive hormones and neuromuscular disease of the gastrointestinal tract. *Digestive Diseases and Sciences* 16:3–13.

Matsuki, S., T. Kotegawa, K. Tsutsumi, K. Nakamura, and S. Nakano. 1999. Pharmacokinetic changes of theophylline and amikacin through the menstrual cycle in healthy women. *Journal of Clinical Pharmacology* 39:1256–1262.

Matthews, K., J. Cauley, K. Yaffe, and J. M. Zmuda. 1999. Estrogen replacement therapy and cognitive decline in older community women. *Journal of the American Geriatric Society* 47:518–523.

Mayer, E. A., B. Naliboff, O. Lee, J. Munakata, and L. Chang. 1999. Review article: gender-related differences in functional gastrointestinal disorders. *Alimentary Pharmacology and Therapeutics* 13(Suppl. 2).65–69.

McCarthy, C. R. 1994. Historical background of clinical trials involving women and minorities. *Academic Medicine* 69:695–698.

McCarthy, M. M., E. H. Schlenker, and D. W. Pfaff. 1993. Enduring consequences of neonatal treatment with antisense oligodeoxynucleotides to estrogen receptor messenger ribonucleic acid on sexual differentiation of rat brain. *Endocrinology* 133:433–439.

McCourt, M. E., V. W. Mark, K. J. Radonovich, S. K. Willison, and P. Freeman. 1997. The effects of gender, menstrual phase, and practice on the perceived location of the midsagittal plane. *Neuropsychologia* 35:717–724.

McCrohon, J. A., A. K. Death, S. Nakhla, W. Jessup, D. J. Handelsman, K.K. Stanley, and D. S. Celermajer. 2000. Androgen receptor expression is greater in macrophages from male than from female donors. A sex difference with implications for atherogenesis. *Circulation* 101:224–226.

McDonough, P. G. 1998. The Y-chromosome and reproductive disorders. *Reproduction, Fertility, and Development* 10:1–16.

McEwen, B. S. 1999. Clinical Review 108: The molecular and neuroanatomical basis for estrogen effects in the central nervous system. *Journal of Clinical Endocrinology and Metabolism* 84:1790–1797.

McEwen, B. S., and S. E. Alves. 1999. Estrogen actions in the central nervous system. *Endocrine Reviews* 20:279–307.

McFadden, D. 1993. A masculinizing effect on the auditory systems of human females having male co-twins. *Proceedings of the National Academy of Sciences of the United States of America* 90:11900–11904.

McGuigan, F. E., D. M. Reid, and S. H. Ralston. 2000. Susceptibility to osteoporotic fracture is determined by allelic variation at the Sp1 site, rather than other polymorphic sites at the COL1A1 locus. *Osteoporosis International* 11:338–343.

McKusick, V. A. 2000. *Online Mendelian Inheritance in Man.* [Online.] National Center for Biotechnology Information. Available: http://www.ncbi.nlm.nih.gov/Omim/ (accessed October 18, 2000).

McMahon, S. B., G. R. Lewin, and P. D. Wall. 1993. Central hyperexcitability triggered by noxious inputs. *Current Opinions in Neurobiology* 3:602–610.

Medzhitov, R., and C. Janeway, Jr. 2000. Innate immunity. *New England Journal of Medicine* 343:338–344.

Meece, J. L., J. Eccles-Parsons, C. M. Kaczala, S. B. Goff, and R. Futterman. 1982. Sex differences in math achievement: toward a model of academic choice. *Psychological Bulletin* 91: 324–348.

Melcher, M., M. Schmid, L. Aagaard, P. Selenko, G. Laible, and T. Jenuwein. 2000. Structure-function analysis of SUV39H1 reveals a dominant role in heterochromatin organization, chromosome segregation, and mitotic progression. *Molecular and Cellular Biology* 20:3728–3841.

Merkatz, R. B., R. Temple, S. Subel, K. Feiden, and D. A. Kessler. 1993. Women in clinical trials of new drugs. A change in Food and Drug Administration Policy. The Working Group on Women in Clinical Trials. *New England Journal of Medicine* 329:292–296.

Merskey, H., and N. Bogduk, eds. 1994. *Classification of Chronic Pain: Descriptions of Chronic Pain Syndromes and Definitions of Pain Terms,* 2nd ed. Seattle: IASP Press.

Mestman, J. H. 1988. Follow-up studies in women with gestational diabetes mellitus: the experience at Los Angeles County/University of Southern California Medical Center. *In: Gestational Diabetes.* P. A. M. Weiss and D. R. Coustan, eds. Vienna, Austria: Springer-Verlag.

Meyer-Bahlburg, H. F. L., R. S. Gruen, M. I. New, J. J. Bell, A. Morishima, M. Shimshi, Y. Bueno, I. Vargas, and S. W. Baker. 1996. Gender change from female to male in classical congenital adrenal hyperplasia. *Hormones and Behavior* 30:319–332.

Miaskowski, C., R. W. Gear, and J. D. Levine. 2000. Sex-related differences in analgesic responses, pp. 209–230. *In: Sex, Gender, and Pain.* R. B. Fillingim, ed. Seattle: IASP Press.

Michael, E., D. A. Bundy, and B. T. Grenfell. 1996. Re-assessing the global prevalence and distribution of lymphatic filariasis. *Parasitology* 112:409–428.

Michnovicz, J. J., R. J. Hershcopf, H. Naganuma, H. L. Bradlow, and J. Fishman. 1986. Increased 2-hydroxylation of estradiol as a possible mechanism for the anti-estrogenic effect of cigarette smoking. *New England Journal of Medicine* 315:1305–1309.

Mihara, K., T. Kondo, A. Suzuki, N. Yasui, U. Nagashima, S. Ono, K. Otani, and S. Kaneko. 2000. Prolactin response to nemonapride, a selective antagonist for D2 like dopamine receptors, in schizophrenic patients in relation to TaqlA polymorphism of DRD2 gene. *Psychopharmacology* 149:246–250.

Miller, E. M. 1998. Evidence from opposite-sex twins for the effects of prenatal sex hormones, pp. 27–58. *In: Males, Females, and Behavior.* L. Ellis and L. Ebertz, eds. Westport, CT: Greenwood Publishing Group, Inc.

Miller, F. W., E. V. Hess, D. J. Clauw, P. A. Hertzman, T. Pincus, R. M. Silver, M. D. Mayes, J. Varga, T. A. Medsger, Jr., and L. A. Love. 2000. Approaches for identifying and defining environmentally associated rheumatic disorders. *Arthritis and Rheumatism* 43:243–249.

Miller, V. M. 1999. Gender and vascular reactivity. *Lupus* 8:409–415.

Miller, W. L. 1996. The adrenal cortex, pp. 1711–1742. *In: Rudolph's Pediatrics*, 20th ed. A. M. Rudolph, J. I. E. Hoffman, C. D. Rudolph, and P. Sagan, eds. Stamford, CT: Appleton and Lange.

Mills, P. J., R. A. Nelesen, M. G. Ziegler, B. L. Parry, C. C. Berry, E. Dillon, and J. E. Dimsdale. 1996. Menstrual cycle effects on catecholamine and cardiovascular responses to acute stress in black but not white normotensive women. *Hypertension* 27:962–967.

Milner, K. A., M. Funk, S. Richards, R. M. Wilmes, V. Vaccarino, and H. M. Krumholtz. 1999. Gender differences in symptom presentation associated with coronary heart disease. *American Journal of Cardiology* 84:396–399.

Miners, J. O., J. Attwood, and D. J. Birkett. 1983. Influence of sex and oral contraceptive steroids on paracetamol metabolism. *British Journal of Clinical Pharmacology* 16:503–509.

Miners, J. O., R. A. Robson, and D. J. Birkett. 1984. Gender and oral contraceptive steroids as determinants of drug glucuronidation: effects on clofibric acid elimination. *British Journal of Clinical Pharmacology* 18:240–243.

Miranda, P., C.L. Williams, and G. Einstein. 1999. Granule cells in aging rats are sexually dimorphic in their response to estradiol. *Journal of Neuroscience* 19:3316–3325.

Mitamura, R., K. Yano, N. Suzuki, Y. Ito, Y. Makita, and A. Okuno. 1999. Diurnal rhythms of luteinizing hormone, follicle-stimulating hormone, and testosterone secretion before the onset of male puberty. *Journal of Clinical Endocrinology and Metabolism* 84:29–37.

Mitamura, R., K. Yano, N. Suzuki, Y. Ito, Y. Makita, and A. Okuno. 2000. Diurnal rhythms of luteinizing hormone, follicle-stimulating hormone, testosterone, and estradiol secretion before the onset of female puberty in short children. *Journal of Clinical Endocrinology and Metabolism* 85:1074–1080.

Mizutani, T., S. Nishiyama, I. Amakawa, K. Mantabe, K. Nakamuro, and N. Terada. 1995. Danazol concentrations in ovary, uterus, and serum and their effect on the hypothalamic-pituitary-ovarian axis during vaginal administration of danazol suppository. *Fertility and Sterility* 63:84–89.

Mogil, J. S. 2000. Interactions between sex and genotype in the mediation and modulation of nociception in rodents, pp. 25–40. *In: Sex, Gender, and Pain*. R. B. Fillingim, ed. Seattle: IASP Press.

Mogil, J. S., L. Yu, and A. I. Basbaum. 2000. Pain genes?: natural variation and transgenic mutants. *Annual Review of Neuroscience* 23:777–811.

Mohiuddin, M. L, K. G. Pursnani, D. A. Katza, J. A. Castell, and D. O. Castell. 1999. Effect of cyclic hormonal changes during normal menstrual cycle on esophageal motility. *Digestive Diseases and Sciences* 44:1368–1375.

Mojaverian, P., M. L. Rocci, Jr., D. P. Conner, W. B. Abrams, and P. H. Vlasses. 1987. Effect of food on the absorption of enteric-coated aspirin: correlation with gastric residence time. *Clinical Pharmacology and Therapeutics* 41:11–17.

Mokdad, A. H., M. K. Serdula, W. H. Dietz, B. A. Bowman, J. S. Marks, and J. P. Koplan. 1999. The spread of the obesity epidemic in the United States, 1991–1998. *Journal of the American Medical Association* 282:1519–1522.

Mokdad, A. H., E. S. Ford, B. A. Bowman, D. E. Nelson, M. M. Engelgau, F. Vinicor, and J. S. Marks. 2000. Diabetes trends in the U.S.: 1990–1998. *Diabetes Care* 23:1278–1283.

Molnár, D., and Y. Schutz. 1997. The effect of obesity, age, puberty, and gender or resting metabolic rate in children and adolescents. *European Journal of Pediatrics* 156:376–381.

Mondal, S., and U. Rai. 1999. Sexual dimorphism in phagocytic activity of wall lizard's splenic macrophages and its control by sex steroids. *General and Comparative Endocrinology* 116:291–298.

Mones, J., I. Carrio, R. Calabuig, M. Estorch, S. Sainz, L. Berna, and F. Vilardell. 1993. Influence of the menstrual cycle and of menopause on the gastric emptying rate of solids in female volunteers. *European Journal of Nuclear Medicine* 20:600–602.

Money, J. A., and A. A. Ehrhardt. 1996. *Man & Woman, Boy & Girl: Gender Identity from Conception to Maturity.* Northvale, NJ: Jason Aronson Inc.

Money, J., J. G. Hampson, and J. L. Hampson. 1955. The examination of some basic sexual concepts: the evidence of human hermaphroditism. *Johns Hopkins Medical Journal* 97:301–319.

Monteleone, P., F. Catapano, A. Tortorella, and M. Maj. 1997. Cortisol response to *d*-fenfluramine in patients with obsessive-compulsive disorder and in healthy subjects: evidence for a gender-related effect. *Neuropsychobiology* 36:8–12.

Montgomery, C., and K. Sherif. 2000. The information problem in women's health: a piece of the solution. *Journal of Women's Health and Gender-Based Medicine* 9:529–536.

Montgomery, S. M., D. L. Morris, R. E. Pounder, and A. J. Wakefield. 1999. Paramyxovirus infections in childhood and subsequent inflammatory bowel disease. *Gastroenterology* 116:796–803.

Moody, M. S. 1997. Changes in scores on the Mental Rotations Test during the menstrual cycle. *Perception and Motor Skills* 84:955–961.

Moore, C. 1990. Comparative development of vertebrate sexual behavior; levels, cascades and webs, pp. 278–299. *In: Issues in Comparative Psychology.* D. A. Dewsbury, ed. New York: Sinauer.

Moore, C. L., and S. A. Rogers. 1984. Contributions of self-grooming to onset of puberty in male rats. *Developmental Psychobiology* 17:243–253.

Moore, C. L., H. Dou, and J. M. Juraska. 1992. Maternal stimulation affects the number of motor neurons in a sexually dimorphic nucleus of the lumbar spinal cord. *Brain Research* 572:52–56.

Moore, J. G., C. Tweedy, P. E. Christian, and F. L. Dizz. 1983. Effect of age on gastric emptying of liquid-solid meals in man. *Digestive Diseases and Sciences* 28:340–344.

Morales, A., J. P. Heaton, and C. C. Carson III. 2000. Andropause: a misnomer for a true clinical entity. *Journal of Urology* 163:705–712.

Morales, A. J., G. A. Laughlin, T. Butzow, H. Maheshwari, G. Baumann, and S. S. Yen. 1996. Insulin somatotropic and luteinizing hormone axes in lean and obese women with polycystic ovary syndrome: common and distinct features. *Journal of Clinical Endocrinology and Metabolism* 81:2854–2864.

Morishima, A., M. M. Grumbach, E. R. Simpson, C. Fisher, and K. Qin. 1995. Aromatase deficiency in male and female siblings caused by a novel mutation and the physiological role of estrogens. *Journal of Clinical Endocrinology and Metabolism* 80:3689–3698.

Morishita, M., M. Miyagi, and Y. Iwamoto. 1999. Effects of sex hormones on production of interleukin-1 by human peripheral monocytes. *Journal Periodontology* 70:757–760.

Mosca, L., S. M. Grundy, D. Judelson, K. King, M. Limacher, S. Oparil, R. Pasternak, T. A. Pearson, R. F. Redberg, S. C. Smith Jr., M. Winton, and S. Zinberg. 1999. Guide to Preventive Cardiology for Women. AHA/ACC Scientific Statement Consensus panel statement. *Circulation* 99:2480–2484.

Mosley, J. R. 2000. Osteoporosis and bone functional adaptation: mechanobiological regulation of bone architecture in growing and adult bone: a review. *Journal of Rehabilitation Research and Development* 37:189–199.

Murabito, J. M., J. C. Evans, M. G. Larson, and D. Levy. 1993. Prognosis after the onset of coronary heart disease. An investigation of differences in outcome between the sexes according to initial coronary disease preesntation. *Circulation* 88:2548–2555.

Nafziger, A. N., M. S. Schwartzman, and J. S. Bertino, Jr. 1989. Absence of tobramycin pharmacokinetic and creatinine clearance variation during the menstrual cycle: implied absence of variation in glomerular filtration rate. *Journal of Clinical Pharmacology* 29:757–763.

Naliboff, B. D., M. M. Heitkemper, L. Chang, and E. A. Mayer. 2000. Sex and gender in irritable bowel syndrome, pp. 327–354. In: *Sex, Gender, and Pain,* R. B. Fillingim, ed. Seattle: IASP Press.

Napirei, M., H. Karsunky, B. Zevnik, H. Stephan, H. G. Mannherz, and T. Moroy. 2000. Features of systemic lupus erythematosus in DNase 1-deficient mice. *Nature Genetics* 25:177–181.

Napolitano, C., S. G. Priori, and P. J. Schwarz. 1994. Torsade de pointes. Mechanisms and management. *Drugs* 47:51–65.

Nathan, L., S. Pervin, and R. Singh. 1999. Estradiol inhibits leukocyte adhesion and transendothelial migration in rabbits in vivo: possible mechanisms for gender differences in atherosclerosis. *Circulation Research* 85:377–385.

Nathanielsz, P. W. 1999. *Life in the Womb: The Origin of Health and Disease.* Ithaca, NY: Promethean Press.

National Cancer Institute, National Institutes of Health. 1986. *Forty-Five Years of Cancer Incidence in Connecticut: 1935–1979.* Monograph 70. NIH Publication No. 86-2652. Washington, DC: U. S. Government Printing Office.

National Center for Health Statistics. 1987. Anthropometric reference data and prevalence of overweight, United States, 1976–1980. In: *Vital and Health Statistics.* M. F. Najjar and M. Rowland, eds. Series 11, No. 238. DHHS Publication No. PHS 87-1688. Public Health Service. Washington, DC: U.S. Government Printing Office.

National Center for Health Statistics. 1996. *Health, United States, 1995.* Publication No. PHS-96-1232. Hyattsville, MD: National Center for Health Statistics.

National Center for Health Statistics. 1999. *Health, United States, 1999, with Health and Aging Chartbook.* Publication No. PHS-99-1232. Hyattsville, MD: National Center for Health Statistics.

National Center for Health Statistics. 2000a. *Health, United States, 2000, with Health and Aging Chartbook.* Publication No. PHS 2000-1232. Hyattsville, MD: National Center for Health Statistics.

National Center for Health Statistics. 2000b. *National Health and Nutrition Examination Survey.* [Online.] Centers for Disease Control and Prevention. Available: http://www.cdc.gov/nchs/nhanes.htm (accessed December 13, 2000).

National Heart, Lung, and Blood Institute, National Institutes of Health. 1998. *Clinical Guidelines for the Assessment, Evaluation, and Treatment of Obesity* [Online]. Available: http://www.nhlbi.nih.gov/guidelines/obesity/ob_home.htm (accessed February 13, 2001).

National Human Genome Research Institute. 2000. *The Human Genome Project.* [Online]. National Institutes of Health. Available: http://www.nhgri.nih.gov:80/HGP/ (accessed November 8, 2000).

National Institutes of Health, Office of Research on Women's Health. 1998. *Women of Color Health Data Book.* NIH Publication No. 98-4247. Bethesda, MD: U.S. Department of Health and Human Services.

National Institutes of Health, Office of Research on Women's Health. 1999a. *Agenda for Research on Women's Health for the 21st Century. A Report of the Task Force on the NIH Women's Health Research Agenda for the 21st Century,* Vol. 1. *Executive Summary.* NIH Publication No. 99-4385. Bethesda, MD.: U.S. Department of Health and Human Services.

National Institutes of Health, Office of Research on Women's Health. 1999b. *Agenda for Research on Women's Health for the 21st Century. A Report of the Task Force on the NIH Women's Health Research Agenda for the 21st Century.* NIH Publication No. 99–4386. Bethesda, MD: U.S. Department of Health and Human Services.

National Institutes of Health, Office of Research on Women's Health. 1999c. *Agenda for Research on Women's Health for the 21st Century. A Report of the Task Force on the NIH Women's Health Research Agenda for the 21st Century,* Vol. 3. *Public Testimony, Bethesda, Maryland, November 1997.* NIH Publication No. 99-4387. Bethesda, MD: U.S. Department of Health and Human Services.

National Institutes of Health, Office of Research on Women's Health. 1999d. *Agenda for Research on Women's Health for the 21st Century. A Report of the Task Force on the NIH Women's Health Research Agenda for the 21st Century,* Vol. 4. *Influences of Sex and Gender on Health. Scientific Meeting and Public Hearing, Philadelphia, Pennsylvania, September 1996.* NIH Publication No. 99-4388. Bethesda, MD: U.S. Department of Health and Human Services.

National Institutes of Health, Office of Research on Women's Health. 1999e. *Agenda for Research on Women's Health for the 21st Century. A Report of the Task Force on the NIH Women's Health Research Agenda for the 21st Century.* Vol. 5. *Sex and Gender Perspectives for Women's Health Research. Scientific Meeting and Public Hearing, New Orleans, Louisiana, June 1997.* NIH Publication No. 99-4389. Bethesda, MD: U.S. Department of Health and Human Services.

National Institutes of Health, Office of Research on Women's Health. 1999f. *Agenda for Research on Women's Health for the 21st Century. A Report of the Task Force on the NIH Women's Health Research Agenda for the 21st Century,* Vol. 6. *Differences Among Populations of Women. Scientific Meeting and Public Hearing, Santa Fe, New Mexico, July 1997.* NIH Publication No. 99-4390. Bethesda, MD: U.S. Department of Health and Human Services.

National Research Council. 1989. *Recommended Dietary Allowances,* 10th ed. Washington, DC: National Academy Press.

National Research Council. 1996. *Guide for the Care and Use of Laboratory Animals.* Washington, DC: National Academy Press.

National Research Council. 2000. *Addressing the Nation's Changing Needs for Biomedical and Behavioral Scientists.* Washington, DC: National Academy Press.

National Research Council and Institute of Medicine. 2000. *From Neurons to Neighborhoods. The Science of Early Childhood Development.* J. P. Shonkoff and D. A. Phillips, eds. Washington, DC: National Academy Press.

Naumova, A. K., M. Leppert, D. F. Barker, K. Morgan, and C. Sapienza. 1998. Parental origin-dependent, male offspring-specific transmission-ratio distortion at loci on the human X chromosome. *American Journal of Human Genetics* 62:1493–1499.

Nehlsen-Cannarella, S., O. Fagoaga, J. Folz, S. Grinde, C. Hinsey, and R. Thorpe. 1997. Fighting, fleeing and having fun: the immunology of physical activity. *International Journal of Sports Medicine* 18(Suppl. 1):S8–S21.

Nelemans, P. J., H. Groenendal, L. A. Kiemeney, F. H. Rampen, D. J. Ruiter, and A. L. Verbeek. 1993. Effect of intermittent exposure to sunlight on melanoma risk among indoor workers and sun-sensitive individuals. *Environmental Health Perspectives* 101:252–255.

Nelson, J. L. 1998. Microchimerism and autoimmune disease. *New England Journal of Medicine* 338:1224–1225.

Nelson, J. L. D. E. Furst, S. Maloney, T. Gooley, P. C. Evans, A. Smith, M. A. Bean, C. Ober, and D. W. Bianchi. 1998. Microchimerism and HLA-compatible relationships of pregnancy in scleroderma. *Lancet* 351:559–562.

Nelson, J. L., K. A. Hughes, A. G. Smith, B. B. Nisperos, A. M. Branchaud, and J. A. Hansen. 1993. Maternal-fetal disparity in HLA class II alloantigens and the pregnancy-induced amelioration of rheumatoid arthritis. *New England Journal of Medicine* 329:466–471.

Nelson, R. J. 1997. The use of genetic "knockout mice" in behavioral endocrinology research. *Hormones and Behavior* 31:188–196.

Nelson, R. J., and S. Chiavegatto. 2000. Aggression in knockout mice. *Institute for Laboratory Animal Research (ILAR) Journal* 41:153–162.

Nelson, R. J., G. E. Demas, P. Huang, M. C. Fishman, V. L. Dawson, T. M. Dawson, and S. H. Snyder. 1995. Behavioral abnormalities in male mice lacking neuronal nitric oxide synthase. *Nature* 378:383–386.

Newman, S. R., J. Butler, E. H. Hammond, and S. D. Gray. 2000. Preliminary report on hormone receptors in the human vocal fold. *Journal of Voice* 14:72–81.

Nichol, K. L., K. L. Margolis, A. Lind, M. Murdoch, R. McFadden, M. Hauge, S. Magnan, and M. Drake. 1996. Side effects associated with influenza vaccination in healthy working adults: a randomized, placebo-controlled trial. *Archives of Internal Medicine* 156:1546–1550.

Nickerson, D. A., S. L. Taylor, K. M. Weiss, A. G. Clark, R. G. Hutchinson, J. Stengard, V. Salomaa, E. Vartiainen, E. Boerwinkle, and C. F. Sing. 1998. DNA sequence diversity in a 9.7-kb region of the human lipoprotein lipase gene. *Nature Genetics* 3:233–240.

Nicklas, B. J., M. J. Toth, and E. T. Poehlman. 1997. Daily energy expenditure is related to plasma leptin concentrations in older African-American women but not men. *Diabetes* 46:1389–1392.

Nicolette, J. 2000. Searching for women's health: a resident's perspective. *Journal of Women's Health & Gender-Based Medicine* 9:697–701.

Nishizawa, S., C. Benkelfat, S. N. Young, M. Leyton, S. Mzengeza, C. De Montigny, P. Blier, and M. Diksic. 1997. Differences between males and females in rates of serotonin synthesis in human brain. 1997. *Proceedings of the National Academy of Sciences of the United States of America* 94:5308–5313.

Nordenstrom, A., A. Servin, A. Larsson, and G. Bohlin. 1999. Psychological follow up of children with congenital adrenal hyperplasia. In: *Neuropsychological Follow-up of Neonatal Screening*. B. A. Berenbaum, chair. Symposium conducted at the 4th Meeting of the International Society for Neonatal Screening, Stockholm, Sweden, June 1999.

Noseworthy, J. H., C. Lucchinetti, M. Rodriguez, and B. G. Weinshenker. 2000. Multiple sclerosis. *New England Journal of Medicine* 343:938–952.

Notarianni, L. J. 1990. Plasma protein binding of drugs in pregnancy and in neonates. *Clinical Pharmacokinetics* 18:20–36.

Nottebohm, F., and A. P. Arnold. 1976. Sexual dimorphism in vocal control areas of the songbird brain. *Science* 194:211–213.

O'Donnell, C. J., K. Lindpaintner, M. G. Larson, V. S. Rao, J. M. Ordovas, E. J. Schaefer, R. H. Myers, and D. Levy. 1998. Evidence for association and genetic linkage of the angiotensin-converting enzyme locus with hypertension and blood pressure in men but not women in the Framingham Heart Study. *Circulation* 97:1766–1772.

O'Farrel, P., J. Murray, P. Huston, C. LeGrand, and K. Adamo. 2000. Sex differences in cardiac rehabilitation. *Canadian Journal of Cardiology* 16:319–325.

Okayasu, I., Y. M. Kong, and N. R. Rose. 1981. Effect of castration and sex hormones on experimental autoimmune thyroiditis. *Clinical Immunology and Immunopathology* 20:240–245.

Olff, M. 1999. Stress, depression and immunity: the role of defense and coping styles. *Psychiatric Research* 85:7–15.

Olweus, D., A. Mattson, D. Schalling, and H. Low. 1980. Testosterone, aggression, physical, and personality dimensions in normal adolescent males. *Psychosomatic Medicine* 42:253–269.

O'Neill, M. J., and R. J. O'Neill. 1999. Whatever happened to SRY? *Cell and Molecular Life Sciences* 56:883–893.

Oppenheimer, E., B. Linder, and J. DiMartino-Nardi. 1995. Decreased insulin sensitivity in prepubertal girls with premature adrenarche and acanthosis nigricans. *Journal of Clinical Endocrinology and Metabolism* 80:614–618.

Ostensen, M. 1999. Sex hormones and pregnancy in rheumatoid arthritis and systemic lupus erythematosus. *Annals of the New York Academy of Sciences* 876:131–143.

O'Sullivan, J. B. 1984. Workshop 4: subsequent morbidity among gestational diabetic women. *In: Carbohydrate Metabolism in Pregnancy and the Newborn*. H. W. Sutherland and J. M. Stowers, eds. Edinburgh: Churchill Livingstone.

Paaby, P., J. Moller-Petersen, C. E. Larsen, and K. Raffn. 1987a. Endogenous overnight creatinine clearance, serum beta 2-microglobulin and serum water during the menstrual cycle. *Acta Medica Scandinavica* 221:191–197.

Paaby, P., J. Brochner-Mortensen, P. Fjeldborg, K. Raffn, C. E. Larsen, and J. Moller-Petersen. 1987b. Endogenous overnight creatinine clearance compared with ^{51}Cr-EDTA clearance during the menstrual cycle. *Acta Medica Scandinavica* 222:281–284.

Pan, W. H., L. B. Cedres, K. Liu, A. Dyer, J. A. Schoenberger, R. B. Shekelle, R. Stamler, D. Smith, P. Collette, and J. Stamler. 1986. Relationship of clinical diabetes and asymptomatic hyperglycemia to risk of coronary heart disease mortality in men and women. *American Journal of Epidemiology* 123:504–516.

Panetta, J., and U. Srinivasan. 1998. Gender-based medicine. *Annual Reports in Medicinal Chemistry* 355–363.

Pardo-Manuel de Villena, F., E. de la Casa-Esperon, T. L. Briscoe, J. M. Malette, and C. Sapienza. 2000. Male-offspring-specific, haplotype-dependent, nonrandom cosegregation of alleles at loci on two mouse chromosomes. *Genetics* 154:351–356.

Parish, R. C., and C. Spivey. 1991. Influence of menstrual cycle phase on serum concentrations of α1 acid glycoprotein. *British Journal of Clinical Pharmacology* 31:197–199.

Parker, W. A. 1984. Effects of pregnancy on pharmacokinetics, pp. 249–268. *In: Pharmacokinetic Basis of Drug Treatment*. L. Z. Benet, N. Massoud, and J. G. Gambertoglio, eds. New York: Raven Press.

Parker, K. L., A. Schedl, and B. P. Schimmer. 1999. Gene interactions in gonadal development. *Annual Review of Physiology* 61:417–433.

Parkman, H. P., A. D. Harris, M. A. Miller, and R. S. Fisher. 1996. Influence of age, gender, and menstrual cycle on the normal electrogastrogram. *American Journal of Gastroenterology* 91:127–133.

Parsons, B., T. C. Rainbow, and B. S. McEwen. 1984. Organizational effects of testosterone via aromatization on feminine reproductive behavior and neural progestin receptors in rat brain. *Endocrinology* 115:1412–1417.

Patterson, F. G. P., C. Holts, and L. Saphire. 1991. Cyclic changes in hormonal, physical, behavioral, and linguistic measures in a female lowland gorilla. *American Journal of Primatology* 24:181–194.

Pedersen, E. A., M. P. Akhter, D. M. Cullen, D. B. Kimmel, and R. R. Recker. 1999. Bone response to in vivo mechanical loading in C3H/HeJ mice. *Calcified Tissue International* 65:41–46.

Pena, C. A., and G. T. Strickland. 1999. Incidence rates of Lyme disease in Maryland: 1993 through 1996. *Maryland Medical Journal* 48:68–73.

Perucca, E., and A. Crema. 1982. Plasma protein binding of drugs in pregnancy. *Clinical Pharmacokinetics* 7:336–352.

Peters, M., B. Laeng, K. Latham, M. Jackson, R. Zaiyouna, and C. Richardson. 1995. A redrawn Vandenberg and Kuse mental rotations test: different versions and factors that affect performance. *Brain Cognition* 28:39–58.

Petri, M., and C. Robinson. 1997. Oral contraceptives and systemic lupus erythematosus. *Arthritis and Rheumatism* 40:797–803.

Petring, O. U., and H. Flachs. 1990. Inter- and intra- subject variability of gastric emptying in healthy volunteers measured by scintigraphy and paracetamol absorption. *British Journal of Clinical Pharmacology* 29:703–708.

Phillips, K., and I. Silverman. 1997. Differences in the relationship of menstrual cycle phase to spatial performance on two- and three-dimensional tasks. *Hormones and Behavior* 32:167–175.

Phipps, W. R., A. M. Duncan, B. E. Merz, and M. S. Kurzer. 1998. Effect of the menstrual cycle on creatinine clearance in normally cycling women. *Obstetrics and Gynecology* 92:585–588.

Phoenix, C. H., R. W. Goy, A. A. Gerall, and W. C. Young. 1959. Organizing action of prenatally administered testosterone propionate on the tissues mediating mating behavior in the female guinea pig. *Endocrinology* 63:369–382.

Piepkorn, M. 2000. Melanoma genetics: an update with focus on the CDKN2A/ARF tumor suppressors. *Journal of the American Academy of Dermatology* 42:705–722.

Pinn, V. W. 2000. NIH studies include women. *USA Today*, May 5, p. 16A.

Pinsky, L., R. P. Erickson, and R. N. Schimke. 1999. *Genetic Disorders of Human Sexual Development*. Oxford: Oxford University Press.

Piquero, K., T. Ando, and K. Sakurai. 1999. Buccal mucosa ridging and tongue indentation: incidence and associated factors. *Bulletin of the Tokyo Dental College* 40:71–78.

Plymate, S. R., D. E. Moore, C. Y. Cheng, C. W. Bardin, M. B. Southworth, and M. J. Levinski. 1985. Sex hormone-binding globulin changes during the menstrual cycle. *Journal of Clinical Enocrinology and Metabolism* 61:993–996.

Poehlman, E. T., and A. Tchernof. 1998. Traversing the menopause: changes in energy expenditure and body composition. *Coronary Artery Disease* 9:799–803.

Prestwood, K. M., A. M. Kenny, C. Unson, and M. Kulldorff. 2000. The effect of low dose micronized 17β-estradiol on bone turnover, sex hormone levels, and side effects in older women: a randomized, double blind, placebo-controlled study. *Journal of Clinical Endocrinology and Metabolism* 85:4462–4469.

Puck, J. M., and H. F. Willard. 1998. X inactivation in females with X-linked disease. *New England Journal of Medicine* 338:325–328.

Quadagno, D. M., R. Briscoe, and J. S. Quadagno. 1977. Effects of perinatal gonadal hormones on selected nonsexual behavior patterns: a critical assessment of the nonhuman and human literature. *Psychology Bulletin* 84:62–80.

Raisman, G., and P. M. Field. 1971. Sexual dimorphism in the preoptic area of the rat. *Science* 173:731–733.

Rao, S., V. Garole, and S. Walawalkar. 1996. Gender differentials in the social impact of leprosy. *Leprosy Review* 67:190–199.

Rappold, G. A. 1993. The pseudoautosomal regions of the human sex chromosomes. *Human Genetics* 92:315–324.

Rautaharju, P. M., S. H. Zhou, S. Wong, H. P. Calhoun, G. S. Berenson, R. Prineas, and A. Davignon. 1992. Sex differences in the evolution of the electrocardiographic QT interval with age. *Canadian Journal of Cardiology* 8:690–695.

Ravelli, A. C. J., J. H. van der Meulen, C. Osmond, D. J. Barker, and O. P. Bleker. 1999. Obesity at the age of 50 y in men and women exposed to famine prenatally. *American Journal of Clinical Nutrition* 70:811–816.

Ray, P. F., R. M. Winston, and A. H. Handyside. 1997. XIST expression from the maternal X chromosome in human male preimplantation embryos at the blastocyst stage. *Human Molecular Genetics* 6:1323–1327.

Raymond, C. S., E. D. Parker, J. R. Kettlewell, L. G. Brown, D. C. Page, K. Kusz, J. Jaruzelska, Y. Reinberg, W. L. Flejter, V. J. Bardwell, B. Hirsch, and D. Zarkower. 1999. A region of human chromosome 9p required for testis development contains two genes related to known sexual regulators. *Human Molecular Genetics* 8:989–996.

Rebiere, I., and C. Galy-Eyraud. 1995. Estimation of the risk of aseptic meningitis associated with mumps vaccination, France, 1991–1993. *International Journal of Epidemiology* 24:1223–1227.

Reed, J. T., R. Ghadially, and P. M. Elias. 1995. Skin type, but neither race nor gender, influence epidermal permeability barrier function. *Archives of Dermatology* 131:1134–1138.

Reidenberg, M. M., and M. Affrime. 1973. Influence of disease on binding of drugs to plasma proteins. *Annals of the New York Academy of Sciences* 226:115–126.

Reigner, B. G., and H. A. Welker. 1996. Factors influencing elimination and distribution of fleroxacin: meta-analysis of individual data from 10 pharmacokinetic studies. *Antimicrobial Agents and Chemotherapy* 40:575–580.

Reiner, W. 2000. Outcomes in gender assignment: cloacal exstrophy. *In: Neonatal Management of Genital Ambiguity.* M. Grumbach, chair. Symposium presented at the Meeting of the Lawson Wilkins Pediatric Endocrine Society, Boston, May 2000.

Reinisch, J. M. 1981. Prenatal exposure to synthetic progestins increases potential for aggression in humans. *Science* 211:1171–1173.

Resnick, S., E. J. Metter, and A. B. Zonderman. 1997. Estrogen replacement therapy and longitudinal decline in visual memory. A possible protective effect? *Neurology* 49:1491–1497.

Resnick, S. M., S. A. Berenbaum, I. I. Gottesman, and T. J. Bouchard. 1986. Early hormonal influences on cognitive functioning in congenital adrenal hyperplasia. *Developmental Psychology* 22:191–198.

Resnick, S. M., I. I. Gottesman, and M. McGue. 1993. Sensation seeking in opposite-sex twins: an effect of prenatal hormones? *Behavior Genetics* 23:323–329.

Rice, M. M., A. B. Graves, S. McCurry, and E. B. Larson. 1997. Estrogen replacement therapy and cognitive function in postmenopausal women without dementia. *American Journal of Medicine* 103:26S–35S.

Riezzo, G., M. Chiloiro, and V. Guerra. 1998. Electrogastrography in healthy children: evaluation of normal values, influence of age, gender and obesity. *Digestive Diseases and Sciences* 43:1646-1651

Riley, J. L., III., M. E. Robinson, E. A. Wise, C. D. Myers, and R. B. Fillingim. 1998. Sex differences in the perception of noxious experimental stimuli: a meta-analysis. *Pain* 74:181–187.

Riley, J. L., III., M. E. Robinson, E. A. Wise, and D. D. Price. 1999. A meta-analytic review of pain perception across the menstrual cycle. *Pain* 81:225–235.

Ringrose, J. H. 1999. HLA-B27 associated spondyloarthropathy, an autoimmune disease based on crossreactivity between bacteria and HLA-B27? *Annals of the Rheumatic Diseases* 58:598–610.

Roberts, L. M., J. Shen, and H. A. Ingraham. 1999. New solutions to an ancient riddle: defining the differences between Adam and Eve. *American Journal of Human Genetics* 65:933–942.

Robinson, M. E., J. L. Riley III, and C. D. Myers. 2000. Psychosocial contributions to sex-related differences in pain responses, pp. 41–68. *In: Sex, Gender, and Pain.* R. B. Fillingim, ed. Seattle: IASP Press.

Roca, P., A. M. Proenza, and A. Palou. 1999. Sex differences in the effect of obesity on human plasma tryptophan/large neutral amino acid ratio. *Annals of Nutrition and Metabolism* 43:145–151.

Rodriguez, I., M. J. Kilborn, X.-K. Liu, J. C. Pezullo, and R. L. Woosley. 2001. Drug-induced QT prolongation in women during the menstrual cycle. *Journal of the American Medical Association* 285:1322–1326.

Rogier, C., A. B. Ly, A. Tall, B. Cisse, and J. F. Trappe. 1999. Plasmodium falciparum clinical malaria in Dielmo, a holoendemic area in Senegal: no influence of acquired immunity on initial symptomatology and severity of malaria attacks. *American Journal of Tropical Medicine and Hygiene* 60:410–420.

Roof, R. L., and E. D. Hall. 2000a. Estrogen-related gender differences in survival rate and cortical blood flow after impact-acceleration head injury in rats. *Journal of Neurotrauma* 17:1155–1169.

Roof, R. L., and E. D. Hall. 2000b. Gender differences in acute CNS trauma and stroke: neuroprotective effects of estrogen and progesterone. *Journal of Neurotrauma* 17:367–388.

Roof, R. L., R. Dudevani, and D. G. Stein. 1993a. Gender influences outcome of brain injury: progesterone plays a protective role. *Brain Research* 607:333–336.

Roof, R. L., A. Zhang, M. M. Glasier, and D. G. Stein. 1993b. Gender-specific impairment on Morris water maze task after entorhinal cortex lesion. *Behavioral Brain Research* 57:47–51.

Rosamond, W. D., L. E. Chambless, A. R. Folsom, L. S. Cooper, D. E. Conwill, L. Clegg, C. H. Wang, and G. Heiss. 1998. Trends in incidence of myocardial infarction and in mortality due to coronary heart disease, 1987–1994. *New England Journal of Medicine* 339:861–867.

Roseboom, T. J., J. H. P. van der Meulen, C. Osmond, D. J. P. Barker, A. C. J. Ravelli, and O. P. Bleker. 2000. Plasma lipid profiles in adults after prenatal exposure to the Dutch famine. *American Journal of Clinical Nutrition* 72:1101–1106.

Rosenberg, L., D. R. Miller, D. W. Kaufman, S. P. Hemrich, S. Van de Carr, P. D. Stolley, and S. Shapiro. 1983. Myocardial infarction in women under 50 years of age. *Journal of the American Medical Association* 250:2801–2806.

Rosenbloom, A. L., J. R. Joe, R. S. Young, and W. E. Winter. 1999. Emerging epidemic of type 2 diabetes in youth. *Diabetes Care* 22:345–354.

Ross, P. D., and W. Knowlton. 1998. Rapid bone loss is associated with increased levels of biochemical markers. *Journal of Bone and Mineral Research* 13:297–302.

Roy, S. D., and G. L. Flynn. 1990. Transdermal delivery of narcotic analgesics: pH, anatomical, and subject differences on cutaneous permeability of fentanyl and sufentanil. *Pharmaceutical Research* 7:842–847.

Ruble, D. N., and C. L. Martin. 1998. Gender development, pp. 933–1016. In: *Handbook of Child Psychology:* Vol. 3. *Social, Emotional, and Personality Development,* 5th ed. W. Damons (series ed.) and N. Eisenberg (vol. ed.), eds. New York: Wiley.

Ruderman, N. B., and C. Haudenschild. 1984. Diabetes as an atherogenic factor. *Progress in Cardiovascular Diseases* 26:373–412.

Russell, T. L., R. R. Berardi, J. L. Barnett, L. C. Dermentzoglou, K. M. Jarvenpaa, S. P. Schmaltz, and J. B. Dressman. 1993. Upper gastrointestinal pH in seventy-nine healthy, elderly North American men and women. *Pharmaceutical Research* 10:187–196.

Sadoshima, S., Y. Nakatomi, K. Fujii, H. Ooboshi, T. Ishitsuka, J. Ogata, and M. Fujishima. 1988. Mortality and histological findings of the brain during and after cerebral ischemia in male and female spontaneously hypertensive rats. *Brain Research* 454:238–243.

Salazar, D. E., D. R. Much, P. S. Nichola, J. R. Seibold, D. Shindler, and P. H. Slugg. 1997. A pharmacokinetic-pharmacodynamic model of *d*-sotalol Q-Tc prolongation during intravenous administration to healthy subjects. *Journal of Clinical Pharmacology* 37:799–809.

Sanders, B., M. P. Soares, and J. M. D'Aquila. 1982. The sex difference on one test of spatial visualization: a nontrivial difference. *Child Development* 53:1106–1110.

Sandstrom, N., J. Kaufman, and S. A. Huettel. 1998. Males and females use different distal cues in a virtual environment navigation task. *Brain Research: Cognitive Brain Research* 6:351–360.

Sanes, J. N., and J. P. Donoghue. 2000. Plasticity and primary motor cortex. *Annual Review of Neuroscience* 23:393–415.

Sankilampi, U., R. Isoaho, A. Bloigu, S. L. Kivela, and M. Leinonen. 1997. Effect of age, sex, and smoking habits on pneumococcal antibodies in an elderly population. *International Journal of Epidemiology* 26:420–427.

Santizo, R. A., S. Anderson, S. Ye, H. Koenig, and D. A. Pelligrino. 2000. Effects of estrogen on leukocyte adhesion after transient forebrain ischemia. *Stroke* 31:2231–2235.

Sapienza, C. 1994. Parental origin effects, genome imprinting, and sex-ratio distortion: double or nothing? *American Journal of Human Genetics* 55:1073–1075.

Sawada, M., N. J. Alkayed, S. Goto, B. J. Crain, R. J. Traystman, A. Shaivitz, R. J. Nelson, and P. D. Hurn. 2000. Estrogen receptor antagonist ICI182,780 exacerbates ischemic injury in female mouse. *Journal of Cerebral Blood Flow and Metabolism* 20:112–118.

Scarr, S., and K. McCartney. 1983. How people make their own environments: a theory of genotype environment effects. *Child Development* 54:424–435.

Schaal, B., R. E. Tremblay, R. Soussignan, and E. J. Susman. 1996. Male testosterone linked to high social dominance but low physical aggression in early adolescence. *Journal of the American Academy of Child and Adolescent Psychiatry* 35:1322–1330.

Schneider, J. E., D. Zhou, and R. M. Blum. 2000. Leptin and metabolic control of reproduction. *Hormones and Behavior* 37:306–326.

Schuetz, E. G., K. N. Furuya, and J. D. Schuetz. 1995. Interindividual variation in expression of P-glycoprotein in normal human liver and secondary hepatic neoplasms. *Journal of Pharmacology and Experimental Therapeutics* 275:1011–1018.

Schumacher, M., H. Coirini, L. M. Flanagan, M. Frankfurt, D. W. Pfaff, and B. S. McEwen. 1992. Ovarian steroid modulation of oxytocin receptor binding in the ventromedial hypothalamus. *Annals of the New York Academy of Sciences* 12:374–386.

Sciore, P., C. B. Frank, and D. A. Hart. 1998. Identification of sex hormone receptors in human and rabbit ligaments of the knee by reverse transcription-polymerase chain reaction: evidence that receptors are present in tissue from both male and female subjects. *Journal of Orthopaedic Research* 16:604–610.

Sehested, A., A. Juul, A. M. Andersson, J. H. Petersen, T. K. Jensen, J. Müller, and N. E. Skakkebaek. 2000. Serum inhibin A and inhibin B in healthy prepubertal, pubertal, and adolescent girls and adult women: relation to age, stage of puberty, menstrual cycle, follicle-stimulating hormone, luteinizing hormone, and estradiol levels. *Journal of Clinical Endocrinology and Metabolism* 85:1634–1640.

Seldin, M. F., C. I. Amos, R. Ward, and P. K. Gregersen. 1999. The genetics revolution and the assault on rheumatoid arthritis. *Arthritis and Rheumatism* 42:1071–1079.

Semenkovich, C. F., and R. E. Ostlund, Jr. 1987. Estrogens induce low-density lipoprotein receptor activity and decrease intracellular cholesterol in human hepatoma cell line G2. *Biochemistry* 26:4987–4992.

Servin, A. 1999. Sex differences in children's play behavior: a biological construction of gender? *In: Comprehensive Summaries of Uppsala Dissertations.* Uppsala, Sweden: Faculty of Social Sciences, Acta Universitatis Upsaliensis..

Shaw, L. J., D. D. Miller, J. C. Romeis, D. Kargl, L. T. Younis, and B. R. Chaitman. 1994. Gender differences in the noninvasive and management of patients with suspected coronary artery disease. *Annals of Internal Medicine* 120:559–566.

Shaywitz, B. A., S. E. Shaywitz, K. R. Pugh, R. T. Constable, P. Skudlarski, R. K. Fulbright, R. A. Bronen, J. M. Fletcher, D. P. Shankweiler, L. Katz, and J. C. Gore. 1995. Sex differences in the functional organization of the brain for language. *Nature* 373: 607–609.

Shaywitz, S. E. 1996. Dyslexia. *Scientific American* 275:98–104.

Shaywitz, S. E., B. A. Shaywitz, J. M. Fletcher, and M. D. Escobar. 1990. Prevalence of reading disability in boys and girls. Results of the Connecticut Longitudinal Study. *Journal of the American Medical Association* 264:998–1002.

Shaywitz, S. E., B. A. Shaywitz, K. R. Pugh, R. K. Fulbright, R. T. Constable, W. E. Mencl, A. M. Lieberman, P. Skudlarski, L. Katz, D. P. Shankweiler, J. M. Fletcher, K. E. Marchione, C. Lacadie, C. Gatenby, and J. C. Gore. 1998. Functional disruption in the organization of the brain for reading in dyslexia. *Proceedings of the National Academy of Sciences of United States of America.* 95:2636–2641.

Shaywitz, S. E., B. A. Shaywitz, K. R. Pugh, R. K. Fulbright, P. Skudlarski, W. E. Mencl, R. T. Constable, F. Naftolin, S. F. Palter, K. E. Marchione, L. Katz, D. P. Shankweiler, J. M. Fletcher, C. Lacadie, M. Keltz, and J. C. Gore. 1999. Effect of estrogen on brain activation patterns in postmenopausal women during working memory tasks. *Journal of the American Medical Association* 281:1197–1202.

Sherwin, B. B. 1997. Estrogen effects on cognition in menopausal women. *Neurology* 48: S21–S26.

Sheifer, S. E., M. R. Canos, K. P. Weinfurt, U. K. Arora, F. O. Mendelsohn, B. J. Gersh, and N. J. Weissman. 2000. Sex differences in coronary artery size assessed by intravascular ultrasound. *American Heart Journal* 139:649–653.

Shoeman, D. W., and D. L. Azarnoff. 1975. Diphenylhydantoin potency and plasma protein binding. *Journal of Pharmacology Experimental Therapy* 195:84–86.

Shriver, S. P., H. A. Bourdeau, C. T. Gubish, D. L. Tirpak, A. L. Davis, J. D. Luketich, and J. M. Siegfried. 2000. Sex-specific expression of gastrin-releasing peptide receptor: relationship to smoking history and risk of lung cancer. *Journal of the National Cancer Institute* 92:24–33.

Shulman, L. E. 1990. The eosinophilia-myalgia syndrome associated with ingestion of L-tryptophan. *Arthritis and Rheumatism* 33:913–917.

Sigurdsson, J. A., C. Bengtsson, L. Lapidus, O. Lindquist, and V. Rafnsson. 1984. Morbidity and mortality in relation to blood pressure and antihypertensive treatment. a 12-year follow-up study of a sample of Swedish women. *Acta Medica Scandinavica* 215:313–322.

Siiteri, P. K., and P. C. MacDonald. 1973. Role of extraglandular estrogen in human endocrinology, pp. 615–629. In: *Handbook of Physiology, Vol. II. Female Reproductive System,* Part I. R. O. Greep and E. B. Astwood, eds. Washington, DC: American Physiological Society.

Siiteri, P. K., and J. D. Wilson. 1974. Testosterone formation and metabolism during male sexual differentiation in the human embryo. *Journal of Clinical Endocrinology and Metabolism* 38:113–125.

Silverman, B. L., B. E. Metzger, N. H. Cho, and C. A. Loeb. 1995. Impaired glucose tolerance in adolescent offspring of diabetic mothers. Relationship to fetal hyperinsulinism. *Diabetes Care* 18:611–617.

Silverman, I., and K. Phillips. 1993. Effects of estrogen changes during the menstrual cycle on spatial performance. *Ethological Sociobiology* 14:257–270.

Simerly, R. B., M. C. Zee, J. W. Pendelton, D. B. Lubahn, and K. S. Korach. 1997. Estrogen receptor-dependent sexual differentiation of dopaminergic neurons in the preoptic region of the mouse. *Proceedings of the National Academy of Sciences of the United States of America* 94:14077–14082.

Simpkins, J. W., G. Rajakumar, Y. Q. Zhang, C. E. Simpkins, D. Greenwald, C. J. Yu, N. Bodor, and A. L. Day. 1997. Estrogens may reduce mortality and ischemic damage caused by middle cerebral artery occlusion in the female rat. *Journal of Neurosurgery* 87:724–730.

Sinclair, A. H. 1998. Human sex determination. *Journal of Experimental Zoology* 281:501–505.

Sinclair, A. H., P. Berta, M. S. Palmer, J. R. Hawkins, B. L. Griffiths, M. J. Smith, J. W. Foster, A. M. Frischauf, R. Lovell-Badge, and P. N. Goodfellow. 1990. A gene from the human sex-determining region encodes a conserved DNA-binding motif. *Nature* 346:240–244.

Sindrup, S. H., and K. Brosen. 1995. The pharmacogenetics of codeine hypoalgesia. *Pharmacogenetics* 5:335–346.

Singh, J., and K. K. Datta. 1997. Measles vaccine efficacy in India: a review. *Journal of Community Diseases* 29:47–56.

Singh, J., A. Kumar, R. N. Rai, S. Khare, D. C. Jain, R. Bhatia, and K. K. Datta. 1999. Widespread outbreaks of measles in rural Uttar Pradesh, India, 1996: high risk areas and groups. *Indian Pediatrics* 36:249–256.

Singhal, S. S., M. Saxena, S. Awasthi, H. Ahman, R. Sharma, and Y. C. Awasthi. 1992. Gender related differences in the expression and characteristics of glutathione *S*-transferase of human colon. *Biochimica et Biophysica Acta* 1171:19–26.

Siracusa, L. D., W. G. Alvord, W. A. Bickmore, N. A. Jenkins, and N. G. Copeland. 1991. Interspecific backcross mice show sex-specific differences in allelic inheritance. *Genetics* 128:813–821.

Skuse, D. H., R. S. James, D. V. Bishop, P. Coppin, P. Dalton, G. Aamodt-Leeper, M. Bacarese-Hamilton, C. Creswell, R. McGurk, and P. A. Jacobs. 1997. Evidence from Turner's syndrome of an imprinted X-linked locus affecting cognitive function. *Nature* 387:705–708.

Smahi, A., G. Courtois, P. Vabres, S. Yamaoka, S. Heuertz, A. Munnich, A. Israel, N. S. Heiss, S. M. Klauck, P. Kioschis, S. Wiemann, A. Poustka, T. Esposito, T. Bardaro, F. Gianfrancesco, A. Ciccodicola, M. D'Urso, H. Woffendin, T. Jakins, D. Donnai, H. Stewart, S.J. Kenwrick, S. Aradhya, T. Yamagata, M. Levy, R. A. Lewis, and D. L. Nelson. 2000. Genomic rearrangement in NEMO impairs NF-kappaB activation and is a cause of incontinentia pigmenti. The International Incontinentia Pigmenti (IP) Consortium. *Nature* 405:466–472.

Smith, E. P., J. Boyd, G. R. Frank, H. Takahashi, R. M. Cohen, B. Specker, T. C. Williams, D. B. Lubahn, and K. S. Korach. 1994. Estrogen resistance caused by a mutation in the estrogen-receptor gene in a man. *New England Journal of Medicine* 331:1056–1060.

Smith, R. B., M. Divoll, W. R. Gillespie, and D. J. Greenblatt. 1983. Effect of subject age and gender on the pharmacokinetics of oral triazolam and temazepam. *Journal of Clinical Pharmacology* 3:172–176.

Smith, S. S., and J. K. Chapin. 1996a. The estrous cycle and the olivo-cerebellar circuit. I. Contrast enhancement of sensorimotor-correlated cerebellar discharge. *Experimental Brain Research* 111:371–384.

Smith, S. S., and J. K. Chapin. 1996b. The estrous cycle and the olivo-cerebellar circuit. II. Enhanced selective sensory gating of responses from the rostral dorsal accessory olive. *Experimental Brain Research* 111:385–392.

Smith, S. S., F. C. Hsu, X. Li, C. A. Frye, D. S. Faber, and R. S. Markowitz. 2000. Oestrogen effects in olivo-cerebellar and hippocampal circuits. *Novartis Foundation Symposium* 230:155–168.

Spear, L. P. 2000. Neurobehavioral changes in adolescence. *Current Directions in Psychological Science* 9:111–114.

Spitzer, J. A. 1999. Gender differences in some host defense mechanisms. *Lupus* 8:380–383.

Spitzer, J. A., and P. Zhang. 1996a. Gender differences in neutrophil function and cytokine-induced neutrophil chemoattractant generation in endotoxic rats. *Inflammation* 20: 485–498.

Spitzer, J. A., and P. Zhang. 1996b. Protein tyrosine kinase activity and the influence of gender in phagocytosis and tumor necrosis factor secretion in alveolar macrophages and lung-recruited neutrophils. *Shock* 6:426–433.

Stanley, J. C., and C. P. Benbow. 1982. Huge sex ratios at upper end. *American Psychologist* 37:972.

Stedman's Medical Dictionary, 26th ed. 1995. Baltimore: Williams & Wilkins.

Stefano, G. B., V. Prevot, and J.-C. Beauvillain. 1999. Estradiol coupling to human monocyte nitric oxide release is dependent on intracellular calcium transients: evidence for an estrogen surface receptor. *Journal of Immunology* 163:3758–3763.

Steffens, D., M. Norton, B. Plassman, J. T. Tschanz, B. W. Wyse, K. A. Welsh-Bohmer, J. C. Anthony, and J. C. Breitner. 1999. Enhanced cognitive performance with estrogen use in demented community-dwelling older women. *Journal of the American Geriatric Society* 47:1171–1175.

Stein, A. D., and L. H. Lumey. 2000. The relationship between maternal and offspring birth weights after maternal prenatal famine exposure: the Dutch Famine Birth Cohort Study. *Human Biology* 72:641–654.

Stein, A. H. 1976. Sex role development, pp. 233–257. In: *Understanding Adolescence*. J. F. Adams, ed. Boston: Allyn & Bacon.

Steingart, R. M., M. Packer, P. Hamm, M. E. Coglianese, B. Gersh, E. M. Geltman, J. Sollano, S. Katz, L. Moye, and L. L. Basta. 1991. Sex difference in the management of coronary artery disease. *New England Journal of Medicine* 325:226–230.

Stensland-Bugge, E., K. H. Bonaa, and I. Njolstad. 2000. Sex differences in the relationship of risk factors to subclinical carotid atherosclerosis measured 15 years later: the Tromso Heart Study. *Stroke* 31:574–581.

Sternberg, W. F., and M. W. Wachterman. 2000. Experimental studies of sex-related factors influencing nociceptive responses: nonhuman animal research, pp. 71–88. In: *Sex, Gender, and Pain*. R. B. Fillingim, ed. Seattle: IASP Press.

Stidham, K. R., J. L. Johnson, and H. F. Seigler. 1994. Survival superiority of females with melanoma. A multivariate analysis of 6383 patients exploring the significance of gender in prognostic outcome. *Archives of Surgery* 129:316–324.

Stones, I., M. Beckmann, and L. Stephens. 1982. Sex-related differences in mathematical competencies of pre-calculus college students. *School Science and Mathematics* 82: 295–299.

Stowers, J. M. 1984. Workshop 5: follow-up of gestational diabetic mothers treated thereafter. In: *Carbohydrate Metabolism in Pregnancy and the Newborn*. H. W. Sutherland and J. M. Stowers, eds. Edinburgh: Churchill Livingstone.

St. Pierre Schneider, B., L. A. Correia, and J. G. Cannon. 1999. Sex differences in leukocyte invasion in injured murine skeletal muscle. *Research in Nursing and Health* 22:243–250.

Stramba-Badiale, M., D. Spagnolo, G. Bosi, and P. J. Schwatz. 1995. Are gender differences in QTc present at birth: MISANAEAS investigators. Multicenter Italian Study on Neonatal Electrocardiography and Sudden Infant Death Syndrome. *American Journal of Cardiology* 75:1277–1278.

Stramba-Badiale, M., S. G. Priori, C. Napolitano, E. H. Locati, X. Vinolas, W. Haverkamp, F. Schulze-Bahr, K. Goulene, and P. J. Schwartz. 2000. Gene-specific differences in circadian variation of ventricular repolarization in the long QT syndrome: a key to sudden death during sleep? *Italian Heart Journal* 1:323–328.

Straus, E. W., and J. P. Raufman. 1989. Meal-stimulated gastrin release in normal men and women. *Journal of the Association for Academic Minority Physicians* 1:9–10.

Strobel A., T. Issad, L. Camoin, M. Ozata, and A. D. Strosberg. 1998. A leptin missense mutation associated with hypogonadism and morbid obesity. *Nature Genetics* 18: 213–215.

Strocchi, E., P. L. Malini, G. Valtancoli, C. Ricci, L. Bassein, and E. Ambrosioni. 1992. Cough during treatment with angiotensin-converting enzyme inhibitors: analysis of prediposing factors. *Drug Investigations* 4:69–72.

Stumpf, H., and J. Stanley. 1998. Standardized tests: still gender based? *Current Directions in Psychological Science* 7:192–196.

Suligoi, B. 1997. The natural history of human immunodeficiency virus infection among women as compared with men. *Sexually Transmitted Diseases* 24:77–83.

Sullivan, E. M., M. A. Burgess, and J. M. Forrest. 1999. The epidemiology of rubella and congenital rubella in Australia, 1992 to 1997. *Communicable Disease Intelligence* 23: 209–214.

Sumner, A. E., H. Kushner, K. D. Sherif, T. N. Tulenko, B. Falkner, and J. B. Marsh. 1999. Sex differences in African-Americans regarding sensitivity to insulin's glucoregulatory and antilipolytic actions. *Diabetes Care* 22:71–77.

Susman, E. J., G. Inoff-Germain, E. D. Nottelman, D. L. Loriaux, G. B. Cutler, and G. P. Chrousos. 1987. Hormones, emotional dispositions, and aggressive attributes in young adolescents. *Child Development* 58:1114–1134.

Suter, P. M., E. Jequier, and Y. Schutz. 1994. Effect of ethanol on energy expenditure. *American Journal of Physiology* 266(4 Pt 2):R1204-R1212.

Swain, A., and R. Lovell-Badge. 1999. Mammalian sex determination: a molecular drama. *Genes and Development* 13:755–767.

Swan, G. E., L. M. Jack, and M. M. Ward. 1997. Subgroups of smokers with different success rates after use of transdermal nicotine. *Addiction* 92:207–217.

Swanson, J. M., S. L. Dibble, and K. Trocki. 1995. A description of the gender differences in risk behaviors in young adults with genital herpes. *Public Health Nursing* 12:99–108.

Tate, C. A., and R. W. Holtz. 1998. Gender and fat metabolism during exercise: a review. *Canadian Journal of Applied Physiology* 23:570–582.

Taurog, J. D., S. D. Maika, N. Satumtira, M. L. Dorris, I. L. McLean, H. Yanagisawa, A. Sayad, A. J. Stagg, G. M. Fox, A. Le O'Brien, M. Rehman, M. Zhou, A. L. Weiner, J. B. Splawski, J. A. Richardson, and R. E. Hammer. 1999. Inflammatory disease in HLA-B27 transgenic rats. *Immunology Review* 169:209–223.

Taylor, R. W., E. Gold, P. Manning, and A. Goulding. 1997. Gender differences in body fat content are present well before puberty. *International Journal of Obesity and Related Metabolic Disorders* 21:1082–1084.

Taylor, S. E. , L. C. Klein, B. P. Lewis, T. L. Grunewald, R. A. Gurung, and J. A. Updegraff. 2000. Biobehavioral responses to stress in females: tend-and-befriend, not fight-or-flight. *Psychological Review* 107:411–429.

Teff, K. L., A. Alavi, J. Chen, M. Pourdehnad, and R. R. Townsend. 1999. Muscarinic blockade inhibits gastric emptying of mixed-nutrient meal: effects of weight and gender. *American Journal of Physiology* 276(3 Pt. 2):R707–R714.

Thelen, E. 1995. Motor development: a new synthesis. *American Psychologist* 50:79–95.

Tilghman, S. M. 1999. The sins of the fathers and mothers: genomic imprinting in mammalian development. *Cell* 96:185–193.

Tobet, S. A., and T. O. Fox. 1992. Sex differences in neuronal morphology influenced hormonally throughout life. In: *Handbook of Neurobiology*. A. A. Gerall, H. Moltz, and I. I. Ward, eds. New York: Plenum Press.

Toung, T. J., R. J. Traystman, and P. D. Hurn. 1998. Estrogen-mediated neuroprotection after experimental stroke in male rats *Stroke* 29:1666–1670.

Trigoso, W. F., J. M. Wesly, D. L. Meranda, and Y. Shenker. 1996. Vasopressin and atrial natriuretic hormone response to hypertonic saline during the follicular and luteal phases of the menstrual cycle. *Human Reproduction* 11:2392–2395.

Troiano, R. P., and K. M. Flegal. 1998. Overweight children and adolescents. Description, epidemiology, and demographics. *Pediatrics* 101:497–504.

Trollfors, B. 1997. Factors influencing antibody responses to acellular pertussis vaccines. *Developments in Biological Standardization* 89:279–282.

Tsao, H., G. S. Rogers, and A. J. Sober. 1998. An estimate of the annual direct cost of treating cutaneous melanoma. *Journal of the American Academy of Dermatology* 38(5 Pt. 1): 669–680.

Tseng, J. E., M. Rodriguez, J. Roe, D. Liu, W. K. Hong, and L. Mao. 1999. Gender differences in *p53* mutational status in small cell lung cancer. *Cancer Research* 59:5666–5670.

Tucci, A., R. Corinaldesi, V. Stanghellini, C. Tosetti, G. DiFebo, G. F. Paparo, O. Vaoli, G. M. Paganelli, A.M. Labate, C. Masci, G. Zoccoli, N. Monettie, and L. Barbara. 1992. Helicobacter pylori infection and gastric function in patients with chronic idiopathic dyspepsia. *Gastroenterology* 103:768–774.

Turnbull, A., and C. Rivier. 1995. Brain-periphery connections: do they play a role in mediating the effect of centrally injected interleukin-1 beta on gonadal function. *Neuroimmunomodulation* 2:224–235.

Turner, R. T. 1999. Mechanical signaling in the development of postmenopausal osteoporosis. *Lupus* 8:388–392.

Udry, J. R., N. M. Morris, and J. Kovenock. 1995. Androgen effects on women's gendered behaviour. *Journal of Biosocial Science* 27:359–368.

Unni, K. K., K. E. Holley, F. C. McDuffie, and J. L. Titus. 1975. Comparative study of NZB mice under germfree and conventional conditions. *Journal of Rheumatology* 2:36–44.

Unruh, A. M. 1996. Gender variations in clinical pain experience. *Pain* 65:123–167.

Unruh, A. M., J. Ritchie, and H. Merskey. 1999. Does gender affect appraisal of pain and pain coping strategies? *Clinical Journal of Pain* 15:31–40.

U.S. Department of Health and Human Services. 1998. Investigational new drug applications and new drug applications, FDA; Final Rule (21 CFR Parts 312 and 314). *Federal Register* 63:6854–6862.

U.S. Food and Drug Administration. 1977. *General Considerations for the Clinical Evaluation of Drugs.* Publication No. HEW (FDA) 77–3040. Washington, DC: U.S. Government Printing Office.

U.S. General Accounting Office. 1990. *National Institutes of Health: Problems in Implementing Policy on Women's Study Populations.* Publication No. GAO/T-HRD-90-38). Washington, DC: U.S. General Accounting Office.

U.S. General Accounting Office. 2000. *Women's Health: NIH Has Increased Its Efforts to Include Women in Research.* Publication No. GAO/HEHS-00-96. Washington, DC: U.S. General Accounting Office.

U.S. Government Printing Office. 1949. *Trials of War Criminals Before the Nuremberg Military Tribunals Under Control Council Law No. 10,* Vol. 2, pp. 181–182. Washington, DC: U.S. Government Printing Office.

U.S. Public Health Service. 1985. Report of the Public Health Service Task Force on Women's Health Issues. *Public Health Reports* 100:73–106.

Uusitalo, M., M. Heikkilä, and S. Vainio. 1999. Molecular genetic studies of Wnt signaling in the mouse. *Experimental Cell Research* 253:336–348.

Vaccarino, V., L. Parsons, N. R. Every, H. V. Barron, and H. M. Krumholz. 1999. Sex-based differences in early mortality after myocardial infarction. *New England Journal of Medicine* 341:217–225.

Vaccarino, V., H. M. Krumholz, J. Yarzebski, J. M. Gore, and R. G. Goldberg. 2001. Sex-based differences in early mortality after myocardial infarction. National Registry Myocardial Infarction 2 Participants. *Annuals of Internal Medicine* 134:173–181.

Valian, V. 1998. *Why So Slow? The Advancement of Women.* Cambridge, MA: The MIT Press.

Vandenbergh, J. G., and C. L. Huggett. 1995. The anogenital distance index, a predictor of the intrauterine position effects on reproduction in female house mice. *Laboratory Animal Science* 45:567–573.

Van Lieshout, E. M., M. Peters, and W. H. Peters. 1998. Age and gender dependent levels of glutathione and glutathione S-transferases in human lymphocytes. *Carcinogenesis* 19:1873–1875.

Van Putten, T., S. R. Marder, and J. Mintz. 1991. Serum prolactin as a correlate of clinical response to haloperidol. *Journal of Clinical Psychopharmacology* 11:357–361.

Venter, J. C., et al. 2001. The sequence of the human genome. *Science* 291:1304–1351.

Vermeulen, A. 2000. Andropause. *Maturitas* 34:5–15.

Vidaver, R. M., B. LaFleur, C. Tong, B. A. Bradshaw, and S. A. Marts. 2000. Women subjects in NIH-funded clinical research literature: lack of progress in both representation and analysis by sex. *Journal of Women's Health and Gender-Based Medicine* 9:495–504.

Vilain, E., and E. R. McCabe. 1998. Mammalian sex determination: from gonads to brain. *Molecular Genetics and Metabolism* 65:74–84.

vom Saal, F. S., M. M. Clark, B. G. Galef, Jr., L. C. Drickamer, and J. G. Vandenbergh. 1999. Intrauterine position phenomenon. In: *Encyclopedia of Reproduction*. E. Knobil and J. D. Neill, eds. New York: Academic Press.

Wachtel, S. S., G. C. Koo, E. E. Zuckerman, U. Hammerling, M. P. Scheid, and E. A. Boyse. 1974. Serological crossreactivity between H-Y (male) antigens of mouse and man. *Proceedings of the National Academy of Sciences of the United States of America* 71:1215–1218.

Walker, P. L., and D. C. Cook. 1998. Brief communication: gender and sex: vive la difference. *American Journal of Physical Anthropology* 106:255–259.

Walle, U. K., S. A. Salle, S. A. Bai, and L. S. Olanoff. 1983. Stereoselective binding of propranolol to human plasma alpha 1-acid glycoprotein albumin. *Clinical Pharmacology and Therapeutics* 34:718–723.

Wallen, K. 1996. Nature needs nurture: the interaction of hormonal and social influences on the development of behavioral sex differences in rhesus monkeys. *Hormones and Behavior* 30:364–378.

Wang, Q., R. Santizo, V. L. Braughman, and D. A. Pelligrino. 1999. Estrogen provides neuroprotection in transient forebrain ischemia through perfusion-independent mechanisms in rats. *Stroke* 30:630–637.

Wareham, K. A., M. F. Lyon, P. H. Glenister, and E. D. Williams. 1987. Age related reactivation of an X-linked gene. *Nature* 327:725–727.

Warner, R. R. 1984. Mating behavior and hermaphroditism in coral reef fish. *American Scientist* 72:128–136.

Warner, R. R., and S. E. Swearer. 1991. Social control of sex change in the bluehead wrasse thalassoma-bifasciatum pisces labridae. *Biological Bulletin* 181:199–204.

Warren, M. P., and A. L. Stiehl. 1999. Exercise and female adolescents: effects on the reproductive and skeletal system. *Journal of the American Medical Women Association* 54:115–120.

Watanabe, M., A. R. Zinn, D. C. Page, and T. Nishimoto. 1993. Functional equivalence of human X- and Y-encoded isoforms of ribosomal protein S4 consistent with a role in Turner syndrome. *Nature Genetics* 4:268–271.

Watkins, P. B., S. A. Wrighton, P. Maurel, E. G. Schuetz, G. Mendez-Picon, G. A. Parker, and P. S. Guzelian. 1985. Identification of an inducible form of cytochrome P-450 in human liver. *Proceedings of the National Academy of Sciences of the United States of America* 82:6310–6314.

Watson, M. S., D. Freije, and H. Donis-Keller. 1992. Identification of a second pseudoautosomal region near the Xq and Yq telomeres. *Science* 258:1784–1787.

Wenger, M. K. 1985. Coronary disease in women. *Annual Reviews of Medicine* 36:285–294.

Wenger, N. K. 1994. Coronary heart disease in women: gender differences in diagnostic evaluation. *Journal of the American Medical Womens Association* 49:181-185, 197.

Wesche, D. L., B. G. Schuster, W. Wen-Xiu, and R. L. Woosley. 2000. Mechanism of cardiotoxicity of halofantrine. *Clinical Pharmacology Therapy* 67:521–529.

Weyer, C., S. Snitker, C. Bogardus, and E. Ravussin. 1999. Energy metabolism in African Americans: potential risk factors for obesity. *American Journal of Clinical Nutrition* 70: 13–20.

White, D. P., N. J. Douglas, C. K. Pickett, J. V. Weil, and C. W. Zwillich. 1983. Sexual influence on the control of breathing. *Journal of Applied Physiology* 54:874–879.

White, P. C., M. I. New, and B. Dupont. 1987. Congenital adrenal hyperplasia. *New England Journal of Medicine* 316:1519–1524.

Wilder, R. L. 1995. Neuroendocrine-immune system interactions and autoimmunity. *Annual Review of Immunology* 13:307–338.

Will, J. C., C. Denny, M. Serdula, and B. Muneta. 1999. Trends in body weight among American Indians: findings from a telephone survey, 1985 through 1996. *American Journal of Public Health* 89:395–398.

Willard, H. F. 2000. The sex chromosomes and X chromosome inactivation. *In: The Metabolic and Molecular Bases of Inherited Disease*, 8th ed. C. R. Scriver, A. L. Beaudet, W. S. Sly, D. Valle, B. Childs, and B. Vogelstein, eds. New York: McGraw-Hill.

Williams, G. H. 1991. Hypertensive vascular disease. *In: Harrison's Principles of Internal Medicine*. J. D. Wilson, E. Braunwald, K. J. Isselbacher, eds. New York: McGraw-Hill.

Wilson, J. D. 1999. The role of androgens in male gender role behavior. *Endocrinology Reviews* 20:726–737.

Wilson, J. D., J. E. Griffin, F. W. George, and M. Leshin. 1981. The role of gonadal steroids in sexual differentiation. *Recent Progress in Hormone Research* 37:1–39.

Wing, L. M., J. O. Miners, D. J. Birkett, T. Foenander, K. Lillywhite, and S. Wanwimolruk. 1984. Lidocaine disposition—sex differences and effects of cimetidine. *Clinical Pharmacology and Therapeutics* 35:695–701.

Witt, D. M., C. S. Carter, and D. H. Walton. 1990. Central and peripheral effects of oxytocin administration in prairie voles (Microtus ochrogaster). *Pharmacology, Biochemistry and Behavior* 37:63–69.

Wolf, M. 1984. Naming, reading, and the dyslexia: a longitudinal overview. *Annals of Dyslexia* 34:87–115.

Wolf, M., and H. Goodglass. 1986. Dyslexia, dysnomia, and lexical retrieval: a longitudinal investigation. *Brain and Language* 28:154–168.

Wong Y., A. Rodwell, S. Dawkins, S. A. Livesey, and I. A. Simpson. 2001. Sex differences in investigation results and treatment in subjects referred for investigation of chest pain. *Heart* 85:149–152.

Woolley, C. S., and B. S. McEwen. 1993. Roles of estradiol and progesterone in regulation of hippocampal dendritic spine density during the estrous cycle in the rat. *Journal of Comparative Neurology* 336:293–306.

World Health Organization. 1998a. *Obesity. Preventing and Managing the Global Epidemic.* Report of a WHO consultation on obesity. Geneva: World Health Organization.

World Health Organization. 1998b. *Gender and Health: Technical Paper*. Geneva: World Health Organization.

Wrighton, S. A., and J. C. Stevens. 1992. The human hepatic cytochromes P450 involved in drug metabolism. *Critical Reviews in Toxicology* 22:1–21.

Xiao, L., and J. B. Becker. 1994. Quantitative microdialysis determination of extracellular striatal dopamine concentration in male and female rats: effects of estrous cycle and gonadectomy. *Neuroscience Letters* 180:155–158.

Xu, P., and Y. W. Chien. 1991. Enhanced skin permeability for transdermal drug delivery: physiopathological and physiocochemical considerations. *Critical Reviews of Therapeutic Drug Carrier Systems* 8:211–236.

Yaffe, K., D. Grady, A. Pressman, and S. Cummings. 1998. Serum estrogen levels, cognitive performance, and risk of cognitive decline in older community women. *Journal of the American Geriatric Society* 46:816–821.

Yamamoto, E. 1999. Studies on sex-manipulation and production of cloned populations in hirame, Paralichthys olivaceus (Temminck et Schlegel). *Aquaculture* 173:235–246.

Yasui, N., T. Kondo, K. Otani, K. Ishida, K. Mihara, A. Suzuki, S. Kaneko, and Y. Inoue. 1998. Prolcotin response to bromperidol treatment in schizophrenic patients. *Pharmacology and Toxicology* 82:153–156.

Yonkers, K. A., J. C. Kando, J. O. Cole, and S. Blumenthal. 1992. Gender differences in pharmacokinetics and pharmacodynamics of psychotropic medicine. *American Journal of Psychiatry* 149:587–589.

Young, M. W. 2000. Circadian rhythms. Marking time for a kingdom. *Science* 288:451–453.

Yung, R., R. Williams, K. Johnson, C. Phillips, L. Stoolman, S. Chang, and B. Richardson. 1997. Mechanisms of drug-induced lupus. III. Sex-specific differences in T cell homing may explain increased disease severity in female mice. *Arthritis and Rheumatism* 40:1334–1343.

Zea-Longa, E., P. R. Weinstein, S. Carlson, and R. Cummins. 1989. Reversible middle cerebral artery occlusion without craniectomy in rats. *Stroke* 20:84–91.

Zucker, K. J. 1999. Intersexuality and gender identity differentiation. *Annual Review of Sex Research* 10:1–69.

Zucker, K. J., S. J. Bradley, G. Oliver, J. Blake, S. Fleming, and J. Hood. 1996. Psychosexual development of women with congenital adrenal hyperplasia. *Hormones and Behavior* 30:300–318.

Zwick, M. E., D. J. Cutler, and A. Chakravarti. 2000. Patterns of genetic variation in Mendelian and complex traits. *Annual Review of Genomics and Human Genetics* 1:387–407.

APPENDIX

A

Data Sources and Acknowledgments

The committee explored various data sources in a concerted effort to cast a broad net for the collection and assessment of information. In addition to reviewing the literature, the committee invited scientific experts to make presentations and commissioned an independent consultant to prepare a background paper. Many of the study sponsors also provided helpful information including published reports, regulations and guidance documents, remarks and testimony from meetings and hearings, and additional literature. The committee also reviewed relevant articles and editorials in the popular press, as well as federal agency and health information sites on the World Wide Web.

LITERATURE REVIEW

The committee was provided with copies of the National Institutes of Health (NIH) *Agenda for Research on Women's Health for the 21st Century* (National Institutes of Health, Office of Research on Women's Health, 1999a–f) before the first committee meeting. That six-volume report provided the committee with a broad base of knowledge and issues on which it could build. The committee expanded its review by conducting numerous literature searches. Search terms used included, but were not limited to, *sex differences* or *gender differences* and each of the following: *biology, immunology, endocrinology, metabolism, physiology, genetics, pharmacology, toxicology, infectious disease, psychology, behavior, animal models,* and *aging.* The sponsors, invited speakers, and other researchers and professionals who consider sex and gender differences in their work also provided literature for the committee's review and consideration.

In addition, Institute of Medicine staff attended professional scientific meetings and symposia during the course of the study to bring back the latest research information for the committee's review. Among the meetings attended were the annual scientific advisory meetings of the Society for Women's Health Research, the Conference on Sex and Gene Expression sponsored by the Society for Women's Health Research, the National Forum of the Centers of Excellence in Women's Health, a Smithsonian Institution seminar entitled Gender Differences in Addiction and Recovery, and a seminar entitled Sex and Gender Analysis in Health Research at the U.S. Department of Health and Human Services.

INVITED PRESENTATIONS

Over the course of the study, the committee received and considered information from organizations and individuals representing many different perspectives on research on sex and gender issues.[1] The committee believed that it was important to receive direct input from researchers whose work has included the analysis of sex and gender differences in health.

At the first four committee meetings, the committee invited experts in various related fields of scientific endeavor to make presentations and have discussions with the committee (Box A-1).

Speakers and topics were chosen to complement, expand upon, and fill gaps in the committee's own collective expertise. Committee members heard presentations and asked questions to explore fully the data, surrounding issues, and unique perspectives that each researcher provided.

TECHNICAL ASSISTANCE

In addition to discussions with the invited speakers, the committee sought additional expert technical assistance over the course of the study. The committee is grateful to the following individuals for their helpful contributions and discussions via phone and e-mail: Philip L. Cohen, University of Pennsylvania; Peter K. Gregersen, North Shore University Hospital; Helen Hobbs, University of Texas Southwestern Medical School; Peter Nathanielsz, Cornell University; J. Lee Nelson, Fred Hutchinson Cancer Research Center; Christopher O'Donnell, Massachusetts General

---

[1]All written materials presented to the committee were reviewed and considered with respect to the committee's four tasks. This material can be examined by the public at 2101 Constitution Avenue, N.W., Room 204, Washington, DC 20418; telephone: (202) 334-3543.

BOX A-1
Invited Presentations

Agenda for Research on Women's Health for the 21st Century, report of the Task Force on the NIH Women's Health Research Agenda for the 21st Century.
Donna Dean
Office of the Director, NIH

Overview of the 9th Annual Scientific Advisory Meeting of the Society for Women's Health Research
Sherry Marts
Society for Women's Health Research

Perspectives on Research on Sex and Gender Differences:
History, Status of Research, Barriers to Progress
Florence Haseltine
National Institute of Child Health and Human Development, NIH

Perspectives on Research on Sex and Gender Differences:
History, Status of Research, Barriers to Progress
Marianne Legato
Columbia University College of Physicians and Surgeons

Sex Hormone Effects
Bruce McEwen
The Rockefeller University

Intrauterine Environment
Peter Nathanielsz
Cornell University

Androgens
William Bremner
University of Washington

Sex and Gender Differences in Cerebrovascular Health
Patricia Hurn
The Johns Hopkins University School of Medicine

Sex and Gender Differences in Musculoskeletal Health
Joan McGowan
National Institute of Arthritis and Musculoskeletal and Skin Diseases, NIH

Sex and Gender Differences in Metabolism
Eric Poehlman
University of Vermont

Sex and Gender Differences in Pharmacokinetics and Pharmacodynamics
Raymond Woosley
Georgetown University Medical Center

Sex and Gender Differences in Aging
Richard Hodes
National Institute on Aging, NIH

Hospital, Harvard Medical School, Allen C. Steere, New England Medical Center.

COMMISSIONED PAPER

To gain a more in-depth perspective on current and potential barriers to the conduct of valid and productive research on sex and gender differences, the committee commissioned an independent consultant to prepare a background paper on this topic for the committee's use. Beth Schachter, a professional science writer and editor with a biomedical research background in cellular and molecular biology and endocrinology, interviewed selected researchers and administrators by phone and e-mail and reviewed relevant articles and editorials in scientific journals and the popular press. That paper provided some of the background for Chapter 6.

APPENDIX

B

Physiological and Pharmacological Differences Between the Sexes

Physiological and pharmacological differences between the sexes are discussed in Chapter 5 (see Table 5-3). Additional examples are presented here in Table B-1, which is a continuation of Table 5-3, as the purpose of understanding sex differences is to achieve better health and health care, and understanding the differences between the sexes in response to therapeutic agents is particularly important in that regard.

TABLE B-1 Receptor, Enzyme, and Structural Differences Between Males and Females

Sex Difference	Clinical Relevance
The dopamine D2 receptor gene has a *Taq*IA restriction fragment length polymorphism that yields two alleles, A1 and A2. Individuals with the A1 allele have a D2 receptor with a lower density and diminished function. Nemonapride, a potent D2 receptor antagonist with antipsychotic activity, increases the plasma prolactin concentration more in females with the A1 allele than males with this polymorphism (Mihara et al., 2000).	Females may be at higher risk than males of adverse events associated with nemonapride-induced hyperprolactinemia.

continued on next page

TABLE B-1 Continued

Sex Difference	Clinical Relevance
The levels of androgen and progesterone receptors present in vocal cords are greater in males than females. Progesterone receptor levels decrease with age (Newman et al., 2000).	May explain why men have deeper voices than women and why women treated with testosterone may develop a deep voice.
Inorganic phosphate pi-class glutathione S-transferase (pI 4.8) is approximately 1.6 times more abundant in the female colon than in the male colon. There are also significant differences between males and females in substrate specificities and inhibition kinetics (Singhal et al., 1992).	Male and female colons may metabolize small organic molecules differently.
Atrial natriuretic peptide (ANP) levels are twofold greater in young women than young men. Levels do not vary during the menstrual cycle. ANP levels are not different in age-matched men and menopausal women. Aldosterone levels are higher in women than men during the luteal phase but not during the preovulatory phase of menses (Clark et al., 1990).	When women are infused with hypertonic saline, ANP levels are increased more during the luteal phase than the follicular phase of the menstrual cycle. Investigators conclude that intravascular volumes were decreased during the luteal phase compared with those during the follicular phase (Trigoso et al., 1996).
Clearance of methylprednisolone is greater in men than women during the late luteal phase of the menstrual cycle. The 50 percent inhibitory concentration for suppression of cortisol secretion is significantly lower in females. No sex differences in net cortisol or helper T-lymphocyte suppression exist. Males had greater net suppression of blood basophil weight (Lew et al., 1993).	More rapid elimination of methylprednisolone by women compensates for their increased sensitivity to methylprednisolone-induced cortisol suppression. The doses given to patients were based on lean body mass.
Blood samples from more men than women (89 versus 48 percent) with stage B-type lymphatic leukemia test positive for the MDR1 (multiple drug resistance) phenotype (Monteleone et al., 1997).	Women have a more benign course of disease, suggesting that sex-dependent differences in drug resistance gene activity may be responsible for at least some of the disease course (Monteleone et al., 1997). In deciding on a treatment for untreated patients, sex and determination of *mdr1* gene expression should be considered in selecting appropriate treatment, including the need to use P-glycoprotein inhibitors.

TABLE B-1 Continued

Sex Difference	Clinical Relevance
d-Fenfluramine is used as a probe for central serotonin activity, such as in patients with obsessive-compulsive disease. In healthy subjects the secretion of a plasma cortisol response to *d*-fenfluramine was blunted in females but not males. The blunted response was more pronounced in female patients than healthy female subjects (Gilmore et al., 1992).	Suggests serotonin dysfunction in female patients with some psychiatric disorders.
Young adults generally discriminate lower concentrations of citric acid and caffeine from water than elderly subjects. Younger subjects also detected suprathreshold concentrations of caffeine significantly more intense than those judged by young males and the elderly (Hyde and Feller, 1981)	These differences may influence the types and quantities of food and drink that people consume.
Young ovulating females excrete more kallikrein in their urine than males and menopausal females. During the follicular phase of the menstrual cycle the levels are similar to those in males and the levels rise during the luteal phase. These sex differences are present in white subjects but not African-American subjects (Kailasam et al., 1998).	The level of renal kallikrein excretion is diminished in essential hypertension. Results suggest that renal kallikrein biosynthesis responses are decreased in African Americans, a group at increased risk for development of hypertension.
Estrogen receptors are higher in varicose segments than nonvaricose segments of the same vein, especially in females. Progesterone receptor levels are denser in the nonvaricose segments of females than in those of males (Mashiah et al., 1999).	It has not been determined if these differences are age related or are associated with an increased incidence of varicosities in females.
Estrogen and progesterone receptor transcripts are expressed in anterial cruciate ligaments of males and females (Sciore et al., 1998). Males have significantly larger knee cartilage than females, independent of body and bone size (Cicuttini et al 1999).	The rate of injury to ligaments in female athletes is greater than that to ligaments in male athletes.

continued on next page

TABLE B-1   Continued

Sex Difference	Clinical Relevance
Platelet phenolsulfotransferase levels have different seasonal profiles in males and females (Marazziti et al., 1998b).	Investigators recommend research into sex-dependent metabolism of the endogenous and exogenous substrates for the enzyme.
A positive relationship between occurrence of buccal mucosa ridging and tongue indentation (signs of bruxism) and sex and age was found, with the relationship found to be more common in females than males (Piquero et al., 1999).	May be associated with a variety of illnesses, e.g., headache and neck stiffness.
Peroxidase activity in tears is higher during the preovulatory and luteal phases of the menstrual cycle. The activity correlates with plasma estradiol levels (Marcozzi et al., 2000).	Is a possible cause for the greater incidence of some ocular diseases, e.g., keratoconjunctivitis sicca (dry eyes), in . females
The dissociation constant (K_d) for paroxetine binding to human platelets is lower in young females than males; the opposite is found in elderly females. The K_d was negatively correlated with age in males (Marazziti et al., 1998a).	These observations suggest that modifications in the serotonin transporter might provide the basis for the increased susceptibility of females to depression.
The ratio of the incidence of irritable bowel syndrome in females:males is 2:1 (Mayer et al., 1999).	Positron emission tomography scans after rectosigmoid balloon distension show differences and may help elucidate the reason for the sex differences.
Obstructive sleep apnea is more prevalent in males than females, but the incidence increases in postmeno-pausal women, suggesting that pro-gesterone may provide protection against the disorder. Jordan et al. (2000) tested this hypothesis and found that one potential mechanism, the poststimulus ventilatory decline, is not different in males and females or in females during the follicular and luteal phases of their menstrual cycles.	
Males receiving a 21-milligram nicotine patch take significantly longer to relapse to smoking than females (Swan et al., 1997).	The biological basis for this difference is unknown.

TABLE B-1 Continued

Sex Difference	Clinical Relevance
Elderly people metabolize the verapamil enantiomer more slowly than young people. Mean arterial pressure and PR interval (an electrocardiogram variable) reduction correlated with S- and R-verapamil levels in blood and are not affected by sex or age (Gupta et al., 1995).	An example of a pharmacokinetic, not a pharmacodynamic, difference.
The endothelial synthesis of nitric oxide from L-arginine is stimulated by acetylcholine. The vasodilating effect of the brachial artery administration of acetylcholine was markedly impaired in hypercholesterolemic males but not hypercholesterolemic females compared with the effect in eucholesterolemic controls. The responses to acetylcholine were normalized by L-arginine in hypercholesterolemic males, whereas the effects were similar in hypercholesterolemic and control women (Chowienczyk et al., 1994).	These responses may account for why hypercholesterolemic females appear to be protected from the adverse effects of nitric oxide production.
Administration of 6 milligrams of bromperidol raises plasma prolactin levels more in females than males and correlates with the levels of bromperidol and its reduced metabolite in plasma (Yasui et al., 1998).	Serum prolactin level increases in males receiving haloperidol have been correlated with the clinical response to this antipsychosis drug (Van Putten et al., 1991). Assuming that the mechanism for the prolactin increases for these drugs is similar in males and females, a smaller dose for females than males may be appropriate.
In healthy subjects a plasma cortisol response to d-fenfluramine is present in females but not males. The response did not differ between patients with obsessive-compulsive disease and control subjects but was significantly reduced in female patients compared with that in female controls (Monteleone et al., 1997).	These results suggest a dysfunction of serotonin transmission in female patients with obsessive-compulsive disease.

continued on next page

TABLE B-1   Continued

Sex Difference	Clinical Relevance
Estrogen binds to the dopamine receptor, providing an explanation of why postmenopausal women are more likely than younger women to experience the dopamine-related side effects of drugs (Dawkins and Potter, 1991; Yonkers et al., 1992).	Binding to receptor probably has an antidopaminergic effect.
Apolipoprotein E genotype differences had no effect on the response to tacrine in patients with mild to moderate Alzheimer's disease, although there was a clear sex difference. Treatment effect size was not different between epsilon 2-3 and epsilon 4 in men but was larger for epsilon 2-3 than epsilon 4 in women (Farlow et al., 1998).	Could significantly improve drug selection for each patient if the effect is substantiated for other drugs.
To satisfactorily dose patients with growth hormone, a dose adjustment method provides the best results since females were less sensitive to growth hormone and larger doses are required to achieve in females the same levels achieved in males (Drake et al., 1998).	Serum insulin-like growth factor type 1 level measurements provide the surrogate endpoint for the appropriate dose.
The incidence of vascular thromboses varies between the sexes. Estrogen beta and androgen receptors are expressed on human megakaryocytes; they are upregulated by 1.5 and 10 nanomoles of testosterone per liter and are down-regulated by 100 nanomoles of testosterone per liter (Khetawat et al., 2000).	The ability of megakaryocytes to respond to testosterone provides a possible mechanism by which sex hormones may mediate sex differences in platelet activity and thrombotic diseases.

APPENDIX

C

Glossary *

Adaptive immunity. Lymphocyte-, macrophage-, or dendritic cell-based systems that encounter, memorize, and recall new antigens (old term: *immunity*).

Allele. Any alternative form of a gene that can occupy a particular chromosomal locus. In
humans and other diploid organisms there are two alleles, one on each chromosome
of a homologous pair.

Aneuploidy. Gain or loss of one or more chromosomes.

Antibody. An immunoglobulin molecule that has a specific amino acid sequence by virtue
of which it interacts with the antigen that induced its synthesis in cells of the lymphoid
series (especially plasma cells) or with an antigen closely related to it.

Antigen. Any substance that is capable under appropriate conditions of inducing a specific
immune response and of reacting with the products of that response, that is, with
specific antibody or specifically sensitized T lymphocytes, or both.

Autoimmunity. A condition characterized by a specific humoral or cell-mediated immune
response against constituents of the body's own tissues (self-antigens or autoantigens).

Autosome. Any chromosome other than a sex chromosome. Humans have 22 pairs of autosomes.

Bioavailability. The fraction of the dose that is absorbed and that reaches the systemic
circulation unaltered by biotransformation.

Biotransformation. The enzymatic conversion of a compound, usually to a more water-
soluble compound.

Body mass index. One of the anthropometric measures of body mass.

Cell. The basic unit of any living organism. It is a small, watery compartment filled with
chemicals and a complete copy of the organism's genome.

---

* Sources for the definitions, in addition to members of the committee, include Dorland's
Illustrated Medical Dictionary (Philadelphia: W.B. Saunders Co., 2000), The On-line Medi-
cal Dictionary (http://www.graylab.ac.uk/); and Glossary of Genetic Terms developed by
National Human Genome Research Institute (http://www.nhgri.nih.gov).

Chromosome. One of the threadlike "packages" of genes and other DNA in the nucleus of a cell. Humans have 23 pairs of chromosomes, 46 in all: 44 autosomes and 2 sex chromosomes. Each parent contributes one chromosome to each pair, so children get half of their chromosomes from their mothers and half from their fathers.

Cytology. The study of cells, their origin, structure, function, and pathology.

Diploid. The number of chromosomes in most cells except the gametes (reproductive cells). In humans, the diploid number is 46.

Disease. Any deviation from or interruption of the normal structure or function of a part, organ, or system of the body as manifested by characteristic symptoms and signs; the etiology, pathology, and prognosis may be known or unknown.

DNA (deoxyribonucleic acid). The chemical inside the nucleus of a cell that carries the genetic instructions required to make living organisms.

Dose-response. The relationship between the dose of a drug and the magnitude or intensity of the response.

Enantiomer. One of a pair of compounds having a mirror-image relationship.

Epigenetic mosaic. Occurs when different cells of the same type within an individual have different "gene expression states," e.g., the two types of cells found in all females, those in which their paternal X chromosome is active and those in which their maternal X chromosome is active.

Exon. The region of a gene that contains the code required to produce the gene's protein. Each exon codes for a specific portion of the complete protein. In some species (including humans), a gene's exons are separated by long regions of DNA (called introns or sometimes "junk DNA") that have no apparent function.

Female. An individual organism of the sex that bears young or that produces ova or eggs.

Gametogenic cells. Producing or favoring the production of germ cells.

Gender. A person's self-representation as male or female or how that person is responded to by social institutions on the basis of the individual's gender presentation. Gender is shaped by environment and experience (see discussion in Chapter 1).

Gene. The functional and physical unit of heredity passed from parent to offspring. Genes are pieces of DNA, and most genes contain the information required to make a specific protein.

Genetics. The study of genes and their heredity.

Genome. All the DNA contained in an organism or a cell, which includes both the chromosomes within the nucleus and the DNA in mitochondria.

Genomic imprinting. The concept that some genes are expressed from only the maternal allele and others are expressed from only the paternal allele.

Genotype. The genetic identity of an individual that does not show as outward characteristics.

Germ line. The sequence of cells in the line of direct descent from zygote to gamete, as opposed to somatic cells (all other body cells). Mutations in germ-line cells are transmitted to progeny; those in somatic cells are not.

Haploid. The number of chromosomes in a sperm or egg cell, half the diploid number. In humans, the haploid number is 23.

Haplotype. 1. A set of alleles of a group of closely linked genes, such as the human leukocyte antigen complex, which is usually inherited as a unit. 2. The genetic constitution of an individual at a set of closely linked genes on a given chromosome.

Hemizygous. Possessing only one instead of a pair of genes of a particular kind.

Heterochromatic. Describes the appearance of certain portions of the genome under a light microscope; usually associated with relatively large portions of the genome in which genes that code for products have been silenced or are absent, such as the inactive X chromosome in females or large amounts of simple sequence repeats associated with centromeres.

Heterozygous. Possessing two different forms of a particular gene, one inherited from each parent.

Homology. The quality of being homologous; the morphological identity of corresponding parts; structural similarity due to descent from a common form.

Homozygous. Possessing two identical forms of a particular gene, one inherited from each parent.

Hormone. A chemical substance that is produced in the body by an organ, cells of an organ, or scattered cells and that has a specific regulatory effect on the activity of an organ or organs. The term was originally applied to substances secreted by endocrine glands and transported in the bloodstream to distant target organs, but later was applied to various substances having similar actions but not produced by special glands.

Immunity. The protection against infectious disease conferred by either the immune response generated by immunization or previous infection or vaccination (active immunity) or transfer of antibody or lymphocytes from an immuno donor (passive immunity).

Infectious disease. A disease caused by a pathogenic microorganism; the etiologic agent may be a bacterium, virus, fungus, or animal parasite and may be transmitted from another host or arise from the host's own indigenous microflora.

Innate immunity. Phagocytic cells that respond to toxic signals with no memory capacity (old term: *inflammation*).

In vitro. Within a glass; observable in a test tube; in an artificial environment.

In vivo. Within the living body.

Locus. The place on a chromosome where a specific gene is located, a kind of address for the gene. The plural is "loci."

Male. An organism of the sex that begets young or that produces spermatozoa.

Meiosis. A special method of cell division, occurring in maturation of the sex cells, by means of which each daughter nucleus receives half the number of chromosomes characteristic of the somatic cells of the species.

Meiotic prophase. The stage of meiosis during which DNA replication, homologous pairing, and recombination (the exchange of portions of maternal and paternal chromosomes, such that children receive portions of both grandparents' chromosomes) occur.

Mitosis. A method of indirect division of a cell, consisting of a complex of various processes, by means of which the two daughter nuclei normally receive identical complements of the number of chromosomes characteristic of the somatic cells of the species. Mitosis, the process by which the body grows and replaces cells, is divided into four phases. (1) Prophase: condensation of replicated chromosomes, disappearance of nuclear membrane, appearance of the achromatic spindle, formation of polar bodies. (2) Metaphase: arrangement of chromosomes in the equatorial plane of the central spindle to form the monaster. Chromosomes separate into exactly similar halves. (3) Anaphase: the two groups of daughter chromosomes separate and move along the fibers of the central spindle, each toward one of the asters, forming the diaster. (4) Telophase: the daughter chromosomes resolve themselves into a reticulum and the daughter nuclei are formed; the cytoplasm then divides, forming two complete daughter cells.

Model (e.g., "animal model"). Any condition found in an animal that is of value in studying a biological phenomenon, e.g., a pathological mechanism of an animal disorder useful in studying human disease.

Mosaicism. The occurrence in an individual of two or more cell populations, derived from a single zygote, with different chromosomal constitutions.

Nondisjunction. Improper separation of chromosomes at nuclear division.

Pharmacodynamics. The study of the biochemical and physiological effects of drugs and the mechanisms of their actions, including the correlation of actions and effects of drugs with their chemical structure; also, such effects on the actions of a particular drug or drugs. Contrast with *pharmacokinetics*.

Pharmacology. The medical science that deals with the discovery, chemistry, effects, uses, and manufacture of drugs.

Pharmacokinetics. The action of drugs in the body over a period of time, including the processes of absorption, distribution, localization in tissues, biotransformation, and excretion.

Phenotype. The total characteristics displayed by an organism under a particular set of environmental factors, regardless of the actual genotype of the organism. Results from interaction between the genotype and the environment.

pKα. The negative logarithm of the ionization constant of an acid (K_α); the buffering power of a buffer system is greatest when its pK_α equals the pH.

Racemic. Made up of two enantiomorphic isomers and therefore optically inactive.

Sex. The classification of living things, generally as male or female, according to their reproductive organs and functions assigned by chromosomal complement (see discussion in Chapter 1).

Sexual dimorphism. Having two different distinct forms of individuals within the same species or two different distinct forms of parts within the same organism. For plants, it could refer to different leaf types, flowers, etc. For animals, it could refer to different coloring, sizes, features, etc. Sexual dimorphism is a common case, in which the two sexes have different shapes, sizes, etc. from each other.

Stochastic effect. Refers to an event that may occur with a known frequency but for which the outcome of any particular event may not be predicted in advance, such as the flip of a coin (which will be a tail 50 percent of the time).

Somatic cells. Usually any cell of a multicellular organism that will not contribute to the production of gametes, i.e., most cells of which an organism is made; not a germ cell.

Spermatogenesis. The process of formation of spermatozoa, including spermatocytogenesis and spermiogenesis.

Therapeutic index. Relationship between the desired and undesired effect(s) of a drug, that is, the benefit/risk ratio.

X chromosome. A sex chromosome. In mammals paired in females (XX), in amphibia paired in males.

Y chromosome. The small chromosome that is male determining in most mammal species and that is found only in the heterogametic sex. Thus, in mammals the male has one Y chromosome and one X chromosome.

Zygote. A single diploid cell resulting from the fusion of male and female gametes (sperm and ovum) at fertilization.

APPENDIX

D

Committee and Staff Biographies

COMMITTEE BIOGRAPHIES

Mary-Lou Pardue, Ph.D. (*Chair*), is the first Boris Magasanik Professor of Biology at the Massachusetts Institute of Technology (MIT) and has been on the MIT faculty for more than 25 years. She earned a bachelor's degree in biology from the College of William and Mary, a master's degree in radiation biology from the University of Tennessee, and a doctoral degree in biology from Yale University. Dr. Pardue is an internationally known cell biologist and geneticist. Her research interests include chromosome structure, especially the structures of telomeres and transposable elements, and the mechanisms by which genes carry out functions and affect the development of higher organisms. Her laboratory has analyzed the molecular mechanisms by which cells respond to stress, especially the heat shock response. She is a past president of the American Society for Cell Biology and the Genetics Society of America. Dr. Pardue is a member of the National Academy of Sciences (NAS). In addition to previous committee service, Dr. Pardue has served as an elected councilor of NAS and as chair of the NAS Section on Genetics.

Daniel L. Azarnoff, M.D., is president of D. L. Azarnoff Associates and senior vice president of Clinical and Regulatory Affairs of Cellegy Pharmaceuticals. He has more than 20 years of academic experience in research and clinical medicine. For 8 years Dr. Azarnoff served as president of research and development for the Searle Pharmaceutical Company, and for the past 14 years he has served as a consultant in drug development. Before joining Searle he was Distinguished Professor of Medicine and Pharmacology and director of the Clinical Pharmacology Toxicology Center at the University of Kansas Medical Center, a job he held for 16 years. He has published more than 175 articles in scientific and medical journals. Dr. Azarnoff is a member of the Institute of Medicine and a fellow of the American Association of Pharmaceutical Scientists, New York Academy of Sciences, American Association for the Advancement of Science, and American College of Physicians. He maintains a teaching appointment at the schools of medicine of the University of Kansas and Stanford University. Dr. Azarnoff has been on the editorial boards of several journals and on committees of the U.S. Food and Drug Administration, World Health Organization, American Medical Association, National Academy of Sciences, Institute of Medicine, and National Institutes of Health, advising them on drugs and drug development.

Sheri Berenbaum, Ph.D., is professor of physiology at the Southern Illinois University School of Medicine. She earned a bachelor's degree in psychology and mathematics from City College of the City University of New York and a doctoral degree in psychology from the University of California, Berkeley, and she completed her fellowship in behavioral genetics at the University of Minnesota. Before joining the faculty at Southern Illinois University she was associate professor of psychology and of psychiatry and behavioral sciences at the University of Health Sciences/ The Chicago Medical School. Before taking her current position, she was professor of behavioral and social sciences at Southern Illinois University. Dr. Berenbaum's research focuses on the development of individual differences in cognition and social behavior, with particular emphasis on the development of sex-typed behaviors, including gender identity. Her laboratory is analyzing the effects of high prenatal levels of androgens in children with congenital adrenal hyperplasia. Dr. Berenbaum recently received the 1999 Faculty University Woman of Distinction Award from Southern Illinois University. She serves on the National Institutes of Health Study Section on Risk Prevention and Health Behavior.

Karen J. Berkley, Ph.D., is McKenzie Professor in the Program of Neuroscience at Florida State University. She also holds appointments as visiting professor and senior clinical fellow at University College, London, and the National Hospital for Neurology and Neurosurgery, Queen Square, London, respectively. She earned a bachelor's degree in biology from Brown University and a doctoral degree in physiology, biophysics, and psychology from the University of Washington. Dr. Berkley's research focuses on the neural mechanisms of pelvic pain, cannabinoid functions within pelvic organs, sex differences in pain, and linking of basic research to the clinic. Dr. Berkley has authored numerous journal articles and book chapters and is on the editorial boards of several leading neuroscience and pain professional journals. She has previously served on the Institute of Medicine Committee on a National Neural Circuitry Database and the U.S. National Committee for the International Brain Research Organization.

Anne Fausto-Sterling, Ph.D., is professor of biology and women's studies in the Department of Molecular and Cellular Biology and Biochemistry at Brown University and has served on the faculty at Brown for more than 20 years. She has been a visiting professor at various universities and colleges in both the United States and Europe. She is a fellow of the American Association for the Advancement of Science and has been the recipient of grants and fellowships in both the sciences and humanities. Her current laboratory research focuses on the evolution and regenerative ability of sexual and asexual systems of reproduction in the group of flatworms known as *Planaria*. She is also the author of scientific publications in the field of *Drosophila* (fruit fly) developmental genetics. Professor Fausto-Sterling has written broadly and critically about the role of race and gender in the construction of scientific theory and the role of such theories in the construction of ideas about race and gender. Her book *Myths of Gender: Biological Theories about Women and Men*, published in 1985 and again in revised form in 1992 (New York: Basic Books) analyzes the biological basis of behavior among men and women. Her new book, *Sexing the Body: Gender Politics and the Construction of Sexuality* (New York: Basic Books), was published in January 2000. This book urges the use of developmental systems theory as a means to move beyond the fruitless attempts to understand sex and gender by using nature-nurture dualism.

Daniel D. Federman, M.D., is senior dean for alumni relations and clinical teaching and the Carl W. Walter Professor of Medicine and Medical Education at Harvard Medical School. He graduated from Harvard College and Harvard Medical School and performed his internship and residency at Massachusetts General Hospital. Dr. Federman conducted research and trained in endocrinology at the National Institutes of Health, the University College Hospital Medical School in London, and Massachusetts General Hospital. He has served as a physician, as chief of the Endocrine Unit, and as associate chief of medical services at the Massachusetts General Hospital and was later Arthur F. Bloomfield Professor of Medicine and chairman of the Department of Medicine at Stanford University Medical School. Beginning in 1977, Dr. Federman served as dean for students and alumni and professor of medicine at Harvard Medical School. He has served as chairman of the Board of Internal Medicine and president of the American College of Physicians. He is a member of the Institute of Medicine (IOM) and recently served as cochair of the IOM

Committee on the Ethical and Legal Issues Relating to the Inclusion of Women in Clinical Studies.

Barbara Ann Gilchrest, M.D., is professor and chair of the Boston University School of Medicine Department of Dermatology. She earned a bachelor's degree from the Massachusetts Institute of Technology in 1967 and a medical degree from Harvard Medical School in 1971, and she completed residencies in internal medicine and dermatology at the Harvard Medical School-affiliated hospitals. She has previously served on the faculties of the Harvard Medical School and Tufts University School of Medicine and as a senior scientist at the U.S. Department of Agriculture Human Nutrition Research Center on Aging at Tufts University. Dr. Gilchrest's research focuses on skin aging and the effects of ultraviolet light on human skin. Dr. Gilchrest is a member of the Institute of Medicine (IOM) and chair of the IOM Section on Internal Medicine, Pathology, and Dermatology.

Melvin M. Grumbach, M.D., is the first Edward B. Shaw Professor of Pediatrics at the University of California, San Francisco, School of Medicine, where he served as chairman of the Department of Pediatrics for more than two decades. He earned a medical degree from the Columbia University College of Physicians and Surgeons and completed a pediatric residency at Babies Hospital, Columbia-Presbyterian Medical Center. After his residency, Dr. Grumbach served as a captain in the U.S. Air Force Medical Corps. He completed a postdoctoral fellowship at the Johns Hopkins University School of Medicine. Before arriving at the University of California, San Francisco, Dr. Grumbach was director of the Pediatric Endocrine Division for 10 years and was associate professor of pediatrics at Columbia University. Dr. Grumbach is a leader in research on the hormonal control of growth and maturation. As an endocrinologist and pediatrician, he has studied the development and function of the human endocrine and neuroendocrine systems from fetal life through puberty, including studies of the endocrinology of growth, puberty, sex differentiation, and disease-causing pathology. He is a past president of the Endocrine Society, the American Pediatric Society, and the Lawson Wilkins Pediatric Endocrine Society and was recently elected honorary president of the International Endocrine Society. His current research focuses on deciphering the unexpected effects in the human of mutations in the gene encoding cytochrome P450 aromatase on growth, bone maturation and density, and sexual development. Dr. Grumbach is a member of the National Academy of Sciences and the Institute of Medicine and is a fellow of the American Academy of Arts and Sciences.

Shiriki Kumanyika, Ph.D., M.P.H., is associate dean for health promotion and disease prevention at the University of Pennsylvania School of Medicine and professor of epidemiology in the Department of Biostatistics and Epidemiology. She earned an M.S. in social work from Columbia University, a Ph.D. in human nutrition from Cornell University, and an M.P.H. from Johns Hopkins University. Before arriving at the University of Pennsylvania, Dr. Kumanyika was professor of nutrition and epidemiology and head of the Department of Human Nutrition and Dietetics at the University of Illinois at Chicago. She has also held prior positions on the nutrition and epidemiology faculties of Pennsylvania State University, Johns Hopkins University, and Cornell University. Her publications reflect more than 20 years of research related to cardiovascular diseases, obesity, nutritional epidemiology, and the health of minority populations, older populations, and women. Dr. Kumanyika was a member of the Institute of Medicine's Committee on Legal and Ethical Issues in the Inclusion of Women in Clinical Studies. From 1996 through 2000 she served as a member of the Advisory Council of the National Institutes of Health's National Heart, Lung, and Blood Institute.

Judith H. LaRosa, Ph.D., R.N., is a professor in the Department of Preventive Medicine and Community Health at the State University of New York (SUNY) Downstate Medical Center at Brooklyn. Before arriving at SUNY Downstate Medical Center at Brooklyn, Dr. LaRosa was a professor in and chair of the Department of Community Health Sciences, Tulane University School of Public Health and Tropical Medicine, director of the Tulane Xavier National Center of Excellence in Women's Health, and associate director of the National Science Foundation's Louisiana Experimental Program to Stimulate Competitive Research. Dr. LaRosa was the first deputy director of the National Institutes of Health's (NIH's) Office of Research on Women's Health. She is coauthor of the legislatively mandated report *National Institutes of Health Guidelines on the Inclusion of Women and Minorities as Subjects in Clinical Research* (Bethesda, MD: U.S. Department of Health and Human Services, 1994). Dr. LaRosa has published extensively in professional and lay journals in the areas of women's health, heart disease, and workplace health promotion and disease prevention. She has coauthored a textbook, *New Dimensions in Women's Health* (New York: Jones and Bartlett, 1994). Dr. LaRosa is a member of the National Institute for Nursing Research's Advisory Council. She has been a member of the Armed Forces Epidemiological Board and the Institute of Medicine's (IOM's) Board on Health Sciences Policy and has served on the IOM Committee on Defense Women's Health Research. Dr. LaRosa recently served on the Office of Research on Women's Health Task Force on the NIH Women's Health Research Agenda for the 21st Century.

Michael D. Lockshin, M.D., is the director of the Barbara Volcker Center for Women and Rheumatic Disease at the Hospital for Special Surgery in New York, New York, and is professor of medicine at the Joan and Sanford I. Weill College of Medicine of Cornell University. He received a bachelor's degree from Harvard College and an M.D. from Harvard Medical School and did his clinical training at Bellevue Hospital and Memorial Sloan-Kettering Hospital, followed by a fellowship at Columbia-Presbyterian Medical Center. As an Epidemic Intelligence Service officer for the Public Health Service Communicable Disease Center, he was assistant professor of epidemiology at the University of Pittsburgh School of Public Health, working on health problems of coal miners. After a fellowship, he joined the Hospital for Special Surgery and Cornell University Medical College, rising to the position of professor of medicine and attending physician. In 1989 he moved to the National Institutes of Health as extramural director and then acting director of the National Institute of Arthritis and Musculoskeletal and Skin Disorders and was then senior adviser to the director of the Clinical Center, National Institutes of Health, before returning to Cornell in 1997. Dr. Lockshin chaired the American Board of Internal Medicine Committee on Rheumatology and has held national offices in and many chairmanships of committees of the Arthritis Foundation and the American College of Rheumatology. He has served on the editorial boards of *Arthritis and Rheumatism, Journal of Rheumatology, Lupus, American Journal of Reproductive Immunology,* and other journals. His research interests include pregnancy and rheumatic disease, antiphospholipid antibody, and other topics related to systemic lupus erythematosus. He convened the first International Conference on Pregnancy and Rheumatic Disease and the first Conference on Gender, Biology, and Human Disease. He is the author of more than 180 scientific papers and textbook chapters and *Guarded Prognosis* (New York: Hill and Wang, 1999).

Jill Panetta, Ph.D., received a doctoral degree in organic chemistry from Dartmouth College and completed postdoctoral work at the University of California, Berkeley. Dr. Panetta joined Eli Lilly & Company in 1982 as senior organic chemist. In 1992 she served as group leader for the Diabetes Medicinal Chemists. She has also served as a member of the Athena Neurosciences/Eli Lilly Alzheimer's Research Team and as a CNS Chemistry Group Leader. Dr. Panetta has recently been appointed research manager for the Lilly Center for Women's Health (LCWH). LCWH research programs focus on enhancing scientific innovation and expertise through basic and clinical research on the causes, treatment, and prevention of diseases that disproportionately or differentially affect women, as well as understanding the complexities of gender-based differences in drug response, metabolism, and safety. Dr. Panetta is the author of more than 80 publications and abstracts and 27 invited lectures and is coinventor on 25 granted U.S. patents. Recently, Dr. Panetta organized and chaired a session on gender-specific drug discovery at the Medicinal Chemistry Gordon Research Conference. She served as a section editor for the Central and Peripheral Nervous System section and the Anti-Inflammatory Section of Expert Opinion on Investigational Drugs and is on the Advisory Board for Current Drugs LTD. She is coeditor of a textbook, *Major Psychiatric Illness in Women: Emerging Treatment and Research* (Washington, DC: American Psychiatric Press), which is in press.

Carmen Sapienza, Ph.D., is professor of pathology and laboratory medicine and associate director of the Fels Institute for Cancer Research and Molecular Biology at Temple University School of Medicine. Before his appointment at Temple, Dr. Sapienza was head of the Laboratory of Developmental Genetics at the Ludwig Institute for Cancer Research (San Diego Branch) and was an associate professor in the Department of Medicine at the University of California, San Diego. Before moving to San Diego, Dr. Sapienza was head of the Laboratory of Developmental Genetics at the Ludwig Institute for Cancer Research in Montreal and an associate professor in the Department of Medicine at McGill University in Montreal. Dr. Sapienza received a B.A. in biology from the University of California, San Diego, an M.S. in oceanography from the University of Maine, and a Ph.D. in biochemistry from Dalhousie University in Halifax. He completed his postdoctoral fellowship at the Howard Hughes Medical Institute in Salt Lake City. An accomplished researcher with more than 60 scientific publications, he is frequently invited to give presentations at both national and international conferences. His current research is concentrated on discovering the genetic rules of genome imprinting. His laboratory was the first to recognize that the process of imprinting is genetically controlled and that the process is controlled by genes that are not, in general, linked to the locus at which the imprinting effect is observed. Dr. Sapienza serves on the editorial boards of the *European Journal of Human Genetics* and *Mammalian Genome* and has been a guest editor for *Developmental Genetics.*

Sally E. Shaywitz, M.D., is codirector, along with Bennett Shaywitz, of the National Institute of Child Health and Human Development-Yale Center for the Study of Learning and Attention and professor of pediatrics at Yale University School of Medicine. Dr. Shaywitz received an M.D. and competed a residency and postdoctoral training in developmental pediatrics at the Albert Einstein College of Medicine. After a 9-year hiatus to care for her children, she joined the Yale faculty. At Yale she initiated the Connecticut Longitudinal Study, a longitudinal study of a representative sample of Connecticut schoolchildren. This study, which is ongoing, has provided the basic modern epidemiological framework for the prevalence, course, conceptual model, and neurobiological changes over time for dyslexia. More recently, she has used functional imaging to study the underlying neurobiology of reading and dyslexia. Her and her husband's work has demonstrated sex differences in brain organization for language; a functional disruption in brain organization for adults and, more recently, for children with dyslexia; the influence of sex hormones (estrogen) on brain organization and reading and language in postmenopausal women; and the functional neural architecture of components of attention in language processing. Current investigations by their laboratory focus on the use of functional imaging and magnetic resonance spectroscopy to study the neurobiology of fluency in reading. She is the author of more than 100 articles in scientific journals and 63 chapters in books. Dr. Shaywitz is a member of the Institute of Medicine and has been awarded the Distinguished Alumnus Award by the Albert Einstein College of Medicine, the Achievement Award in Women's Health by the Society for Women's Health Research, and the Sidney Berman Award of the American Academy of Child and Adolescent Psychiatry. She recently served on the National Research Council's Committee on the Prevention of Reading Difficulties in Young Children and serves on the National Academy of Sciences' Committee on Women in Science and Engineering.

John G. Vandenbergh, Ph.D., is a professor in the Department of Zoology at North Carolina State University. He received a B.A. degree from Montclair State College and an M.S. degree from Ohio University and completed a Ph.D. at Pennsylvania State University. He spent 3 years studying the behavior and endocrinology of free-ranging rhesus monkeys in Puerto Rico as a scientist with the National Institutes of Health, U.S. Public Health Service. He then moved to North Carolina and joined the research program at Dorothea Dix Hospital, a large mental hospital. There he studied the relationship between hormones and behavior in rodents, monkeys, and humans. Next he moved to North Carolina State University to become head of the Department of Zoology. After leading the department through a major growth period, he left administration to focus on teaching and managing a research program in behavioral endocrinology. Twenty-one graduate students have received advanced degrees under his direction, and nine postdoctoral fellows have completed training in his laboratory. He has published two books, 26 chapters in books, and 78 articles in scientific journals. He is a present or past member of several editorial and research boards. Currently he serves as a member of the Board of the North Carolina Association for Biomedical Research, as a member of the Council of the Institute for Laboratory Animal Research (National Research Council, National Academies), and as a consulting scientist to the U.S. Environmental Protection Agency.

Huntington F. Willard, Ph.D., is the Henry W. Payne Professor and chairman of the Department of Genetics at Case Western Reserve University and director of the Center for Human Genetics at Case Western Reserve University and University Hospitals of Cleveland. He is also president and director of The Research Institute of University Hospitals of Cleveland. Dr. Willard did his early training in genetics at Harvard University and received a Ph.D. in 1979 from the Department of Human Genetics at Yale University. After a postdoctoral fellowship at Johns Hopkins University, Dr. Willard held appointments in the Department of Medical Genetics at the University of Toronto and in the Department of Genetics at Stanford University. Dr. Willard's research focuses on aspects of the molecular structure and function of human chromosomes and the human genome. His goal is to understand the chromosomal mechanisms involved in gene control or implicated in genetic disorders, including the mechanisms of X-chromosome inactivation. He has been a member of the American Society of Human Genetics since 1975 and is currently President of that Society. He is also an original member of the Human Genome Organization. Dr. Willard serves on the Mammalian Genetics Study Section of the National Institutes of Health (NIH) and in the past has served as chairman of the Mental Retardation and Developmental Disabilities Research Committee of NIH. He has served on the editorial boards of numerous journals and is currently coeditor of *Human Molecular Genetics*. Dr. Willard is coauthor of *Genetics in Medicine* (Philadelphia: W. B. Saunders), a widely used medical and graduate student textbook, now published in its sixth edition.

Board on Health Sciences Policy Liaison

Mary Woolley is the President of Research!America, a nonprofit, membership-supported, grassroots public education and advocacy organization committed to making health-related research a much higher national priority. Under her leadership, Research!America's membership has more than tripled as it has earned the attention and respect of research, media, and community leaders with its signature public opinion surveys, advocacy resource materials, and public service advertising campaigns. Ms. Woolley received a B.S. from Stanford University and an M.A. from San Francisco State University. She studied advanced management at the University of California, Berkeley. In her early career, Ms. Woolley served as San Francisco project director for the then largest-ever National Institutes of Health-funded clinical trial, the Multiple Risk Factor Intervention Trial. In 1981 she became administrator of the Medical Research Institute of San Francisco and in 1986 was named the institute's executive director and chief executive officer. Ms. Woolley serves on the University of California, Berkeley, School of Public Health Dean's Council and the board of the Lovelace Respiratory Research Institute and is a founding member of the Board of Associates of the Whitehead Institute for Biomedical Research. She is a member of the Institute of Medicine and is a fellow of the American Association for the Advancement of Science. Ms. Woolley has served as president of the Association of Independent Research Institutes, editor of the *Journal of the Society of Research Administrators*, a reviewer for the National Institutes of Health and National Science Foundation, and a consultant to several research organizations. Ms. Woolley has a 20-year editorial and publication history on science advocacy and research-related topics. Her op-ed pieces and letters to the editor are published in newspapers from coast to coast; and she has been published in *Science, Nature, Issues in Science and Technology, New England Journal of Medicine, The Scientist*, and other research-oriented periodicals. She is a sought-after speaker and is frequently interviewed by science, news, and policy journalists. For her work on behalf of medical research, she has been awarded the Distinguished Contribution to Research Administration Award from the Society for Research Administrators, the American Hospital Association Silver Touchstone Award for Public Affairs Programming, the Columbia University College of Physicians and Surgeons Dean's Award for Distinguished Service, the Federation of American Societies for Experimental Biology Special Award for Science Advocacy, and the Friends of the National Institute for Nursing Research's Health Advocacy Award.

IOM STAFF

Theresa M. Wizemann, Ph.D., is a senior program officer for the Board on Health Sciences Policy at the Institute of Medicine and served as the study director for *Exploring the Biological Contributions to Human Health.* She earned a bachelor's degree in medical technology from Douglass College of Rutgers University and master's and doctoral degrees in microbiology and molecular genetics, jointly from Rutgers University and the University of Medicine and Dentistry of New Jersey. She did a postdoctoral fellowship in infectious diseases at The Rockefeller University in New York. Dr. Wizemann came to the Institute of Medicine from the Office of Senator Edward M. Kennedy, Senate Committee on Health Education, Labor and Pensions, where she handled various health and science policy issues as a congressional fellow. Before the fellowship, she led a vaccine research team at MedImmune, Inc., a leading biotechnology company in Maryland. Dr. Wizemann has expertise in microbiology, immunology, and infectious diseases and has a particular interest in women's and children's health.

Thelma L. Cox is a project assistant for the Board on Health Sciences Policy. During her more than 10 years at the Institute of Medicine (IOM) she has also provided assistance to the Division of Health Care Services and the Division of Biobehavioral Sciences and Mental Disorders. Ms. Cox has worked on several IOM reports, including *Designing a Strategy for Quality Review and Assurance in Medicare; Evaluating the Artificial Heart Program of the National Heart, Lung, and Blood Institute; Federal Regulation of Methadone Treatment; Legal and Ethical Issues Relating to the Inclusion of Women in Clinical Studies; Review of the Fialuridine (FIAU/FIAC) Clinical Trials;* and *Cancer Research Among Minorities and the Medically Underserved.* She has received the National Research Council Recognition Award and two IOM Staff Achievement Awards.

Andrew Pope, Ph.D., is director of the Board on Health Sciences Policy at the Institute of Medicine. With expertise in physiology and biochemistry, his primary interests focus on environmental and occupational influences on human health. Dr. Pope's previous research activities focused on the neuroendocrine and reproductive effects of various environmental substances on food-producing animals. During his tenure at the National Academy of Sciences and since 1989 at the Institute of Medicine, Dr. Pope has directed numerous reports on topics that include injury control, disability prevention, biological markers, neurotoxicology, indoor allergens, and the enhancement of environmental and occupational health content in medical and nursing school curricula. Most recently, Dr. Pope directed studies on National Institutes of Health priority-setting processes, fluid resuscitation practices in combat casualties, and organ procurement and transplantation.

Sarah Pitluck was a research associate for the Board on Health Sciences Policy at the Institute of Medicine (IOM). Ms. Pitluck helped support IOM's Committee on Understanding the Biology of Sex and Gender Differences and the Roundtable on Environmental Health Sciences, Research, and Medicine. She received an undergraduate degree in political science at Washington University in St. Louis, Missouri, before completing a master's degree in public policy and public administration at the London School of Economics and Political Science. Ms. Pitluck's master's thesis addressed the sources of divergent policies toward screening for prostate cancer in the United States and the United Kingdom. Additional IOM studies with which she assisted were *Fluid Resuscitation: State of the Science for Treating Combat Casualties and Civilian Injuries; Organ Procurement and Transplantation Policy: Assessing Current Policies and the Potential Impact of the DHHS Final Rule; Managed Care Systems and Emerging Infections: Challenges and Opportunities for Strengthening Surveillance, Research, and Prevention;* and *Rational Therapeutics for Infants and Children.* She resigned from the IOM staff on June 5, 2000.

Index